A New Look at
Tumour Immunology

CANCER SURVEYS

Advances and Prospects in Clinical, Epidemiological and Laboratory Oncology

Published for the

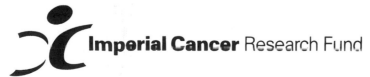

Imperial Cancer Research Fund

A New Look at Tumour Immunology

Guest Editors
A J McMichael
W F Bodmer

COLD SPRING HARBOR LABORATORY PRESS 1992

CANCER SURVEYS
A New Look at Tumour Immunology
Volume 13

Cover and book design by Leon Bolognese & Associates, Inc.

All Cold Spring Harbor Laboratory Press publications may be ordered directly from Cold Spring Harbor Laboratory Press, 10 Skyline Drive, Plainview, New York 11803-9729. Phone: Continental US & Canada 1-800-843-4388; all other locations (516) 349-1930. FAX: (516) 349-1946.

Contents

A New Look at
Tumour Immunology

Introduction

WALTER BODMER • ANDREW McMICHAEL

New discoveries clarifying the mechanism of T cell immune recognition, together with major advances in the identification of specific genetic changes in tumours and observations on changes in the expression of HLA class I determinants on tumours, have dramatically transformed the nature of tumour immunology. It is now possible to envisage a precise understanding of the basis for immune response to tumours and so approach, in an organized way, strategies for exploiting the immune system for treatment, and even prevention, of cancers. The papers in this issue provide a valuable survey of the current state of knowledge and ideas concerning T cell immune responses to tumours—ranging from the description of the basic mechanisms of immune response to reviews of approaches to immunotherapy and the clinical evidence for immune response to human tumours.

The most important advance in our understanding of the nature of T cell immune recognition of cellular determinants is the demonstration that the recognized targets are processed protein antigens, which can be represented in in vitro assays by short oligopeptide sequences from the relevant protein. These are presented by HLA molecules on the cell surface. The structure of the HLA class I molecule, established by Bjorkman, Wiley and Strominger, shows where peptides are held in the cleft of the HLA molecule so that they are available for recognition by the T cell receptor. Specific peptides, characteristically eight or nine aminoacids long, can be eluted from the HLA molecules of target cells, and this provides a totally new approach for the potential identification of T cell target antigens. Particularly relevant is the finding that peptides presented by class I HLA molecules are usually derived from cytoplasmic proteins; thus, the immune system can respond to internal changes in transformed cells. These advances are reviewed by McMichael, using response to influenza virus as a model. The response to virus induced tumours is the basis for Melief and Kast's analysis of the role of peptides in T cell recognition and the approaches that can be envisaged for peptide vaccination. The oncogenic Epstein-Barr virus (EBV), as discussed by Rickinson and colleagues, provides another valuable model for the analysis of T cell responses and possible mechanisms of escape through mutations that lead to the loss of viral epitopes. This is, of course, only possible so long as the mutations do not at the same time lead to a loss of the transformed phenotype. Such an escape mechanism will only be effective if there is at most one or a very small number of potentially recognizable immune targets. When this is not the case, escape must occur by mutations affecting general immune mechanisms such as the expression of HLA class I molecules or necessary accessory molecules to T cell recognition such as LFA3.

The first human cell line to show complete loss of surface expression of HLA-A,B,C was the Burkitt lymphoma derived cell line Daudi. Early studies, which indicated that the basis for this lack of expression was lack of production of β_2-microglobulin, led to the suggestion that this reflected escape from T cell immune response to EBV determinants during the outgrowth of the lymphoma (Arce-Gomez et al, 1978). It was then pointed out by Brodsky et al (1979) that these ideas could be generalized to other tumours. Thus, tumours that produced variants with lowered or altered expression of HLA-A,B,C or β_2-microglobulin would be the ones against which there must have been a T cell response to a tumour determinant. Since then, there have been many observations on human and other tumours of changes in HLA class I expression and discussions of the evidence this provides for T cell immune attack against tumours. The papers by Kaklamanis and Hill and Möller and Hämmerling provide an up to date survey of data on HLA changes in tumours and the variety of mechanisms by which these can arise. Each genetic step during tumour progression must be selected for, if it is present in all, or at least a high percentage of the cells in a tumour. Thus, if two mutational steps are needed to eliminate completely HLA-A,B,C expression, as is the case if this happens through recessive mutations knocking out the function of both versions of the β_2-microglobulin gene (as in the Daudi cell line), then the first mutation must itself confer selective advantage. This is because the probability of a first mutation, by chance, sweeping through the population of cells followed by a second mutation, even if advantageous, will be very small. It is not surprising therefore that, as shown by Smith et al (1988) and others, loss of expression of single alleles is a commoner event than overall loss of expression of all HLA class I products. From the point of view of escape from T cell attack, the mutational mechanisms by which HLA expression is changed are largely irrelevant, and this is both consistent with, and can account for, the evidence for a variety of mechanisms by which these changes in expression may occur.

Möller and Hämmerling indicate that in their data, there is no apparent correlation between the changes in HLA expression and tumour prognosis, although other studies have suggested that such correlations might exist. However, it is not necessarily surprising that the immune response to a tumour, signalled by a change in HLA expression, has no major effect on its outcome. Primary immune responses to specific changes in tumours may take some time to be established, by which time the tumour may be so large that outgrowth of immune resistant variants is not a limitation to the growth of the tumour, much as in the case of the development of resistance to conventional chemotherapy. This explanation is consistent with the observation, discussed by Oliver and Nouri, that in immunosuppressed transplant patients, the tumours that grow out are overwhelmingly those with a viral aetiology, specifically EBV related lymphoproliferation and HPV associated skin and other cancers, and not the common carcinomas, for which there is no evidence for a viral aetiology. This is easily explained by the fact that immune response to a virus is likely to be much more readily established than that to tumour specific or associated cellular determinants, so that the immune system may play a much greater part in the prognosis of virally associated cancers than those that have no viral aetiology. This, incidentally, is a strong argument against the suggestion that behavioural factors may have a major influence on the incidence and prognostic outcome of cancers through their effect on immune response.

The lack of prognostic significance of immune response for the common carcinomas does not imply that immune therapy or vaccination might not be effective. It is entirely possible, given better approaches for the recognition of potential targets for T cell attack on tumours, that stimulation of the specific immune response at a sufficiently early stage during tumour development could have therapeutic value and that vaccination against such determinants might be effective in preventing the onset of a cancer. As will increasingly be the case in the future, the biological characterization of a tumour will not so much predict prognosis but determine it through the development of therapeutic approaches targeted to particular biological properties.

Knuth *et al* and Boon *et al* show how it is possible to obtain cytotoxic T lymphocytes (CTL) that are specific for tumours and how these can then be used to clone tumour specific target antigens. Boon and his colleagues have very clearly established their elegant approach to cloning using mouse model systems and tumour negative variants induced with relatively high levels of mutagens. The difference in the human situation is that the induction of human tumours is presumably not associated with high levels of mutagen, and so the problem of bystander mutations that could be targets for T cell attack is likely to be insignificant. Boon and Knuth's groups have isolated CTL for human melanomas and through this have cloned a melanoma specific antigen which is a considerable achievement (Van der Bruggen *et al*, 1991). The results suggest that potential targets may not only be novel mutations in proteins, such as in *p53* and the *ras* oncogenes, but may also be normal genes that are abnormally expressed or expressed at higher levels as a result of the action of mutated oncogenes or transforming viruses. It seems entirely possible that changed levels of expression, such as happen as a result of *p53* mutations, or changes in the rate of turnover of a protein could generate novel processed peptides that can be recognized by the immune system but that are not due to mutations in that protein and do not necessarily relate to a protein that is expressed only in a particular tumour. It may also be possible that the products of mutated recessive or suppressor oncogenes could be recognized as abnormal. For example, a nonsense mutation that prevents the formation of a functional product may still allow the synthesis of a partial protein product that is rapidly turned over and so enters, relatively effectively, a processing pathway creating determinants for T cell recognition that might not be created by the normal full length functional product.

Schirrmacher and Oliver and Nouri discuss, from different angles, approaches that have been taken to vaccination against tumours in mouse models and even in humans. Schirrmacher emphasizes the importance of help in the induction of primary responses and also emphasizes the need for proper immunological monitoring of patients involved in any immune therapy trials. Oliver and Nouri review cases of spontaneous regression that may be considered as evidence for occasional affects of immune response on prognosis. They also discuss some of the approaches to immunotherapy using interleukin-2 (IL-2) as a non-specific stimulus of the immune system. A more promising approach, as discussed by Melief and Kast, appears to be to incorporate IL-2 or other lymphokines into autologous tumours to be used as a source of material for vaccination, after appropriate inactivation.

Elution of peptides bound to HLA molecules on tumour cells appears to be a very promising approach to the identification of T cell targets on tumours. There seems little doubt that in the relatively near future this, or other approaches, such as those taken by Boon and Knuth and their colleagues, will lead to the proper identification of tumour specific or associated antigens recognized by T cells that may form the basis for active immunotherapy and eventually for genuine anti-tumour vaccination.

References

Arce-Gomez B, Jones EA, Barnstaple CJ, Solomon E and Bodmer WF (1978) The genetic control of HLA-A and B antigens in somatic cell hybrids: requirement for beta 2-microglobulin. *Tissue Antigens* 11 96–112

Brodsky FM, Parham P, Barnstaple CJ, Crumpton MJ and Bodmer WF (1979) Monoclonal antibodies for analysis of the HLA system. *Immunological Reviews* 47 3–61

Smith MEF, Bodmer WF and Bodmer JG (1988) Selective loss of HLA-A,B,C locus products in colorectal adenocarcinoma. *Lancet* i 823–824

Van der Bruggen P, Traversari C, Chomez P *et al* (1991) A gene encoding an antigen recognised by cytolytic T-lymphocyte on a human melanoma. *Science* 254 1643–1647

Cytotoxic T Lymphocytes and Immune Surveillance

ANDREW McMICHAEL

Institute of Molecular Medicine, John Radcliffe Hospital, Oxford OX3 9DU

Introduction
Specificity of CTL
Processing of antigens recognized by CTL
T cell receptors
Function of CTL
HLA polymorphism
Immune surveillance
Summary

INTRODUCTION

Cytotoxic T lymphocytes (CTL) are a subpopulation of T lymphocytes that carry the CD8 surface glycoprotein and recognize foreign antigen in association with class I molecules of the major histocompatibility complex (MHC). They were first identified as causing lysis of allogeneic target cells in vitro in mixed lymphocyte reactions (Cerottini and Brunner, 1974). Considerable insight into their natural function came from experiments showing that they contribute a major part of defence to virus infections (Gardner *et al*, 1974; Askonas *et al*, 1982). Cytotoxic T lymphocytes were shown to kill virus infected autologous cells with a crucial role for class I MHC (Zinkernagel and Doherty, 1975). Since then, there has been extensive study of CTL specific for viruses (Bangham and McMichael, 1989), including oncogenic viruses (Leclerc *et al*, 1973; Plata *et al*, 1975; Blank *et al*, 1976; Moss *et al*, 1978; Gooding and O'Connell, 1983; Kast *et al*, 1989). Tumour specific CTL have also been demonstrated in tumours not caused by viruses (Leclerc *et al*, 1973; Mukherji and McAlister, 1983; Slavin *et al*, 1986; Herin *et al*, 1987; De Plaen *et al*, 1988; Anichini *et al*, 1989; Knuth *et al*, 1989a,b; Van den Eynde *et al*, 1989; Wolfel *et al*, 1989; Crowley *et al*, 1991). Taken together, these findings indicate that CTL have an important role in immune surveillance by identifying and eliminating abnormal cells. Although CD8+ CTL are thought to be primarily responsible, CD4+ T cells, restricted by class II MHC molecules, can also have cytolytic activity. This is, however, not a constant feature of such cells in vitro, and lytic activity has not been demonstrated in vivo for CD4+ cells as it has for CD8+ cells.

This review discusses recent information on the specificity of CTL and evidence for their function in vivo. Although much of the data have come from studies of virus specific CTL, these can be regarded as models for tumour specific T cells.

SPECIFICITY OF CTL

Zinkernagel and Doherty (1975) demonstrated that CTL specific for viral antigens would only lyse histocompatible infected target cells. This specificity was mapped to class I MHC and was a property of CTL demonstrable in many or all systems (Bangham and McMichael, 1989). Recognition of self MHC was exquisitely specific: mutant HLA or H-2 molecules differing in one to four aminoacids could be distinguished (McMichael *et al*, 1988).

The nature of this MHC restriction was hard to understand until the nature of virus specificity was revealed. The first clues came from the study of influenza specific CTL clones, which distinguished between virus subtypes (Bennink *et al*, 1982; Townsend and Skehel, 1982). Using reassorted viruses, it was possible to map specificity to viral proteins, which surprisingly were internal and not expressed intact on the surfaces of infected cells (Bennink *et al*, 1982; Townsend and Skehel, 1982). The specificity of one such clone for nucleoprotein was confirmed by transfection of the *NP* gene into target cells (Townsend *et al*, 1985b), and subsequently it was shown that nucleoprotein was a major target antigen for both murine (Townsend *et al*, 1985b) and human influenza specific CTL (Gotch *et al*, 1987a). Other internal proteins could also be recognized, whereas specificity for surface glycoproteins was a minor component (Townsend *et al*, 1985b). These results were puzzling, because of the lack of expression of these proteins on cell surfaces, until it was shown that fragments of nucleoprotein could be presented to CTL, suggesting that some form of antigen processing was occurring within cells (Townsend *et al*, 1985a). This was shown most clearly by the finding that synthetic peptides added to uninfected cells could sensitize them for lysis by virus specific CTL (Townsend *et al*, 1986). The role of MHC then became clear when it was found that MHC type determined the peptide epitope to which CTL responded (McMichael *et al*, 1986, 1988; Townsend *et al*, 1986). This effect is very striking in outbred humans, with the majority of individuals with given MHC types responding to the same peptides despite diverse genetic backgrounds.

These results coincided with the determination of the crystal structure of HLA-A2 (Bjorkman *et al*, 1987a,b). The first two domains fold to form a groove, bounded by two long α helices on either side and an eight stranded β pleated sheet floor containing unidentified electron density. This was thought to be a mixture of peptides, and further crystallographic analysis of HLA-A2, A68 and B27 has clearly confirmed this (Jardetsky *et al*, 1991; Madden *et al*, 1991; Saper *et al*, 1991). Nearly all of the genetic polymorphism in HLA class I molecules was found in aminoacids that contributed to the groove, explaining why different MHC molecules bind and present different peptides.

Recently, peptides have been eluted from purified class I MHC molecules (Falk *et al*, 1990, 1991; Van Bleek and Nathenson, 1990). The majority of peptides were nonamers, and mixed peptides were eluted from a preparation of purified class I molecules. However, sequencing has revealed shared amino-acids at particular positions that can be defined as anchor residues, suggesting that they are involved in binding to a particular class I molecule. The anchor residues defined in this way agree with the known peptide epitopes from viral antigens (Fig. 1). The concept of anchor residues in the peptide is complementary to fine structural information on class I molecules: this has revealed that pockets in the groove contain side chains of peptide residues (Garrett *et al*, 1989; Saper *et al*, 1991).

A specific example illustrates how close we are to understanding peptide–class I MHC association. HLA-A2 presents a peptide derived from influenza matrix protein to CTL. This was originally identified as peptide sequence 55–73 (Gotch *et al*, 1987b), which was quickly narrowed down to 57–68 (Gotch *et al*, 1988). By altering peptide sequence, it was possible to show that most of the specificity resided in aminoacids 59–66 (Gotch *et al*, 1988). Recent analysis of nonamer peptides indicates that peptide 58–66 is the most likely natural peptide (Morrison *et al*, in press) because it sensitizes target cells at concentrations an order of magnitude lower than other peptides around this sequence. Study of HLA-A2 molecules in which single point mutations were made by site directed mutagenesis has revealed that the following naturally polymorphic aminoacids in HLA-A2 have some role in peptide binding: residues 9, 45, 62–63, 66, 70, 74, 114, 116, 152 and 156 (McMichael *et al*, 1988; Moots *et al*, 1991); the positions of these aminoacids are illustrated in Fig. 2. Most of these residues contribute to the pockets, some of which admit peptide side chains. A recent and very informative finding is that a peptide based on the matrix peptide 58–68 aminoacid sequence with an arginine substituted for leucine at position 66 was very poorly presented by HLA-A2 but very well presented by an HLA-A2 mutant molecule with aspartic acid instead of tyrosine at position 116 (Fig. 2) (Latron *et al*, in press). Other combinations of altered peptide and mutant HLA-A2 molecules did not give this result. This finding indicates that the poor presentation of the peptide with the arginine substitution is compensated by changing tyrosine in the floor at position 116 to a smaller negatively charged aspartic acid. This implies that these two aminoacids are close enough to form a salt bridge, and because aminoacid 116 is at the right hand end of the groove and residue 66 is at the carboxyl end of the peptide, this result orientates the peptide from left to right, as shown in Fig. 2.

Two of the pockets, recently defined, known as the A and F pockets, are at either end of the groove, and both contain conserved tyrosine and serine residues (Saper *et al*, 1991). In the crystal structure of HLA-B27, it has been shown that the aminoterminal of peptide hydrogen bonds in the A pocket and the carboxyterminal bonds in the F pocket. As these pockets are conserved in all known HLA class I sequences, the results strongly support the view that the

HLA A2

Eluted peptides:

```
          1 2 3 4 5 6 7 8 9
            L         V
            M     E   V     K
              K
          I   A G I   I A E L
          L   Y P K   L Y S
          F   F D Y   T H
          K   P T N
          M   M G
          Y   S F
          V   R V
              H
```

Epitope peptides:

	1	2	3	4	5	6	7	8	9
Influenza matrix	G	I	L	G	F	V	F	T	L
Influenza N NP	L	L	G	E	F	Y	N	Q	M
HIV pol	E	L	A	E	N	R	E	I	L
HIV gag	E	L	R	S	L	Y	N	T	V

HLA B27

Eluted peptides:

	1	2	3	4	5	6	7	8	9
Human histone H3	R	R	Y	Q	K	S	T	E	L
Human hsp 89a	R	R	I	K	E	I	V	K	K
Human hsp 89ß	R	R	V	K	E	V	V	K	K
Human elong f. 2	R	R	W	L	P	A	G	D	A
Human ATP dep helicase	R	R	S	K	E	I	T	V	R
Ribosomal protein	G	R	I	D	K	P	I	L	K
Ribosomal protein L28	F	R	Y	N	G	L	I	H	R
-	K	R	F	E	G	L	T	Q	R
-	R	R	F	T	R	P	E	H	-
-	R	R	I	S	G	V	D	R	Y
-	A	R	L	F	G	I	R	A	K

Epitope peptides:

	1	2	3	4	5	6	7	8	9
Influenza NP	S	R	Y	W	A	I	R	T	R
HIV gag	K	R	W	I	I	L	G	L	N	K

Fig. 1. Peptides and motifs presented by HLA-A2 and B27. Shown are peptide sequences derived from eluted peptides from HLA-A2 (Falk *et al*, 1991) and B27 (Jardetsky *et al*, 1991); sequences are given in the single letter aminoacid code. For HLA-A2, the aminoacids found at each position in the eluted peptide pool are given; those in bold type are the dominant residues at a given position. For HLA-B27, the sequences of the eluted purified peptides are given and, where known, the origin of the peptide; in some positions, the aminoacid is derived from the probable peptide sequence (see Jardetsky *et al*, 1991 for details). Under each list of eluted peptides are the sequences of known virus derived peptide epitopes that are known to be presented to CTL. Key anchor residues are shown in bold type. Note the correspondence between these positions in the eluted and epitope peptides

influenza matrix peptide is also oriented in this way. If the hydrogen bonding hydroxyl groups are mutated from tyrosine to phenylalanine, peptide presentation is impaired, emphasizing the importance of these binding sites (Latron F,

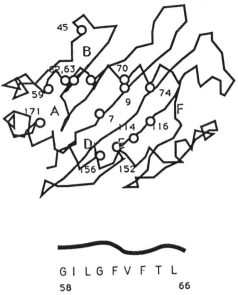

G I L G F V F T L
58   66

Fig. 2. Peptide binding groove of HLA-A2 showing aminoacid residues known to be critical in binding of presenting peptides. Also indicated are the positions of the A-F pockets (Saper *et al*, 1991); note that the C pocket is closed in HLA-A2 (Garrett *et al*, 1989). Critical residues in the A pocket are: 7 F, 59 F, 171 F (all conserved); in the B pocket 45 M, 6 E, 66 K, H 70; in the D pocket L 156; in the E pocket H 114 and V 156; and in the F pocket Y 116. Other residues in these pockets have not yet been mutagenized and tested. Below the HLA-A2 backbone, the influenza matrix peptide (to scale) is shown. Replacing the leucine at position 66 in the peptide gave a peptide that was presented much more effectively by HLA-A2, with tyrosine at residue 116 replaced by aspartic acid; this orients the nonamer peptide in the groove from left (aminoterminal) to right (carboxyterminal)

Moots R, McMichael AJ and Strominger JL, unpublished). Crystallographic analysis of the HLA-A2 groove has also shown that there is a relatively large pocket, known as the B pocket, that admits an isoleucine or leucine side chain (Saper *et al*, 1991). Mutation of aminoacid 45 in the pocket destroys peptide presentation (Morrison *et al*, in press). The crystal suggests that the side chain of the second aminoacid fits into this groove, and this is consistent with our orientation of the peptide within the groove. Thus, all of the results, functional data, crystallographic analysis and eluted peptide sequences agree and provide a fairly clear picture of the peptide-HLA complex.

Other peptides presented by HLA-A2 appear to show similar motifs within a nonamer sequence. A general rule is emerging that characterizes peptides that bind to HLA-A2 and elicit CTL responses. Similar rules can be deduced for other class I HLA molecules. For instance, peptides that are presented by HLA-B27 have positively charged arginine at residue 2 and nearly always have lysine or arginine at residue 9 (Huet *et al*, 1990; Jardetsky *et al*, 1991); B27 has a negatively charged B pocket and a negatively charged aspartic acid at residue

116 (Madden *et al*, 1991). Therefore, it should not be long before candidate antigenic peptides can be predicted from the aminoacid sequence of the foreign peptide for particular class I MHC molecules. The ability of these peptides to elicit CTL responses could be tested by culturing T lymphocytes with peptide pulsed antigen presenting cells and looking for growth of effector CTL. The potential of such peptides can also be tested by measuring their ability to stabilize newly folded class I MHC molecules (see below) (Elvin *et al*, 1991). Thus, as mutations associated with tumour cells are defined, it should be possible to predict and test whether these can elicit specific CTL responses.

PROCESSING OF ANTIGENS RECOGNIZED BY CTL

Most, or perhaps all, of the peptides in class I molecules that stimulate CTL responses originate from proteins that reside in the cytoplasm of the cell. Even surface glycoproteins may enter the class I antigen processing pathway because small amounts may fail to be translocated into the secretory pathways. It has been found that normal expression of class I MHC molecules depends on their association with peptides (Ljunggren *et al*, 1990; Townsend *et al*, 1990). Mutant cell lines have been described where class I heavy chains are present in the endoplasmic reticulum (ER) but surface expression is very low (Townsend *et al*, 1989b; Cerundolo *et al*, 1990). Surface expression of class I molecules can be enhanced in these cells by incubation with peptide. This is thought to stabilize empty class I molecules that come out at the cell surface but that are normally rapidly degraded. Townsend and colleagues have shown that class I molecules will fold in the absence of peptide but that the peptide is required for stabilization of such molecules in the ER (Townsend *et al*, 1989a, 1990; Cerundolo *et al*, 1991a). Thus, peptide is an integral part of a mature class I MHC molecule. Some of the abnormal genes in the mutant cell lines map to the MHC itself (Spies and DeMars, 1991). Two putative peptide transporter genes have recently been mapped in the class II region of H2 and HLA gene complexes (Deverson *et al*, 1990; Monaco *et al*, 1990; Spies *et al*, 1990; Trowsdale *et al*, 1990). Furthermore, in one mutant cell line with a phenotype similar to those previously described, one of these transporter genes contains a point mutation (Spies and DeMars, 1991). In addition, a proteasome gene maps in this region (Brown *et al*, 1991; Glynne *et al*, 1991). Proteasomes are complexes of proteolytic enzymes present in the cytoplasm and are attractive candidates for the protein degrading enzymes. Therefore, it appears that the MHC controls the whole process by which proteins are degraded in the cytoplasm to peptides that are transported into the ER, where they stabilize newly folded class I MHC molecules (Fig. 3). It is not clear whether the peptides are transported into the ER as nonamers or whether they are clipped to nonamers once there, before or after they have bound to the class I MHC molecules. Measurements of binding affinities and on-rates indicate that non-

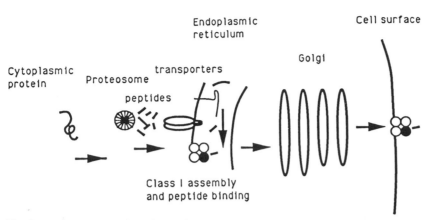

Fig. 3. Antigen processing of cytoplasmic proteins. Protein is thought to be digested by cytoplasmic proteosomes to peptide fragments which are transported into the endoplasmic reticulum by ADP binding cassette proteins. There, the peptides associate with newly synthesized class I molecules and the folded and stable heavy chain-β_2m-peptide complex is translocated to the cell surface through the Golgi complex where glycosylation is completed. Components of the proteosome complex and two transporters map in the MHC in the class II region (Deverson *et al*, 1990; Monaco *et al*, 1990; Trowsdale *et al*, 1990; Brown *et al*, 1991; Glynne *et al*, 1991)

amers bind with much higher affinity, with faster on-rates and slower off-rates than longer peptides (Cerundolo *et al*, 1991b).

Recent results indicate that there can be genetic polymorphism in the processing pathways. In the PVG R8 rat strain, Livingstone *et al* (1989) described class I modifying (CIM) genes, which appear to deliver different peptides to the same class I molecule; such genes mapped in the MHC and may be identical to the peptide transporter or proteasome genes described above. In humans, we have recently found a similar HLA linked polymorphism that modifies presentation of viral peptide epitopes by HLA-B27 (Pazmany *et al*, 1992) and other class I genes (Rowland-Jones S, Sutton J, Hill A, Rosenberg W and McMichael AJ, unpublished). Thus, the dominant role of class I MHC in selecting peptide epitopes can be modified by other HLA linked polymorphisms. This means that individuals with a given MHC type may be divisible into two or more subgroups that select and present different peptide epitopes.

It is not clear at this stage whether different tissues might present different peptides, derived from the same proteins. Differential tissue expression of the processing genes has not been explored. Similarly, their expression in tumour cells will be important to analyse, particularly where the HLA class I phenotype of a tumour resembles that of the RMA-S mutant cell line (see Kaklamanis and Hill in this issue). More subtly, if the processing phenotype of a tumour cell is modified, a new set of self peptides to which the individual is not tolerant may be generated, and these could be capable of eliciting CTL responses. Such peptide epitopes would not have to contain mutant sequences.

T CELL RECEPTORS

The T cell receptors are made up of two chains, α and β, both of which have variable joining and plus junctional diversity segments between the variable and constant regions (Davis and Bjorkman, 1989). CTL specific for class I restricted epitopes have been analysed (Rupp et al, 1985; Moss et al, 1991). In some cases, they are highly restricted in heterogeneity in both α and β chains (Moss et al, 1991). In other examples, either α or β may be restricted in heterogeneity (Moss P and Bowness P, unpublished). On the whole, CTL responses to a single peptide epitope are polyclonal by this analysis and by analysis of fine specificity of clones (McMichael et al, 1988). However, "polyclonal" in this context means more than six clones, and the responses are far less heterogeneous than, for instance, antibody responses to haptens. The restricted heterogeneity of CTL to certain epitopes does expose them to therapeutic modulation by antibody or superantigens. The mouse mammary tumour (retro) viruses, which encode superantigens in their 3′ long terminal repeat (LTR) regions and which are integrated in the mouse genomes, profoundly affect the T cell receptor repertoire of mice (Sato et al, 1986; Dyson et al, 1991; Frankel et al, 1991; Marrack et al, 1991). It is not clear how this relates to immunity to this tumour at this stage. Neither is it clear whether such integrated superantigens exist in humans.

FUNCTION OF CTL

CTL responses are normal components of the immune reaction. However, the level of CTL response is dependent on the nature of the antigen. Soluble protein antigens given by injection do not elicit strong CTL responses (Wraith and Askonas, 1985), although such proteins can if given within cells (Moore et al, 1988; Carbone and Bevan, 1989) or in particulate form as an immune complex (Randall and Young, 1987). Foreign proteins that are part of a virus elicit strong CTL responses. Proteins in other intracellular microorganisms can elicit CTL; this has been demonstrated for intracellular bacteria (Aggarwal et al, 1990) and for intracellular protozoal parasites (Romero et al, 1989). Foreign cells elicit CTL responses, as do mutant cells or experimental self cells transfected with foreign genes.

An important function of CTL is control of virus infections. There is substantial evidence to support this. For instance, CTL clones given to mice lethally infected with influenza virus or respiratory syncytial virus can clear lung infections; antibody alone cannot do this (Yap and Ada, 1978; Lin and Askonas, 1981; Cannon et al, 1988). T cell deficient mice, infected with a virus such as influenza, are more likely to die, and survivors do not clear virus; this can be reversed by giving CTL (Wells et al, 1981). In in vitro models, CTL can clear human immunodeficiency virus (HIV) (Walker et al, 1986; Brinchmann et al, 1990; Kannagi et al, 1990) and Epstein-Barr virus (EBV) from cultured cells (Moss et al, 1978).

Evidence for the role of CTL in human infections in vivo is less direct. CTL levels have correlated with protection against infection with influenza virus (McMichael *et al,* 1983) and respiratory syncytial virus (Isaacs *et al,* 1990) in volunteer studies. Cytomegalovirus specific CTL have been correlated with control of this infection after bone marrow transplantation (Quinnan *et al,* 1982). CTL activity is strong against EBV, and diminished CTL activity is associated with outgrowth of EBV positive lymphomas (Crawford *et al,* 1980; Rowe *et al,* 1991). A less direct but highly persuasive argument comes from situations where virus escapes from CTL control. Pircher *et al* (1990) infected mice transgenic for a CTL receptor specific for an epitope of lymphocytic choriomeningitis virus and obtained a mutant virus with an altered epitope sequence. In this model system, virus therefore escaped from CTL control. In natural infections, a recent study (Phillips *et al,* in press) has shown that mutations are relatively frequent in epitopes of HIV presented by HLA-B8 in HLA-B8+ but not B8− individuals. Peptides representing these mutant sequences were not recognized by CTL from the patients, and there was further evidence in these patients of an unstable CTL response, switching from one epitope to another. These data argue for escape mutation occurring in HIV, but this must be dependent on the HLA type of the infected individuals because the virus might tolerate variation in some regions (ie epitopes) and not others. The results also point to a protective role for CTL in HIV infection; other evidence for this is that the CTL responses are strong during the latent phase of infection but decline when acquired immunodeficiency syndrome (AIDS) develops. Overall, it appears that CTL control or eliminate virus infections. Antibody is much less efficient at doing this and, indeed, is more efficient at selecting escape mutants (Reitz *et al,* 1988). The role of antibody in virus infections is more important in prophylaxis, neutralizing virus and preventing reinfection.

There is a strong body of evidence that tumour cells can also escape from CTL control in vitro (Maryanski *et al,* 1982; De Plaen *et al,* 1988; Knuth *et al,* 1989a,b). This has been demonstrated for CTL specific for melanoma cell lines and is discussed elsewhere in this issue. Conversely, the mutant P815 cell line that is rejected on transfer into mice elicits strong CTL responses and differs in one aminoacid in the peptide epitope that the CTL see. There is no direct evidence that such events occur in vivo, but there seems to be no reason why they should not.

One issue that arises is whether an escape mutation in one epitope can offer a tumour or a virus selective advantage when other epitopes that co-elicit CTL responses may be unchanged. For viruses, this would be unlikely if a cell was infected with multiple viral particles, only one of which had a mutation in one epitope. With a retrovirus where a cell may have a low number of integrated copies, a change in one epitope, given that the total number of epitopes eliciting CTL responses is small, could easily confer a selective advantage on that virus. If the CTL responses are extremely strong, this may be unlikely, but if the CTL responses are borderline, as may happen if the total response is less strong or perhaps in certain sites in the body, then selective advantage, albeit slight, may give mutant virus the edge. Similarly, in tumour cells, mutation in one epitope in a single gene may give a cell population an advantage, making the cells slightly less susceptible to destruction by CTL. This concept is not very different from considerations of selective advantage offered by single mutations in multicellular organisms.

A related alteration may be in expression of HLA antigens themselves or of adhesion molecules. Some viruses can downregulate class I MHC molecules (Signas *et al*, 1982; Schrier *et al*, 1983; Andersson *et al*, 1985) or alter expression of adhesion molecules (Gregory *et al*, 1988). This must give the virus some advantage in evading CTL responses. Similarly, tumour cells frequently express class I MHC molecules abnormally (Gopas *et al*, 1989; Momberg *et al*, 1989a,b; Smith *et al*, 1989) and often show abnormal expression of adhesion molecules (Vanky *et al*, 1990). These issues are discussed elsewhere in this issue. Whether or not they are driven by CTL responses, a consequence must be that total CTL responses are impaired. These could be some of many factors that contribute to tumour growth spread.

HLA POLYMORPHISM

HLA class I antigens are extremely polymorphic. This implies that there is a parallel polymorphism in peptide epitopes selected and presented to CTL. The available evidence strongly supports this. It is widely believed that HLA polymorphism has been driven by infectious disease and that certain HLA types confer resistance to particular infectious diseases and therefore have selective advantages. Until recently, little real evidence for this existed. There is a clear example in chickens, namely Marek's disease (Briles *et al*, 1977), in which a particular allele confers resistance. There is less strong evidence that certain HLA types protected against typhoid and yellow fever in Dutch settlers in Surinam (De Vries *et al*, 1979). In a recent study, Hill *et al* (1991) showed that HLA-B53 and HLA-DR1302 confer resistance to severe malaria. The resistance offered by B53 may contribute to its relatively high frequency in subsaharan Africa compared to Europe. There should be many other examples where HLA contributes to resistance to disease, but the type of study required to demonstrate this is daunting because very large numbers of patients must be investigated to demonstrate statistically significant reductions in frequency of relatively rare alleles. The absence of such data does not weaken the hypothesis. It is less clear whether resistance to malignancy can play a part in the generation of HLA polymorphism. Because malignant diseases tend to occur in elderly populations, selective forces are much less strong than those operating in infectious diseases of childhood. However, one consequence of HLA polymorphism is that, by chance, certain HLA types may confer resistance or susceptibility to particular tumours. Examples of this are sparse, although an association between the HLA-B5 cross reactive group and resistance to Hodgkin's lymphomas was one of the earliest, albeit weak, associations described between HLA and disease (Amiel, 1967).

IMMUNE SURVEILLANCE

It is now clear that the primary function of CTL is to monitor cell surfaces for abnormal peptides presented by class I MHC molecules. Normal self peptides should have made reactive T cells tolerant, either by clonal deletion or by clonal anergy. Preliminary evidence suggests that CTL can detect as few as 200 foreign peptide molecules on a target cell (Christinck *et al*, 1991), and CTL are therefore extremely sensitive to changes within the environment of potential target cells. These may include not only expression of foreign or abnormal proteins, derived from viruses or by mutation, but also altered processing to generate different self peptides. An array of cell surface molecules, such as the LFA adhesion molecules, CD2-LFA3 and CD8 as well as class I MHC T cell receptor, are accessories to this surveillance process. The challenge now in relation to cancer research is to elucidate the role of CTL in tumours of major importance and to learn how to manipulate them for prophylaxis and therapy.

SUMMARY

Cytotoxic T lymphocytes recognize peptide fragments of cytoplasmic proteins presented by class I MHC molecules. Recently, these peptides have been shown to be short, usually nonamers, and their binding to particular class I molecules is now well understood. There is also detailed understanding of how proteins are processed to generate antigenic peptides and some knowledge of the T lymphocyte receptors involved. CTL have been shown to be important in controlling virus infections, including those that cause tumours. CTL have also been demonstrated against other tumours, and their activity may lead to the abnormalities of MHC class I molecule expression that are frequently observed on tumours. The overall role of CTL is probably to survey body cells for abnormalities, including those induced by virus infection and mutation, and to destroy potentially harmful cells.

References

Aggarwal A, Kumar S, Jaffe R, Hone A, Gross M and Sadoff J (1990) Oral salmonella: malaria circumsporozoite recombinants induce CD8+ cytotoxic T cells. *Journal of Experimental Medicine* **172** 1083–1090

Amiel J L (1967) Study of the leucocyte phenotypes in Hodgkins disease. *Histocompatibility Testing* **3** 14–24

Andersson M, Paabo S, Nilsson T and Peterson PA (1985) Impaired intracellular transport of class I MHC antigens as a possible means for adenovirus to evade immune surveillance. *Cell* **43** 215

Anichini A, Mazzocchi A, Fossati G and Parmiani G (1989) Cytotoxic T lymphocyte clones from peripheral blood and from tumor site detect intratumor heterogeneity of melanoma cells: analysis of specificity and mechanisms of interaction. *Journal of Immunology* **142** 3692–3701

Askonas BA, McMichael AJ and Webster RG (1982) The immune response to influenza virus and the problem of protection against infection, In: Beare AS (ed). *Basic and Applied Influenza Research*, pp 157–188, CRC Press, Boca Raton, Florida

Bangham CRM and AJ McMichael (1989) T-cell immunity to viruses, In: Feldmann M, Lamb J and Owen MJ (eds). *T Cells*, pp 281–310, John Wiley and Sons, New York

Bennink JR, Yewdell J and Gerhard W (1982) A viral polymerase involved in recognition of influenza virus-infected cells by a cytotoxic T cell clone. *Nature* **296** 75–76

Bjorkman P, Saper M, Samraoui B, Bennett W, Strominger J and Wiley D (1987a) The foreign antigen binding site and T cell recognition regions of class I histocompatibility antigens. *Nature* **329** 512–519

Bjorkman P, Saper M, Samraoui B, Bennett W, Strominger J and Wiley D (1987b) Structure of human class I histocompatibility antigen, HLA-A2. *Nature* **329** 506–511

Blank KJ, Freedman HA and Lilly F (1976) T-lymphocyte response to Friend virus-induced tumor cell-lines in mice congenic at H-2. *Nature* **260** 250–252

Briles WE, Stone HA and Cole RK (1977) Marek's disease: effects of B histocompatibility alloalleles in resistant and susceptible chicken lines. *Science* **195** 193–195

Brinchmann JE, Gaudernack G and Vartdal F (1990) CD8+ T cells inhibit HIV replication in naturally infected CD4+ T cells: evidence for a soluble inhibitor. *Journal of Immunology* **144** 2961–2966

Brown MG, Driscoll J and Monaco JJ (1991) Structural and serological similarity of MHC-linked LMP and proteosome (multicatalytic proteinase) complexes. *Nature* **353** 365–357

Cannon MJ, Openshaw PJM and Askonas BA (1988) Cytotoxic cells clear virus but augment lung pathology in mice infected with respiratory syncytial virus. *Journal of Experimental Medicine* **168** 1163–1168

Carbone FR and Bevan MJ (1989) Induction of ovalbumin-specific cytotoxic T cells by in vivo peptide immunization. *Journal of Experimental Medicine* **169** 603–12

Cerottini J-C and Brunner KT (1974) Cell mediated cytotoxicity, allograft rejection and tumour immunity. *Advances in Immunology* **18** 67–132

Cerundolo V, Alexander J, Anderson K *et al* (1990) Presentation of viral antigen controlled by a gene in the major histocompatibility complex. *Nature* **345** 449–452

Cerundolo V, Elliott T, Bastin J, Rammensee H-G and Townsend A (1991a) The binding affinity and dissociation rates of peptides for class I major histocompatibility complex molecules. *European Journal of Immunology* **21** 2069–2076

Cerundolo V, Tse AGD, Salter RD, Parham P and Townsend A (1991b) CD8 independence and specificity of cytotoxic T lymphocytes restricted by HLA Aw68 1. *Proceedings of the Royal Society Series B* **244** 169–177

Christinck ER, Luscher MA, Barber BH and Williams DB (1991) Peptide binding to class I MHC on living cells and quantitation of complexes required for CTL lysis. *Nature* **352** 67–70

Crawford DH, Thomas JA, Janossy G *et al* (1980) Epstein-Barr virus nuclear antigen positive lymphoma after cyclosporin A treatment in patients with renal allograft. *Lancet* **i** 1355–1356

Crowley NJ, Darrow TL, Quinn-Allen MA and Seigler HF (1991) MHC-restricted recognition of autologous melanoma by tumor-specific cytotoxic T cells: evidence for restriction by a dominant HLA allele. *Journal of Immunology* **146** 1692–1699

Davis MM and Bjorkman PJ (1989) T-cell receptor genes and T-cell recognition. *Nature* **334** 395–402

De Plaen E, Lurquin C, Van Pel A *et al* (1988) Immunogenic (tum-) variants of mouse tumor P815: cloning of the gene of tum- antigen P91A and identification of the tum- mutation.

Proceedings of National Academy of Sciences of the USA **85** 2274–227

Deverson EV, Gow JR, Coadwell WJ, Monaco JJ, Butcher GW and Howard JC (1990) MHC class II region encoding proteins related to the multidrug resistance family of transmembrane transporters. *Nature* **348** 738–741

De Vries RR, Khan PM Bernini LF, Van Loghem E and Van Rood (1979) Genetic control of survival in epidemics. *Journal of Immunogenetics* **6** 271–287

Dyson PJ, Knight AM, Fairchild S, Simpson E and Tomonari K (1991) Genes encoding ligands for deletion of V70 1 T cells cosegregate with mammary tumour virus genomes. *Nature* **349** 531–533

Elvin J, Cerundolo V, Elliot T and Townsend A (1991) A quantitative assay of peptide-dependent class I assembly. *European Journal of Immunology* **21** 2025–2032

Falk K, Rotzschke O and Rammensee H-G (1990) Cellular peptide composition governed by major histocompatibility complex class I molecules. *Nature* **348** 248–251

Falk K, Rotzschke O, Stevanovic S, Jung G and Rammensee H-G (1991) Allele specific motifs revealed by sequencing of self peptides eluted from MHC molecules. *Nature* **351** 290–296

Frankel WN, Rudy C, Coffin JM and Huber BT (1991) Linkage of Mls genes to endogenous mammary tumour viruses of inbred mice. *Nature* **349** 526–529

Gardner I, Bowern NA and Blanden RV (1974) Cell-mediated cytotoxicity against ectromelia virus infected target cells: II identification of effector cells and analysis of mechanisms. *European Journal of Immunology* **4** 68–72

Garrett TPJ, Saper MA, Bjorkman PJ, Strominger JL and Wiley DC (1989) Specificity pockets for the side chains of peptide antigens in HLA-Aw68. *Nature* **342** 692

Glynne R, Powis SH, Beck S, Kelly A, Kerr L-A and Trowsdale JA (1991) Proteosome-related gene between the two ABC transporter loci in the class II region of the human MHC. *Nature* **353** 357–360

Gooding LR and O'Connell KA (1983) Recognition by cytotoxic T lymphocytes of cells expressing fragments of the SV40 tumour antigen. *Journal of Immunology* **131** 2580–2586

Gopas J, Rager-Zisman B, Bar-Eli M, Hammerling GJ and Segal S (1989) The relationship between MHC antigen expression and metastasis. *Advances in Cancer Research* **53** 89–115

Gotch FM, McMichael AJ, Smith GL and Moss B (1987a) Identification of the virus molecules recognised by influenza specific cytotoxic T lymphocytes. *Journal of Experimental Medicine* **165** 408–416

Gotch F, Rothbard J, Howland K, Townsend A and McMichael A (1987b) Cytotoxic T lymphocytes recognise a fragment of influenza virus matrix protein in association with HLA-A2. *Nature* **326** 881–882

Gotch FM, McMichael AJ and Rothbard J (1988) Recognition of influenza A matrix protein by HLA-A2 restricted cyotoxic T lymphocytes: use of analogues to orientate the matrix peptide in the HLA A2 binding site. *Journal of Experimental Medicine* **168** 2045–2058

Gregory CD, Murray RJ, Edwards CF and Rickinson AB (1988) Downregulation of cell adhesion molecules LFA-3 and ICAM-1 in Epstein-Barr virus-positive Burkitt's lymphoma underlies tumor cell escape from virus-specific T cell surveillance. *Journal of Experimental Medicine* **167** 1811–1824

Herin M, Lemoine C, Weynants P *et al* (1987) Production of stable cytolytic T-cell clones directed against autologous human melanomas. *International Journal of Cancer* **39** 390–396

Hill AVS, Allsopp CEM, Kwiatkowski D *et al* (1991) Common West African HLA antigens are associated with protection from severe malaria. *Nature* **352** 595–600

Huet S, Nixon DF, Rothbard J, Townsend ARM, Ellis SA and McMichael AJ (1990) Structural homologies between two HLA B27 restricted peptides suggest residues important for interaction with HLA B27. *International Immunology* **2** 311

Isaacs D, McDonald NE, Bangham CRM, McMichael AJ, Higgins PG and Tyrrell DAJ (1990) The specific cytotoxic T-cell response of adult volunteers to infection with respiratory syncitial virus. *Immunology and Infectious Diseases* **1** 5–12

Jardetsky T, Lane WS, Robinson RA, Madden DR and Wiley DC (1991) Identification of self peptides bound to purified HLA-B27. *Nature* **353** 326–329

Kannagi M, Masuda T, Hattori T *et al* (1990) Interference with human immunodeficiency virus (HIV) replication by CD8+ T cells in peripheral blood leukocytes of asymptomatic HIV carriers in vitro. *Journal of Immunology* **64** 3399–3406

Kast WM, Offringa R, Peters PJ *et al* (1989) Eradication of adenovirus E1-induced tumors by E1A-specific cytotoxic T lymphocytes. *Cell* **59** 603–614

Knuth A, Danowski B, Oettgen HF and Old LJ (1989a) T-cell-mediated cytotoxicity against autologous malignant melanoma: analysis with interleukin 2-dependent T-cell cultures. *Proceedings of the National Academy of Sciences of the USA* **81** 3511–3515

Knuth A, Wolfel T, Klehmann E, Boon T and Meyer zum Buschenfelde K-H (1989b) Cytolytic T-cell clones against an autologous human melanoma: specificity study and definition of three antigens by immunselection. *Proceedings of the National Academy of Sciences of the USA* **86** 2804–2808

Latron F, Moots R, Rothbard J *et al* Positioning of a peptide in the cleft of HLA A2 by complementing amino acid changes. *Proceedings of the National Academy of Sciences of the USA* (in press)

Leclerc JC, Gomard E, Plata F and Levy J-P (1973) Cell-mediated immune reaction against tumours induced by oncornaviruses II Nature of effector cells in tumour-cell cytolysis. *International Journal of Cancer* **11** 426–432

Lin Y and Askonas BA (1981) Biological properties of an influenza A virus specific killer T cell clone. *Journal of Experimental Medicine* **154** 225–234

Livingstone AM, Powis SJ, Diamond AG, Butcher GW and Howard JC (1989) A trans-acting major histocompatibility complex-linked gene whose alleles determine gain and loss changes in the antigenic structure of a classical class I molecule. *Journal of Experimental Medicine* **170** 777–795

Ljunggren HG, Stam NJ, Ohlen C *et al* (1990) Empty MHC class I molecules come out in the cold. *Nature* **346** 476–80

McMichael AJ, Gotch FM, Noble GR and Beare PAS (1983) Cytotoxic T-cell immunity to influenza. *New England Journal of Medicine* **309** 13–17

McMichael A, Gotch F and Rothbard J (1986) HLA B37 determines an influenza A virus nucleoprotein epitope recognized by cytotoxic T lymphocytes. *Journal of Experimental Medicine* **164** 1397–1406

McMichael AJ, Gotch FM Santos-Aguado J and Strominger JL (1988) Effect of mutations and variations of HLA-A2 on recognition of a virus peptide epitope by cytotoxic T lymphocytes. *Proceedings of the National Academy of Sciences of the USA* **85** 9194–1006

Madden DR, Gorga JC, Strominger JL and Wiley DC (1991) The structure of HLA-B27 reveals nonamer self-peptides bound in an extended conformation. *Nature* **353** 221–325

Marrack P, Kushnir E and Kappler J (1991) A maternally inherited superantigen encoded by a mammary tumour virus. *Nature* **349** 524–526

Maryanski JL, Van Snick J, Cerottini J-C and Boon T (1982) Immunogenic variants obtained by mutagenesis of mouse mastocytoma P815 III. Clonal analysis of the syngeneic cytolytic T lymphocyte response. *European Journal of Immunology* **12** 401–406

Momberg F Degener T Bacchus E Moldenhauer G and Hammerling GJ (1989a) Loss of HLA-ABC and de novo expression HLA-D in colorectal cancer. *International Journal of Cancer* **37** 179–184

Momberg F, Ziegler A, Harpprecht J, Moller P, Moldenhauer G and Hammerling GJ (1989b) Selective loss of HLA-A or HLA-B antigen expression in colon carcinoma. *Journal of Immunology* **142** 352–358

Monaco J, Cho S and Attaya M (1990) Transport protein genes in the murine MHC: possible implications for antigen processing. *Science* **250** 1723–1726

Moore MW, Carbone FR and Bevan MJ (1988) Introduction of soluble protein into the class I pathway of antigen presentation. *Cell* **54** 777–785

Moots RJ, Matsui M, Pazmany L, McMichael AJ and Frelinger JA (1991) A cluster of mutations in the HLA A2 alpha2 helix abolishes peptide recognition by T cells. *Immunogenetics* **34** 141–148

Morrison J, Elvin J, Latron F *et al* Identification of the nonamer peptide from influenza A matrix protein and the role of pockets of HLA A2 in its recognition by cytotoxic T lymphocytes. *European Journal of Immunology* (in press)

Moss DJ, Rickinson AB and Pope JH (1978) Long term T cell mediated immunity to Epstein-Barr virus in man I Complete regression of virus-induced transformation on cultures of seropositive donor leukocytes. *International Journal of Cancer* **22** 662–668

Moss PAH, Moots RJ, Rosenberg WMC, Rowland-Jones SJ, McMichael AJ and Bell JI (1991) Extensive conservation of alpha and beta chains of the human T cell antigen receptor recognizing HLA-A2 and influenza matrix peptide. *Proceedings of the National Academy of Sciences of the USA* **88** 8987–8981

Mukherji B and McAlister TJ (1983) Clonal analysis of cytotoxic T cell response against human melanoma. *Journal of Experimental Medicine* **158** 240–245

Pazmany L, Rowland-Jones S, Huett S *et al* Genetic modulation of antigen presentation by HLA B27 molecules. *Journal of Experimental Medicine* (in press)

Phillips RE, Rowland-Jones S, Nixon DF *et al* Human immunodeficiency virus genetic variation that can escape cytotoxic T cell recognition. *Nature* (in press)

Pircher H, Moskphidis A, Rohrer U, Burki K, Hengartner H and Zinkernagel RM (1990) Viral escape by selection of cytotoxic T cell-resistant variants in vivo. *Nature* **346** 629–233

Plata F, Cerottini JC and Brunner KT (1975) Primary and secondary in vitro generation of cytolytic T lymphocytes in the murine sarcoma virus system. *European Journal of Immunology* **5** 227–233

Quinnan GV, Kirmani N, Rook AH *et al* (1982) Cytotoxic T cell in cytomegalovirus infection: HLA restricted T lymphocyte and non-T lymphocyte cutotoxic responses correlate with recovery from cytomegalovirus infection on bone-marrow transplant recipients. *New England Journal of Medicine* **307** 7–13

Randall RE and Young DF (1987) Humoral and cytotoxic T cell responses to internal and external structural proteins of Simian virus 5 induced by immunization with solid matrix antibody and antigen complexes. *Journal of General Virology* **69** 2505

Reitz MS, Wilson, Nangle C, Gallo RC and Robert-Guroff M (1988) Generation of a neutralization resistant variant of HIV-1 is due to selection for a point mutation in the envelope gene. *Cell* **54** 57–63

Romero P, Maryanski JL, Corradin G, Nussenzweig R, Nussenzweig V and Zavala F (1989) Cloned cytotoxic T cells recognize an epitope in the circumsporozoite protein and protect against malaria. *Nature* **341** 323–326

Rowe M, Young LS, Crocker J, Stokes H, Henderson S and Rickinson AB (1991) Epstein-Barr virus (EBV)-associated lymphoproliferative disease in the SCID mouse model: implications for the pathogenesis of EBV-positive lymphomas in man. *Journal of Experimental Medicine* **173** 147–158

Rupp FH, Acha-Orbea H, Hengartner H, Zinkernagel R and Joho R (1985) Identical V β T cell receptor genes used in alloreactive cytotoxic and antigen plus I-A specific helper T cells. *Nature* **315** 425

Saper MA, Bjorkman PJ and Wiley DC (1991) Refined structure of the human histocompatibility antigen HLA-A2 at 2.6 Å resolution. *Journal of Molecular Biology* **219** 277–319

Sato T, Sato N, Takahashi S, Koshiba H and Kikuchi K (1986) Specific cytotoxicity of a long-term cultures T-cell clone on human autologous mammary cancer cells. *Cancer Research* **46** 4384–4389

Schrier PL, Bernards R, Vaessen RTMJ, Houweling A and van der Eb AJ (1983) Expression of class I major histocompatibility antigens switched off by highly oncogenic adenovirus 12 in transformed rat cells. *Nature* **305** 771–775

Signas C, Katze M, Persson H and Philipsson L (1982) An adenovirus glycoprotein binds heavy chain of class I transplantation antigens from man and mouse. *Nature* **299** 175–178

Slavin SF, Lackman RD, Ferrone S, Kiely PE and Mastrangelo MJ (1986) Cellular immune response to human sarcomas: cytotoxic T cell clones reactive with autologous sarcomas I development phenotype and specificity. *Journal of Immunology* **137** 3042–3048

Smith ME, Marsh SGE, Bodmer JG, Gelsthorpe K and Bodmer WF (1989) Loss of HLA-ABC allele products and lymphocyte functioassociated antigen-3 in colorectal neoplasia. *Proceedings of the National Academy of Sciences of the USA* **86** 5557–5561

Spies and DeMars R (1991) Restored expression of major histocompatibility class I molecules by gene transfer of a putative peptide transporter. *Nature* **351** 323–325

Spies T, Bresnahan M, Bahram S *et al* (1990) A gene in the major histocompatibility complex class II region controlling the class I antigen presentation pathway. *Nature* **348** 744–747

Townsend ARM and Skehel JJ (1982) Influenza A specific cytotoxic T cell clones that do not recognise viral glycoproteins. *Nature* **300** 655

Townsend ARM, Gotch FM and Davey J (1985a) Cytotoxic T cells recognise fragments of influenza nucleoprotein. *Cell* **42** 457–467

Townsend ARM, McMichael AJ and Brownlee GG (1985b) *Recognition of the Viral Nucleoprotein by Influenza A Specific Cytotoxic T Cells,* Humana Press, London

Townsend A, Rothbard J, Gotch F, Bahadur B, Wraith D and McMichael A (1986) The epitopes of influenza nucleoprotein recognized by cytotoxic T lymphocytes can be defined with short synthetic peptides. *Cell* **44** 959–968

Townsend A, Ohlen C, Bastin JL Junggren HG, Foster L and Karre K (1989a) Association of class I major histocompatibility heavy and light chains induced by viral peptides. *Nature* **340** 443–448

Townsend A, Ohlen C, Foster L, Bastin JL, Junggren HG and Karre K (1989b) A mutant cell in which association of class I heavy and light chains is induced by viral peptides. *Cold Spring Harbor Symposia on Quantative Biology* **1** 299–308

Townsend A, Elliott T, Cerundolo V, Foster L, Barber B and Tse A (1990) Assembly of MHC class I molecules analyzed in vitro. *Cell* **62** 285–295

Trowsdale J, Hanson I, Mockridge I, Beck S, Townsend ARM and Kelly A (1990) Sequences encoded in the class II region of the MHC related to the ABC superfamily of transporters. *Nature* **348** 741–744

Van Bleek GM and Nathenson SM (1990) Isolation of an endogenously processed immunodominant viral peptide from the class I H2Kb molecule. *Nature* **348** 213

Van den Eynde B, Hainaut P, Herin M *et al* (1989) Presence on a human melanoma of multiple antigens recognized by autologous CTL. *International Journal of Cancer* **44** 634–640

Vanky F, Wang P, Patarroyo M and Klein E (1990) Expression of the adhesion molecule ICAM-1 and major histocompatibility complex class I antigens on human tumor cells is required for their interaction with autologous lymphocytes in vitro. *Cancer Immunology and Immunotherapy* **31** 19–27

Walker CM, Moody DJ, Stites DP and Levy JA (1986) CD8+ lymphocytes can control HIV infection in vitro by suppressing virus replication. *Science* **234** 1563–1566

Wells MA, Ennis FA and Albrecht P (1981) Recovery from a viral respiratory infection II Passive transfer of immune spleen cells to mice with influenza pneumonia. *Journal of Immunology* **126** 1042–1046

Wolfel T, Klehmann E, Muller C *et al* (1989) Lysis of human melanoma cells by autologous cytolytic T cell clones Identification of human histocompatibity leukocyte antigen A2 as a restriction element for three different antigens. *Journal of Experimental Medicine* **170** 797–810

Wraith DC and Askonas BA (1985) Induction of influenza A virus cross-reactive cytotoxic T cells by a nucleoprotein/haemagglutin preparation. *Journal of General Virology* **66** 1327

Yap KL and Ada GL (1978) Transfer of specific cytotoxic T lymphocytes protects mice inoculated with influenza virus. *Nature* **273** 238–240

Zinkernagel RM and Doherty PC (1975) H-2 compatibility requirement for T-cell mediated lysis of target cells infected with lymphocytic choriomeningitis virus. *Journal of Experimental Medicine* **141** 1427–1436

The author is responsible for the accuracy of the references.

Identification of Tumour Rejection Antigens Recognized by T Lymphocytes

T BOON[1] • **E DE PLAEN**[1] • **C LURQUIN**[1] • **B VAN DEN EYNDE**[1]
P VAN DER BRUGGEN[1] • **C TRAVERSARI**[1] • **A AMAR-COSTESEC**[2]
A VAN PEL[1]

[1]*Ludwig Institute for Cancer Research, Brussels Branch, 74 avenue Hippocrate,
B-1200 Brussels, Belgium, and Cellular Genetics Unit, Université Catholique de Louvain;*
[2]*International Institute of Molecular and Cellular Pathology, University of Louvain,
B-1200 Brussels*

Introduction
Tum⁻ antigens and tum⁻ mutations
    Tum⁻ antigens recognized by CTL
    Genes encoding tum⁻ antigens
    Genomic mutations and immune surveillance
A tumour rejection antigen of mouse tumour P815
    Tumour rejection antigens defined on P815
    Absence of mutation on gene P1A
    Discussion
Transfection of a human gene coding for an antigen recognized on a
melanoma by autologous CTL
Summary

INTRODUCTION

Rodent tumours induced with chemical carcinogens elicit immune responses that lead to the rejection of secondary tumour grafts in syngeneic animals (Gross, 1943; Prehn and Main, 1957; Klein *et al*, 1960). The relevant antigens are different for every tumour (Basombrio, 1970). They have been named tumour specific transplantation antigens (TSTA), and similar antigens are observed on tumours induced by ultraviolet irradiation (Kripke, 1974). Virus induced mouse tumours also express antigens that correspond to viral products (Sjögren *et al*, 1961; Khera *et al*, 1963; Klein and Klein, 1964). Other tumours, especially spontaneous tumours, appear to be completely incapable of inducing immune rejection responses (Hewitt *et al*, 1976; Middle and Embleton, 1981). This finding led to the suggestion that TSTA might constitute a

Cancer Surveys Volume 13: *A New Look at Tumour Immunology*
© 1992 Imperial Cancer Research Fund. 0-87969-370-3/92. $3.00 + .00

laboratory artefact restricted to tumours induced with very high doses of carcinogen. However, immunogenic tumour variants derived from spontaneous tumours by mutagen treatment are capable of eliciting a specific immune protection against the original tumours (Van Pel *et al*, 1983). Similar results have been obtained with other non-immunogenic tumours by transfection of a gene coding for a viral antigen or for interleukin-2 (Fearon *et al*, 1988, 1990). This indicates that spontaneous or induced non-immunogenic tumours also express antigens that are potential targets for immune responses. To what extent these antigens must be absolutely specific for the tumour is not entirely clear, as will be seen below. We therefore prefer the name "tumour rejection antigens" rather than "tumour specific transplantation antigens".

It is now generally accepted that T lymphocytes are the key element of the specific immune responses that can lead to tumour rejection (Rouse *et al*, 1972; Kripke and Fisher, 1976; Kripke, 1981). For several tumour systems, it is possible to obtain from syngeneic animals highly specific cytolytic T lymphocytes (CTL), which can be used to define tumour rejection antigens rigorously (Leclerc *et al*, 1973; Boon *et al*, 1980; Brunner *et al*, 1980). Stable CTL clones with high activity and specificity have been obtained (Uyttenhove *et al*, 1983). They have proved to be extremely useful for the identification of multiple antigens expressed by the same tumour cell.

The nature of tumour rejection antigens has proved difficult to elucidate because no antibodies have been obtained that recognized specifically the antigenic molecules. This is not surprising considering the overwhelming evidence that T lymphocytes recognize short antigenic peptides presented in a groove formed by the external domains of major histocompatibility complex (MHC) class I or class II molecules (Allen *et al*, 1984; Bjorkman *et al*, 1987; Townsend and Bodmer, 1989). This has prevented the isolation of tumour rejection antigens by immunoprecipitation, a difficulty that applies not only to these antigens but also to minor histocompatibility antigens. Biochemical fractionation of tumour cell extracts to obtain purified tumour rejection antigens has been attempted by several groups. The fractions were tested for their ability to immunize mice so as to make them resistant to tumour challenge. Thus, an immunogenic protein was isolated from MethA, a methylcholanthrene induced sarcoma (Ullrich *et al*, 1986; Moore *et al*, 1987). This protein proved to be a heat shock protein. With a similar approach, two proteins have been isolated from two methylcholanthrene induced sarcomas. Each induces an immunity that is specific for its sarcoma of origin. The genes coding for these proteins have been isolated, but the basis for the diversity of these antigens has not yet been elucidated (Srivastava *et al*, 1986, 1987, 1988).

We have developed a genetic approach aimed at cloning the genes producing antigens recognized by CTL. We applied it first to elucidate the nature of tum⁻ antigens, which are expressed by tumour cells treated with mutagen. The same method ensured the identification of a tumour rejection antigen of mouse tumour P815. We present here a summary of these results and also discuss an approach aimed at identifying a human tumour rejection antigen.

TUM⁻ ANTIGENS AND TUM⁻ MUTATIONS

Tum⁻ Antigens Recognized by CTL

Exposure of mouse tumour cell lines to chemical mutagens generates at very high frequency tumour cell variants that are no longer able to form progressive tumours in syngeneic animals (Boon, 1983). These variants have accordingly been named "tum⁻", in contrast to the original tumorigenic "tum⁺" cell line. The tum⁻ variants are stable, but the tum⁻ phenotype is rarely absolute: most tum⁻ variants produce progressive tumours in a small fraction of the injected animals (Uyttenhove et al, 1980). Tum⁻ variants have been obtained from many different mouse tumour cell lines, including a teratocarcinoma (Boon and Kellermann, 1977), mastocytoma P815 (Uyttenhove et al, 1980), radiation induced or spontaneous leukaemias (Van Pel and Boon, 1982; Van Pel et al, 1983) and other tumours (Bonmassar et al, 1970; Frost et al, 1983; Zbar et al, 1984; Altevogt et al, 1985). More recently, tum⁻ variants were obtained by ultraviolet irradiation (Hostetler et al, 1986).

The failure of tum⁻ variants to form tumours appears to be the consequence of an immune rejection response, because these variants form progressive tumours in mice that have been immunosuppressed by sublethal irradiation (Van Pel et al, 1979). Mice that have rejected a tum⁻ variant usually have a higher degree of resistance against a challenge with the same variant than against any other tum⁻ variant derived from the same tumour cell line (Boon and Van Pel, 1978). This was the first evidence that most tum⁻ variants express new transplantation antigens that are specific for each variant. The specific immune memory can be transferred adoptively with T lymphocytes (Boon and Kellermann, 1977).

We have analysed in vitro the response directed against tum⁻ variants derived from mastocytoma P815, a tumour obtained by methylcholanthrene treatment of a DBA/2 ($H-2^d$) mouse. When spleen cells of DBA/2 mice that have rejected a tum⁻ variant are stimulated in vitro with the same variant, very active populations of CTL are produced, and these show preferential lysis on the immunizing variant (Boon et al, 1980). This confirmed that tum⁻ variants express "tum⁻" antigens specific for each individual variant. Analysis of more than 15 independent tum⁻ variants showed that none of their tum⁻ antigens were present on more than one variant, nor was any cross reaction observed among these antigens. The repertoire of the tum⁻ antigens is therefore quite large (Boon, 1983), like that of the antigens observed on the methylcholanthrene induced tumours.

Stable CTL clones that show strict specificity for the immunizing P815 tum⁻ variant have been obtained. These CTL clones provided a very important tool for the analysis of tum⁻ antigens, namely the immune selection of antigen loss variants (Maryanski and Boon, 1982; Maryanski et al, 1982). By incubation of some tum⁻ variants with the appropriate anti-tum⁻ CTL clones, stable secondary variants resistant to the CTL can be selected. In many instances, these cells are still sensitive to other CTL clones that are specific for the same tum⁻ variant. These CTL clones can then be used in turn to select resistant variants, and the results indicate that many tum⁻ variants express several tum⁻ antigens that can be lost independently of each other. In addition, antigen loss variants have provided proof that the tum⁻ antigens defined by CTL cause the immune rejection of the tum⁻ variants. When antigen loss variants selected in vitro were injected into DBA/2 mice, we observed that they had regained the ability to form progressive tumours (Maryanski and Boon, 1982). The converse was also observed: most of the rare tumours obtained after injection of tum⁻ variants were found to have become resistant to the CTL clones directed against at least one of the tum⁻ antigens of the injected variants (Maryanski *et al*, 1983). These observations demonstrate beyond reasonable doubt that antigens recognized by CTL are relevant in vivo, and they justify attempts to isolate the genes that code for these antigens. We undertook to clone these genes from tum⁻ variants of P1, a clonal line isolated from P815.

Genes Encoding tum⁻ Antigens

The first gene isolated was the gene coding for tum⁻ antigen P91A, an antigen expressed by tum⁻ variant P91. To clone the genes that determine the expression of this antigen, we resorted to an approach based on gene transfection and detection of antigen expressing transfectants with CTL (Wölfel *et al*, 1987). By transfecting P815 tum⁺ cells with a cosmid library prepared with the DNA of a cell expressing tum⁻ antigen P91A, we obtained transfectants expressing this antigen, and from these transfectants, we recovered a cosmid carrying the encoding gene (De Plaen *et al*, 1988). Northern blots hybridized with a probe derived from gene P91A revealed a single mRNA species. The band was of equal intensity for the mRNA of tum⁻ variant P91 and for that of P815 cells, which do not express the antigen (Lurquin *et al*, 1989). The expression of antigen P91A is therefore not due to the activation of a silent gene.

The structure of gene P91A is shown in Fig. 1. It consists of 12 exons spread over 14 kb (Lurquin *et al*, 1989). The complete sequence has been obtained. It is unrelated to any sequence presently recorded in the main data banks. Confirmation for the relevance of this gene was provided by the study of three "escaping" tumours obtained with tum⁻ variant P91. These variants, which had lost the expression of gene P91A, all showed deletions in the tum⁻ allele of the gene (Lurquin *et al*, 1989).

A sequence comparison of the normal and tum⁻ alleles of gene P91A indicated that they differ by a point mutation in an exon (Fig. 1). This "tum⁻" mutation consists of a G to A transition, which changes an arginine into a histidine in the product of the main open reading frame of the gene (De Plaen *et al*, 1988). This mutation appears to be the only difference distinguishing the normal from the antigenic allele.

Genes coding for tum⁻ antigens P35B and P198, expressed by other tum⁻ variants of P815, have also been cloned (Sibille *et al*, 1990; Szikora *et al*, 1990).

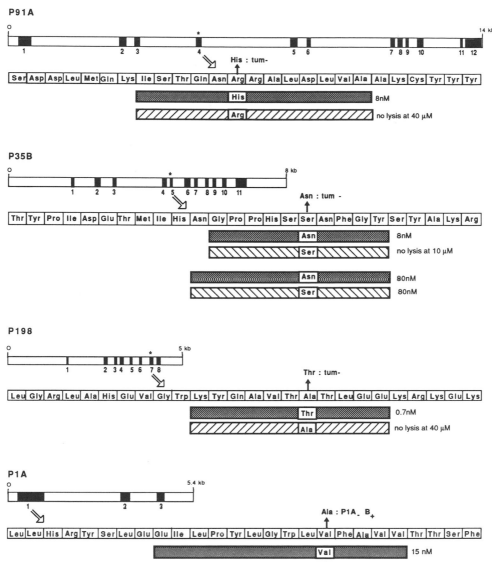

Fig. 1. Genes coding for mouse tum⁻ antigens P91A, P35B and P198 and for tumour rejection antigen P1A. Exons are marked in black. Asterisks indicate locations of tum⁻ mutations. Concentrations of antigenic peptides shown are those that provide half maximum lysis with the appropriate CTL (μM/l). The aminoacids encoded by the relevant exons are also given, with the changes directed by the tum⁻ mutations

The study of the tum⁻ alleles of these genes also revealed that they differ from their normal counterpart by a point mutation in an exon (Fig. 1). These genes are also expressed equally in the relevant tum⁻ variant and in other P815 cells. The general structures and the sequences of the three tum⁻ genes isolated so far are completely unrelated. These genes show no homology with any gene so far recorded in data banks.

The main open reading frame of gene P91A encodes a protein of 529 aminoacid residues (60 kDa; Lurquin *et al*, 1989). Subcellular fractionation of mouse liver, 3T3 fibroblasts, and P815 cell lines indicates that this protein is cytosolic, a finding consistent with the fact that its primary aminoacid sequence contains no endoplasmic reticulum targeting signal (Amar-Costesec *et al*, 1990). This subcellular location is not surprising, since CTL recognize influenza antigens corresponding to viral proteins that remain inside the cell (Townsend *et al*, 1986). We examined whether we could identify a small peptide that would render P1 cells sensitive to lysis by anti-P91A CTL. In our search for this peptide, we were guided by the location of the tum⁻ mutation. A short peptide corresponding to the sequence surrounding this mutation made P1 cells sensitive to anti-P91A CTL at a concentration of approximately 10 nmol/l (Fig. 1). In confirmation of previous transfection experiments, studies with fibroblasts that expressed either K^d, D^d or L^d demonstrated that this P91A peptide is associative with L^d.

Studies with P91A peptides enabled us to understand the role of the tum⁻ mutation. A priori, this mutation should be able to influence the production of the antigenic peptide, its ability to associate with the L^d molecule (ie the aggretope of the peptide) or the epitope presented to T cells by the peptide-MHC complex. Having defined the antigenic P91A peptide, we prepared the homologous peptide corresponding to the normal allele of the gene. This peptide did not induce lysis by anti-P91A CTL, nor did it compete with the mutant peptide. Moreover, we found that the mutant peptide competed effectively to prevent a cytomegalovirus derived peptide from inducing lysis by CTL directed against an L^d associative cytomegalovirus antigenic peptide. The normal peptide did not compete, indicating that it did not bind to L^d (Lurquin *et al*, 1989). We conclude that the P91A tum⁻ mutation generates the aggretope of the antigen, but we cannot exclude an influence on the epitope.

Antigenic peptides corresponding to the sequence surrounding the tum⁻ mutation were also obtained for genes P35B and P198 (Fig. 1). They associate with D^d and K^d, respectively. For antigen P198, the effect of the mutation appears to be different from that of P91A: here, a new epitope is introduced on a peptide that is already capable of binding to the K^d presenting molecule (Sibille *et al*, 1990). Presumably, the complex between this normal peptide and K^d corresponds either to a hole in the T cell repertoire or to T cell clones that have been deleted by natural tolerance. For antigen P35B, we were surprised to find that a peptide with the normal sequence provoked lysis with a half maximum value of approximately 80 nmol/l. However, no lysis was produced with a shorter normal peptide corresponding to the most active peptide derived from the mutant sequence. This suggests either that peptides active at concentrations above 80 nmol/l do not have a physiological role or that not all possible peptides, in this instance the longer one, are produced inside the cell in a manner that enables them to be effectively presented. Using a procedure described recently (Lie *et al*, 1990), we have found that the shorter peptide with the normal sequence cannot increase the surface exposure of D^d, suggesting that it lacks the adequate aggretope.

Genomic Mutations and Immune Surveillance

The identification of tum⁻ genes and mutations provides a plausible explanation for the high frequency and stability of tum⁻ variants. They are stable because they are point mutants. They are extremely frequent and diverse because the tum⁻ mutations arise in a large number of different genes. These mutations generate new antigenic peptides, either by enabling them to bind to an MHC class I molecule or by generating new epitopes on peptides that are already capable of binding but are not recognized by the T cell repertoire, possibly because of natural tolerance. It is worth noting that point mutations generating new peptides are also involved in the generation of minor histocompatibility antigen MTF (Fischer Lindahl *et al*, in press).

Our results suggest that mutations occurring throughout the mammalian genome can produce new antigenic peptides recognized by some members of the adult T cell repertoire. There is thus an elaborate presentation mechanism, which confers to T lymphocytes the potential of monitoring the integrity of the mammalian genome. This provides a basis for the longstanding concept of immune surveillance (Burnet, 1970). In our opinion, however, it would be mistaken to believe that cells are eliminated whenever they acquire a mutation. It is likely that cells expressing a new antigen must accumulate in large numbers before they can elicit a T cell response (Old and Boyse, 1964). Perhaps these cells must also express several new antigens, so that different T cells can reinforce each other, for instance by interleukin secretion.

A TUMOUR REJECTION ANTIGEN OF MOUSE TUMOUR P815

Tumour Rejection Antigens Defined on P815

Clonal cell line P1, which was derived from tumour P815, expresses several antigens recognized by CTL of the syngeneic DBA/2 mice (Uyttenhove *et al*, 1980). From mice immunized either with living cells of P815 tum⁻ variants or with irradiated P1 cells, stable CTL clones have been obtained that lyse P815 and do not lyse other syngeneic tumours or normal DBA/2 cells. A panel of these CTL clones was used to select P1 cells that are resistant in vitro. Antigen loss variants resistant to some CTL and not to others were obtained, and in this way, three distinct antigens could be defined. We also observed that P1 cells injected intraperitoneally sometimes undergo a nearly complete rejection, followed by a long stationary state, during which a small number of tumour cells survive in the peritoneal cavity (Uyttenhove *et al*, 1980). Eventually, the tumour cells invariably resume their growth and kill the animal. This "tumour dormant state" has been observed in at least one other tumour system (Weinhold *et al*, 1979). When these escaping P815 cells were analysed for their sensitivity to the panel of anti-P815 CTL, we found that one of the three antigens defined by in vitro selection could be "split": one of the antigen loss variants obtained in vivo (P1.istA⁻) had lost only one of two antigens that were invariably lost together in the antigen loss variants selected in vitro. This brought the number of distinct P815 tumour rejection antigens to four: P815A, B, C and D; A and B are usually lost together. The observation that P815A and B are lost by tumour cells that escape tumour rejection in vivo provided a rigorous demonstration that these antigens have a significant role in the anti-tumoral response occurring in vivo.

Absence of Mutation on Gene P1A

To isolate the gene coding for tumour rejection antigen P815A, we transfected DNA of the P1 cell line into an A⁻B⁻ antigen loss variant of P815. Transfectants expressing antigen P815A were obtained. All of them also expressed P815B, confirming the close linkage between these two antigens and suggesting that they were encoded by the same gene. Transfectants were also obtained with a cosmid library, and from these, a gene was retrieved that was able to transfer the expression of antigens P815A and P815B (Van den Eynde *et al*, 1991). Transfection studies carried out with fibroblasts expressing K^d, D^d or L^d demonstrated that antigens P815A and P815B were both presented to the CTL by the L^d molecule.

The structure and complete sequence of gene P1A have been determined (see Fig. 1). They proved to be completely different from those of the three tum⁻ genes. No significant homology was found in gene data banks, except with sequences that code for an acidic domain present in two nucleolar proteins. When the sequence of gene P1A cloned from tumour cells was compared with that of the equivalent gene cloned from normal cells of the same mouse strain, no difference was found (Van den Eynde *et al*, 1991). In confirmation of this, the gene isolated from normal tissue transfers the expression of antigens P815A and P815B as well as the gene cloned from P815 cells. The antigens produced by gene P1A are therefore not the result of a mutation affecting the gene expressed by the tumour.

Because the antigenicity of gene P1A is not due to a point mutation, there was no easy guide in the search for the antigenic peptide. However, analysis of the gene carried by the P1A⁻B⁺ antigen loss variant (P1.istA⁻) indicated that it differed by a point mutation in exon 1 (Lethé B, Van den Eynde B and Boon T, unpublished). Synthetic peptides corresponding to the normal version of the sequences surrounding this mutation were prepared, and one of them proved to be capable of causing lysis by anti-P815A CTL (Fig. 1). Surprisingly, this peptide also sensitized cells to the anti-P815B CTL. These results suggest that these two CTL recognize two different epitopes on the same peptide.

The expression of gene P1A has been analysed with northern blots and RNase protection. The level of transcription is high in P815, but it is undetectable in normal tissues of adult mice, such as liver, spleen and bone marrow. Because P815 was originally described as a mastocytoma, we also tested a number of mast cell lines for expression of the gene (Van den Eynde *et al*, 1991). Mast cell line MC/9 and short term cultures of mast cells isolated from mouse bone marrow were negative on northern blots. In contrast, a strong signal was obtained with L138.8A, a mast cell line derived from Balb/c bone marrow by culture in medium containing interleukin-3. We took advantage of the fact that Balb/c and DBA/2 mice share the H-2^d haplotype to test the sensitivity of L138.8A to lysis by anti-P815 CTL clones. A high level of lysis was observed with anti-A and anti-B CTL. We conclude that tumour rejection antigens P815A and B result from the expression by tumour P815 of a gene that is silent in normal adult tissues but may also be active in other tumours of similar origin.

Discussion

Mice that have rejected P815 cells do not show any obvious health impairment. How can antigens that are encoded by normal genes elicit an immune rejection response against the tumour without severe autoimmune consequences? A first explanation may be provided by the longstanding notion of "oncofetal" antigens, implying that tumours re-express fetal antigens that have disappeared from all normal cells before the establishment of natural tolerance—hence, the absence of tolerance and the absence of autoimmune consequences of the response, since no normal cell of the adult animal would express these antigens. An alternative explanation is that gene P1A is expressed by mast cell precursors located in the bone marrow at a brief stage of their differentiation. These cells would not by themselves induce an immune response because of their small number and dispersion. The anti-tumoural response might eliminate some of these precursor cells, but after the rejection of the tumour, the active effector T cells would become resting memory cells, and mast cell differentiation could resume without damage.

There is as yet no evidence that antigens P815A and B can elicit a T cell response on their own. P815 appears to express at least two other antigens recognized by CTL. One cannot exclude that a response against these antigens creates conditions that strongly facilitate the response against antigens A and B. This would be in line with the observation that tum⁻ variants derived from non-immunogenic tumours elicit a response directed against an antigen present on these tumours (Van Pel *et al*, 1983).

TRANSFECTION OF A HUMAN GENE CODING FOR AN ANTIGEN RECOGNIZED ON A MELANOMA BY AUTOLOGOUS CTL

For human neoplasms, several groups have observed that autologous mixed lymphocyte-tumour cell cultures (MLTC) frequently generate responder lymphocytes that lyse the autologous tumour cells and do not lyse natural killer targets, autologous Epstein-Barr virus (EBV)-transformed B cells or autologous fibroblasts (Anichini *et al*, 1987). This response has been particularly well studied in melanomas with MLTC that have been carried out either with peripheral blood cells or with tumour infiltrating lymphocytes (Mukherji and MacAlister, 1983; Knuth *et al*, 1984; Hérin *et al*, 1987; Topalian *et al*, 1988).

From MLTC responder cells, it has been possible to derive stable CTL clones that appear to be completely specific for the tumour cells (Mukherji and Mac Alister, 1983; Hérin *et al*, 1987; Knuth *et al*, 1989). The analysis of potential rejection antigens by autologous cytolytic T lymphocytes is reviewed by Knuth *et al* (this issue).

Using a panel of autologous CTL, we have been able to demonstrate the existence of four different stable antigens on melanoma cell line MZ2-MEL (Van den Eynde *et al*, 1989). We have initiated an approach aimed at isolating the gene that codes for one of these antigens, namely MZ2-E. As a first step, we attempted to obtain a transfectant expressing this antigen. We used as DNA recipient cell a variant of MZ2-MEL, which had been selected with an anti-E CTL clone for the loss of antigen E. This variant was then cotransfected with genomic DNA of the original MZ2-MEL melanoma line and with selective plasmid pSVtkneoβ. Geneticin resistant transfectants were obtained, and these transfectants were then screened for their ability to stimulate the anti-E CTL clone to produce tumour necrosis factor. One transfectant expressing antigen E was identified among 66 000 drug resistant transfectants. When this cell was submitted to immunoselection with the anti-E CTL clone, a resulting antigen loss variant was found to have lost several of the transfected pSVtkneoβ sequences. This indicated that the gene coding for the antigen had been integrated in the vicinity of pSVtkneoβ sequences, as expected for cotransfected DNA. This result suggests that the approach that has been used to isolate genes coding for antigens recognized on mouse tumours by CTL may be extended to human tumours.

SUMMARY

On the basis of the results reviewed here, there are two major mechanisms whereby tumour rejection antigens may arise. The first mechanism is mutational. Point mutations occurring in a large variety of genes may produce new antigenic peptides, either by providing them with the ability to bind to MHC class I molecules or by providing them with a new epitope (Fig. 2). The second mechanism is the activation of a gene that is silent in normal tissues and for which no strong natural tolerance has been established.

Plausible candidates for the mutational mechanism are the "tumour specific transplantation antigens" observed on methylcholanthrene induced tumours and tumours induced by ultraviolet light. The diversity of these antigens appears to be very large, like that of the tum⁻ antigens. Moreover, these tumours have been obtained with high doses of carcinogens, which are proven mutagens. On the other hand, a P815 tumour rejection antigen appears to arise through the activation of a silent gene, and it may turn out that this is the rule for most tumour rejection antigens. It is our hope that other genes coding for mouse and human tumour rejection antigens will soon be identified, so that it will become clear whether the activational mechanism is the

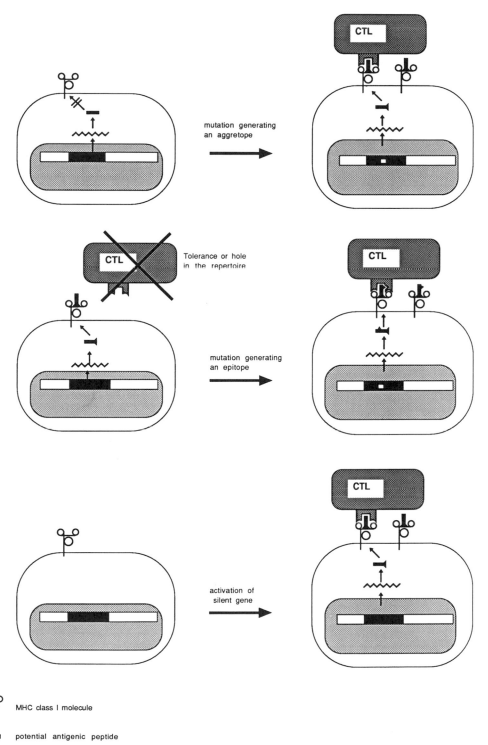

mutation generating
an aggretope

Tolerance or hole
in the repertoire

mutation generating
an epitope

activation of
silent gene

qʘ
P̕   MHC class I molecule

▬   potential antigenic peptide

Fig. 2. Possible mechanisms for the production of antigens recognized by T lymphocytes on tumour cells. See the text for explanation

rule or the exception. In our view, this is a crucial issue. Insofar as tumour rejection antigens result from mutations, they may be highly specific for every individual tumour. The tumour specific nature of these antigens would then be easily ascertained. However, active immunization of cancer patients would require that a tumour cell line be obtained from each patient, a most unpractical prospect. If, on the other hand, production of tumour rejection antigens results from the activation of a normal gene, then there is a good probability that the same gene may be activated in many different tumours, being perhaps preferentially shared by tumours of the same histological type. This would probably not result in the expression of the same antigen in all these tumours, because the patients would differ in their presenting molecules, which are determined by their HLA haplotype. However, a subset of the tumours expressing the same "tumour rejection" gene should share the same class I restricting element, so that all of these patients could be immunized with a cell that would express the gene and carry the appropriate HLA molecule. In other words, the identification of patients suitable for immune intervention may become possible at an early stage of their disease by means of HLA typing and using the polymerase chain reaction to analyse small tumour cell samples for expression of various genes known to code for tumour rejection antigens.

References

Allen PM, Strydom D and Unanue ER (1984) Processing of lysozyme by macrophages: identification of the determinant recognized by two T cell hybridomas. *Proceedings of the National Academy of Sciences of the USA* **81** 2489–2493

Altevogt P, Von Hoegen P, Leidig S and Schirrmacher V (1985) Effects of mutagens on the immunogenicity of murine tumor cells: immunological and biochemical evidence for altered cell surface antigens. *Cancer Research* **45** 4270–4277

Amar-Costesec A, Godelaine D, Verlant V, Van Pel A and Beaufay H (1990) The class I-restricted tum⁻ antigen P91A derives from a bona fide cytosolic protein. *Journal of Cell Biology* **111** 481a

Anichini A, Fossati G and Parmiani G (1987) Clonal analysis of the cytolytic T-cell response to human tumors. *Immunology Today* **8** 385–389

Basombrio M (1970) Search for common antigenicity among twenty-five sarcomas induced by methylcholanthrene. *Cancer Research* **30** 2458–2462

Bjorkman PJ, Saper MA, Samraoui B, Bennett WS, Strominger JL and Wiley DC (1987) The foreign antigen binding site and T cell recognition regions of class I histocompatibility antigens. *Nature* **329** 512–518

Bonmassar E, Bonmassar A, Vadlamudi S and Goldin A (1970) Immunological alteration of leukemic cells in vivo after treatment with an antitumor drug. *Proceedings of the National Academy of Sciences of the USA* **66** 1089–1095

Boon T (1983) Antigenic tumor cell variants obtained with mutagens. *Advances in Cancer Research* **39** 121–151

Boon T and Kellermann O (1977) Rejection by syngeneic mice of cell variants obtained by mutagenesis of a malignant teratocarcinoma cell line. *Proceedings of the National Academy of Sciences of the USA* **74** 272–275

Boon T and Van Pel A (1978) Teratocarcinoma cell variants rejected by syngeneic mice: protection of mice immunized with these variants against other variants and against the original malignant cell line. *Proceedings of the National Academy of Sciences of the USA* **75** 1519–1523

Boon T, Van Snick J, Van Pel A, Uyttenhove C and Marchand M (1980) Immunogenic variants obtained by mutagenesis of mouse mastocytoma P815 II T lymphocyte-mediated cytolysis. *Journal of Experimental Medicine* **152** 1184–1193

Brunner K, MacDonald R and Cerottini J-C (1980) Antigenic specificity of the cytolytic T lymphocyte (CTL) response to murine sarcoma virus-induced tumors II Analysis of the clonal progeny of CTL precursors stimulated in vitro with syngeneic tumor cells. *Journal of Immunology* **124** 1627–1634

Burnet FM (1970) A certain symmetry: histocompatibility antigens compared with immunocyte receptors. *Nature* **226** 123–126

De Plaen E, Lurquin C, Van Pel A *et al* (1988) Immunogenic (tum⁻) variants of mouse tumor P815: cloning of the gene of tum⁻ antigen P91A and identification of the tum⁻ mutation. *Proceedings of the National Academy of Sciences of the USA* **85** 2274–2278

Fearon ER, Itaya T, Hunt B, Vogelstein B and Frost P (1988) Induction in a murine tumor of immunogenic tumor variants by transfection with a foreign gene. *Cancer Research* **48** 2975–2980

Fearon ER, Pardoll DM, Itaya T *et al* (1990) Interleukin-2 production by tumor cells bypasses T helper function in the generation of an antitumor response. *Cell* **60** 397-403

Fischer Lindahl K, Hermel E, Loveland BE and Wang C-R Maternally transmitted antigen of mice: a model transplantation antigen. *Annual Review of Immunology* **9** (in press)

Frost P, Kerbel R, Bauer E, Tartamella-Biondo R and Cefalu W (1983) Mutagen treatments as a means for selecting immunogenic variants from otherwise poorly immunogenic malignant murine tumors. *Cancer Research* **43** 125–132

Gross L (1943) Intradermal immunization of C3H mice against a sarcoma that originated in an animal of the same line. *Cancer Research* **3** 326–333

Hérin M, Lemoine C, Weynants P *et al* (1987) Production of stable cytolytic T-cell clones directed against autologous human melanoma. *International Journal of Cancer* **39** 390–396

Hewitt H, Blake E and Walder A (1976) A critique of the evidence for active host defence against cancer based on personal studies of 27 murine tumors of spontaneous origin. *British Journal of Cancer* **33** 241–259

Hostetler LW, Ananthaswamy HN and Kripke ML (1986) Generation of tumor-specific transplantation antigens by UV radiation can occur independently of neoplastic transformation. *Journal of Immunology* **137** 2721–2725

Khera KS, Ashkenasi A, Rapp F and Melnick JL (1963) Immunity in hamsters to cells transformed in vitro among the papovaviruses. *Journal of Immunology* **91** 604–613

Klein E and Klein G (1964) Antigenic properties of lymphomas induced by the Moloney agent. *Journal of the National Cancer Institute* **32** 547–568

Klein G, Sjögren H, Klein E and Hellström KE (1960) Demonstration of resistance against methylcholanthrene-induced sarcomas in the primary autochthonous host. *Cancer Research* **20** 1561–1572

Knuth A, Danowski B, Oettgen HF and Old L (1984) T-cell-mediated cytotoxicity against autologous malignant melanoma: analysis with interleukin-2-dependent T-cell cultures. *Proceedings of the National Academy of Sciences of the USA* **81** 3511–3515

Knuth A, Wölfel T, Klehmann E, Boon T and Meyer zum Büschenfelde K-H (1989) Cytolytic T-cell clones against an autologous human melanoma: specificity study and definition of three antigens by immunoselection. *Proceedings of the National Academy of Sciences of the USA* **86** 2804–2808

Kripke ML (1974) Antigenicity of murine skin tumors induced by ultraviolet light. *Journal of the National Cancer Institute* **53** 1333–1336

Kripke ML (1981) Immunologic mechanism in UV radiation carcinogenesis. *Advances in Cancer Research* **34** 69–106

Kripke ML and Fisher MS (1976) Immunologic parameters of ultraviolet carcinogenesis. *Jour-*

nal of the National Cancer Institute **57** 211–215

Leclerc JC, Gomard E, Plata F and Levy JP (1973) Cell-mediated immune reaction against tumors induced by oncornaviruses II Nature of the effector cells in tumor-cell cytolysis. *International Journal of Cancer* **11** 426–432

Lie W-R, Myers NB, Gorka J, Rubocki RJ, Connolly JM and Hansen TH (1990) Peptide ligand-induced conformation and surface expression of the Ld class I MHC molecule. *Nature* **344** 439–441

Lurquin C, Van Pel A, Mariamé B *et al* (1989) Structure of the gene coding for tum⁻ transplantation antigen P91A: a peptide encoded by the mutated exon is recognized with Ld by cytolytic T cells. *Cell* **58** 293–303

Maryanski JL and Boon T (1982) Immunogenic variants obtained by mutagenesis of mouse mactocytoma P815 IV Analysis of variant-specific antigens by selection of antigen-loss variants with cytolytic T cell clones. *European Journal of Immunology* **12** 406–412

Maryanski JL, Van Snick J, Cerottini J-C and Boon T (1982) Immunogenic variants obtained by mutagenesis of mouse mastocytoma P815 III Clonal analysis of the syngeneic cytolytic T lymphocyte response. *European Journal of Immunology* **12** 401–406

Maryanski JL, Marchand M, Uyttenhove C and Boon T (1983) Immunogenic variants obtained by mutagenesis of mouse mastocytoma P815 VI Occasional escape from host rejection due to antigen-loss secondary variants. *International Journal of Cancer* **31** 119–123

Middle J and Embleton M (1981) Naturally arising tumors of the inbred WAB/Notrat strain II Immunogenicity of transplanted tumors. *Journal of the National Cancer Institute* **67** 637–643

Moore SK, Kozak C, Robinson EA, Ullrich SJ and Appella E (1987) Cloning and nucleotide sequence of the murine hsp84 cDNA and chromosome assignment of related sequences. *Gene* **56** 29–40

Mukherji B and MacAlister TJ (1983) Clonal analysis of cytotoxic T cell response against human melanoma. *Journal of Experimental Medicine* **158** 240–245

Old LJ and Boyse EA (1964) Immunology of experimental tumors. *Annual Review of Medicine* **15** 167–186

Prehn RT and Main JM (1957) Immunity to methycholanthrene-induced sarcomas. *Journal of the National Cancer Institute* **18** 769–778

Rouse BT, Röllinghoff M and Warner NL (1972) Anti-θ serum-induced suppression of the cellular transfer of tumour-specific immunity to a syngeneic plasma cell tumour. *Nature New Biology* **238** 116–117

Sibille CP, Chomez C, Wildmann A *et al* (1990) Structure of the gene of tum⁻ transplantation antigen P198: a point mutation generates a new antigenic peptide. *Journal of Experimental Medicine* **172** 35–45

Sjögren HO, Hellström I and Klein G (1961) Resistance of polyoma virus-immunized mice to transplantation of established polyoma tumors. *Experimental Cell Research* **23** 204–208

Srivastava PK, Deleo AB and Old LJ (1986) Tumor rejection antigens of chemically induced sarcomas of inbred mice. *Proceedings of the National Academy of Sciences of the USA* **83** 3407–3411

Srivastava PK, Chen Y-T and Old LJ (1987) 5′-structural analysis of genes encoding polymorphic antigens of chemically induced tumors. *Proceedings of the National Academy of Sciences of the USA* **84** 3807–3811

Srivastava PK, Kozak CA and Old LJ (1988) Chromosomal assignment of the gene encoding the mouse tumor rejection antigen gp96. *Immunogenetics* **28** 205–207

Szikora JP, Van Pel A, Brichard V *et al* (1990) Structure of the gene of tum⁻ transplantation antigen P35B: presence of a point mutation in the antigenic allele. *EMBO Journal* **9** 1041–1050

Topalian SL, Solomon D, Davis FP *et al* (1988) Immunotherapy of patients with advanced cancer using tumor-infiltrating lymphocytes and recombinant interleukin-2: a pilot study. *Journal of Clinical Oncology* **6** 839–853

Townsend A and Bodmer H (1989) Antigen recognition by class I-restricted T lymphocytes. *Annual Review of Immunology* **7** 601–624

Townsend A, Rothbard J, Gotch F, Bahadur G, Wraith D and McMichael A (1986) The epitopes of influenza nucleoprotein recognized by cytotoxic T lymphocytes can be defined with short synthetic peptides. *Cell* **44** 959–968

Ullrich SJ, Robinson EA, Law LW, Willingham M and Appella E (1986) A mouse tumor-specific transplantation antigen is a heat shock-related protein. *Proceedings of the National Academy of Sciences of the United States of the USA* **83** 3121–3125

Uyttenhove C, Van Snick J and Boon T (1980) Immunogenic variants obtained by mutagenesis of mouse mastocytoma P815 I Rejection by syngeneic mice. *Journal of Experimental Medicine* **152** 1175–1183

Uyttenhove C, Maryanski J and Boon T (1983) Escape of mouse mastocytoma P815 after nearly complete rejection is due to antigen-loss variants rather than immunosuppression. *Journal of Experimental Medicine* **157** 1040–1052

Van den Eynde B, Hainaut P, Hérin M *et al* (1989) Presence on a human melanoma of multiple antigens recognized by autologous CTL. *International Journal of Cancer* **44** 634–640

Van den Eynde B, Lethé B, Van Pel A, De Plaen E and Boon T (1991) The gene coding for a major tumor rejection antigen of tumor P815 is identical to the normal gene of syngeneic DBA/2 mice. *Journal of Experimental Medicine* **173** 1373–1384

Van Pel A and Boon T (1982) Protection against a nonimmunogenic mouse leukemia by an immunogenic variant obtained by mutagenesis. *Proceedings of the National Academy of Sciences of the USA* **79** 4718–4722

Van Pel A, Georlette M and Boon T (1979) Tumor cell variants obtained by mutagenesis of a Lewis lung carcinoma cell line: immune rejection by syngeneic mice. *Proceedings of the National Academy of Sciences of the USA* **76** 5282–5285

Van Pel A, Vessière F and Boon T (1983) Protection against two spontaneous mouse leukemias conferred by immunogenic variants obtained by mutagenesis. *Journal of Experimental Medicine* **157** 1992–2001

Weinhold K, Miller D and Wheelock E (1979) The tumor dormant state: comparison of L5178Y cells used to establish dormancy with those that emerge after its termination. *Journal of Experimental Medicine* **149** 745–757

Wölfel T, Van Pel A, De Plaen E, Lurquin L, Maryanski JL and Boon T (1987) Immunogenic (tum⁻) variants obtained by mutagenesis of mouse mastocytoma P815 VIII Detection of stable transfectants expressing a tum⁻ antigen with a cytolytic T cell stimulation assay. *Immunogenetics* **26** 178–187

Zbar B, Sukumar S, Tanio Y, Terata N and Hovis J (1984) Antigenic variants isolated from a mutagen-treated guinea pig fibrosarcoma. *Cancer Research* **44** 5079–5085

The authors are responsible for the accuracy of the references.

T Cell Responses to Human Malignant Tumours

A KNUTH • T WÖLFEL • K-H MEYER ZUM BÜSCHENFELDE

I Medizinische Klinik und Poliklinik, Johannes-Gutenberg-Universität, Langenbeckstrasse 1, D-6500 Mainz, Germany

INTRODUCTION

The search for human cancer antigens that trigger a specific autologous immune response has been pursued with serum antibodies and T lymphocytes. The most compelling evidence, to date, for the existence of human tumour antigens that induce a specific autologous antibody response in patients comes from studies of Old and colleagues, which demonstrated serum autoantibodies with specificity for autologous cancer cells (Old 1981; Furukawa *et al*, 1989). It is now clear that cellular antigens are recognized by T cells in a way that is quite different from the recognition of cell surface antigens by antibodies. Firstly, T cells were found to recognize antigens at the cell surface in association with surface proteins encoded by the major histocompatibility complex (MHC) (Zinkernagel and Doherty, 1979). Then, antigen recognition by T cells was shown to be mediated, in general, through intracellular processing of protein antigens into small peptides, which are presented in a small groove of the MHC protein at the cell surface (Townsend *et al*, 1986; Bjorkman *et al*, 1987; Garrett *et al*, 1989; Townsend and Bodmer 1989; Falk *et al*, 1991). This explains why antigenic determinants relevant for T lymphocyte recognition usually do not at the same time induce an antibody response in the host. This also means, however, that antibody to immunoprecipitate and characterize these antigens is not readily available. The identification and characterization of tumour rejection antigens recognized by T lymphocytes have been carried furthest in experimental animal systems (reviewed in Boon *et al*, this issue). Here, we summarize our and others' experiences in detecting and dissecting human tumour antigens that elicit an autologous T lymphocyte response.

CYTOLYTIC T LYMPHOCYTES (CTL) IN MELANOMA

Since the early 1970s, evidence has been accumulating that patients with malignant melanoma respond immunologically to their tumours (Hellström and Hellström 1974; Clark *et al*, 1977). The first extensive analysis of cytolytic activity found in peripheral blood mononuclear cells (PBMC) against auto-logous melanoma cells established in permanent tissue culture was published by Livingston *et al* (1979). Of 32 patients, 18 consistently showed autologous reactivity, which appeared to correlate with more limited disease and better prognosis. Cellular immunology took an unprecedented leap forward with the characterization of T cell markers by means of monoclonal antibodies and the production of T cell growth factors and other cytokines with recombinant DNA technology, starting in the later 1970s. Subsequently, numerous reports were published on cytolytic and regulatory T lymphocyte functions in vitro after stimulation with autologous tumour cells from cancer patients. The key issue in cancer immunology remains the definition of unique cancer antigens that elicit an immune response in the tumour bearing host.

Derivation of CTL

T cell cultures and clones for use as probes for the detection of cancer antigens have been derived from different sources and in different tumour systems. The vast majority of studies (reviewed in Anichini *et al*, 1987) describe PBMC as a source of effector lymphocytes. Freshly isolated PBMC from cancer patients have been tested in autologous systems by many groups, including ours (Mukherji and MacAlister, 1983; Knuth *et al*, 1984; Hérin *et al*, 1987). Depending on the assay systems used, in particular the time of effector and target cell incubations, little or no cytolytic activity was detected with freshly isolated PBMC against autologous tumour target cells, even at high effector cell to target cell ratios.

To approach standards set by Old and colleagues (1981), systematic analysis of CTL responses to autologous tumour cells required large enough numbers of CTL to test specific reactions against a broad panel of targets in repeated tests. For a rigorous specificity analysis, including cold target inhibition, not only effector lymphocytes but also target cells should be available in sufficient quantity, preferentially established in tissue culture and cloned for the study of target antigens. There are obvious limitations with tissue culture, since not all tumour targets are easily established in vitro. Moreover, tissue culture itself has inherent disadvantages, for example the possible introduction of artefacts, contamination with virus or mycoplasma and outgrowth of non-representative target cell populations from the primary tumour cell culture.

Mixed lymphocyte-tumour cell cultures (MLTC) have proved useful in initiating CTL cultures from PBMC and eliciting specific CTL (Mukherji and MacAlister, 1983; Knuth et al, 1984). Briefly, PBMC are separated from peripheral blood on density gradients and mixed with irradiated or drug treated stimulator tumour cells. Although endogenous interleukin-2 (IL-2) is released from lymphocytes upon stimulation with tumour targets, exogenous IL-2 at low concentrations is generally necessary to maintain growth of stimulated lymphocytes without impairing the specificity of responder CTL. Repeated antigen stimulation at regular intervals and growth factors are the driving forces for an actively growing population of CTL (Hérin et al, 1987). In this way, CTL cultures and CTL clones can be generated in sufficient quantity for a rigorous specificity analysis.

Other ways of generating CTL cultures with lytic activity on autologous tumour target cells include stimulation with pooled allogeneic lymphocytes (MLC) from healthy donors and activation with IL-2 alone (Zarling et al, 1978; Vose and Bonnard, 1982; Parmiani et al, 1985). Although lymphocyte proliferation and lytic activity will be induced this way, induction of specificity for autologous tumour targets has generally been insufficient. Lymphokine activated killer cells (LAK) will not be discussed in this context (Grimm et al, 1982).

In the late 1980s, much attention was paid to mononuclear cell infiltrates in and around tumour sites. For T lymphocytes recovered from those specimens by scraping or by enzyme treatment of tumour specimens, sometimes with subsequent density gradient centrifugation, the term "tumour infiltrating lymphocytes" (TIL) was coined. The presence of TIL in tumour tissue is assumed to indicate a host response against the tumour. Although freshly separated TIL generally have low cytolytic activity against tumour target cells, further propagation in IL-2 may generate highly cytolytic effector cells that in some instances have been shown to have specificity for the autologous tumour target cells (Topalian et al, 1989). However, culture conditions for the in vitro propagation of TIL are different from those generally applied to PBMC stimulated in MLTC. IL-2 concentrations used for TIL are generally 10–50 times higher and, owing to the presence of fresh tumour cells in early cultures of TIL, conditions required for in vitro restimulation are quite different from those required for standard MLTC. Instead of waiting for residual tumour cells to disappear gradually from early TIL cultures, some workers have used density gradient centrifugation to separate lymphocytes and tumour cells for restimulation at regular intervals with irradiated autologous tumour cells (Anichini et al, 1989). Other workers reported that MLTC carried out with TIL derived from melanoma specimens generated specific effector cells earlier than PBMC-MLTC (Itoh et al, 1988). In most reports, however, the activity of TIL is described as highly cytolytic for a broader range of fresh and cultivated tumour cells, resembling the broad activity of LAK cells. Whether

TIL are a special effector cell entity with a particular pattern of cytolytic activity and specificity or resemble PBMC exposed to tumour is not yet clear. Miescher *et al* (1986) compared lectin stimulation of TIL and PBMC in microculture systems. They found with TIL a suppressed proliferative response to lectin stimulation as compared to PBMC, suggesting suppressive effects of tumour cells. Conversely, when PBMC were exposed to tumour cells, a similarly reduced lectin response was observed. The main obstacle to specificity studies with TIL is that fresh tumour tissue is generally not available for extensive analysis of putative tumour antigens expressed on these targets.

Specificity Analysis of CTL

Specificity analysis of CTL against human cancer cells supposedly expressing cancer associated antigens is hindered by major ethical and strategic difficulties. Firstly, it is impossible to test the lytic activity of CTL on a wide variety of autologous normal cells. In melanoma, for example, it is not easy to obtain melanocyte cultures, from which melanomas are thought to arise, for unlimited testing. Secondly, whether cancer associated antigens recognized by CTL, if they exist, are truly tumour rejection antigens cannot be tested in vivo, as was done in experimental animal systems. The only reasonable way to overcome these obstacles will be to clone genes coding for CTL defined human cancer antigens. A first approach to this goal is covered by Boon *et al* in this issue.

Until a human CTL defined cancer antigen is cloned and sequenced, the search for tumour specific antigens will continue with the limited means available. Three categories of targets for specificity analysis are available at the present time. Autologous targets will mostly be limited to fibroblasts, Epstein-Barr virus transformed B cells (EBV-B cells), melanocytes and cultures of normal kidney epithelial cells in the case of renal cancer. The second category consists of allogeneic tumour target cells established from other cancer patients, preferentially HLA typed to encounter HLA restricted recognition of antigens by CTL. A third category consists of targets such as K562 cells that are sensitive to "natural killer" cell activity.

Lytic specificity of CTL is usually tested in 4-hour assays measuring chromium-51 release from targets after a lethal hit encounter with a CTL. Competitive inhibition with non-labelled or cold targets resembles absorption studies known in serology. CTL are probes with exquisite specificity, not only triggering a lytic event but also capable of a specific proliferative response to re-exposure with the respective antigen. Since CTL generated in MLTC are usually polyclonal, a thorough specificity analysis will require tests with CTL clones, preferentially on cloned target cell populations. Below, we outline our and other laboratories' approaches at defining tumour antigens with CTL clones.

Our strategy for obtaining stable CTL clones was described by Hérin *et al*

(1987). In brief, culture conditions after MLTC with irradiated melanoma targets as stimulator cells included restimulation of responder lymphocytes with autologous melanoma at regular intervals in the presence of human recombinant IL-2 in low concentrations (25 units/ml). For cloning, CTL were seeded at limiting dilutions in IL-2 containing media with allogeneic irradiated EBV-B cells as feeder cells. CTL clones generated were restimulated at regular intervals with autologous melanoma cells in the presence of feeder cells and tested for reactivity with autologous melanoma and a panel of control targets.

Several laboratories have described stable CTL clones with a tumour restricted pattern of reactivity, mostly from melanoma patients (Mukherji and MacAlister, 1983; Knuth et al, 1984; Hérin et al, 1987; Mukherji et al, 1989) but also from patients with other cancers, such as sarcoma (Slovin et al, 1986), breast cancer (Sato et al, 1986), B lymphoma (Yssel et al, 1984) and ovarian carcinoma (Ferrini et al, 1985). Whereas non-cloned CTL cultures tend to lose their specific cytolytic activity, CTL clones can be maintained in culture for several months, retaining a specific pattern of reactivity upon restimulation with antigen expressing cells at regular intervals (Knuth et al, 1984; Hérin et al, 1987).

In 1976, Carey et al established a cell line, SK-MEL-29, from a patient, AV, who had recurrent metastatic melanoma. Our own studies in this patient were prompted by the observations of Livingston et al (1979), who detected in PBMC preparations from the patient strong cytolytic reactions with autologous melanoma cells in a 40 hour ^{3}H-labelled proline retention assay (Bean et al, 1973). After various treatments, including surgery, chemotherapy and repeated treatments with irradiated autologous and allogeneic melanoma cell vaccines, grown in tissue culture, the patient, now 38, remains clinically free of disease, although adequate surgical margins never were obtained.

After an initial analysis of this patient's CTL response to autologous melanoma cells, we successfully established CTL clones that preferentially lysed autologous tumour cells but not other autologous target cells (such as EBV-B cells or fibroblasts) or allogeneic target cells (Knuth et al, 1984). With more advanced techniques for establishing stable long term CTL cultures (Hérin et al, 1987), we extended our study to investigation of AV CTL activity against autologous and allogeneic targets (Knuth et al, 1989). We established a panel of CTL clones with restricted reactivity both to autologous tumour cell clones and to non-cloned tumour cells in culture and confirmed the restricted reactivity by testing against a broad panel of HLA typed allogeneic target cell lines sharing HLA class I allospecificities with AV/SK-MEL-29. We also tested the clones for "natural killer" like phenomena. There was no lysis of any target cell except the autologous tumour clones. The specificity analysis consisted of assays of direct cytolytic activity, as well as stimulation assays for proliferative responses. The CTL clones established in this study were exclusively of a CD3+/CD8+ phenotype, in agreement with the finding of HLA class I restricted lysis demonstrated by blocking with a monoclonal antibody against a monomorphic HLA class I determinant. Others have also found CD3+/CD4+ CTL clones reactive with autologous tumours, suggesting an HLA class II restricted pattern of target cell recognition (Hérin *et al*, 1987).

From patient MZ-2 with advanced metastatic melanoma, we established a tumour cell line that was mutagenized with N-methyl-N-nitro-N-nitrosoguanidine (MNNG) based on a rationale and an approach for experimental tumour systems outlined by Boon *et al* in this issue. In a collaboration between Boon and our laboratory patient, MZ-2 repeatedly received mutagenized autologous tumour cell clones that had been exposed to lethal irradiation. After surgical tumour resection, the patient experienced an intra-abdominal recurrence early in the course of autologous tumour cell vaccination. After a few weeks of immune stimulation, however, the tumour stopped growing, and it gradually disappeared over the next few weeks. The patient remains alive and well with no evidence of disease more than 8 years later. Thus, patient MZ-2 is a second example of a remarkable clinical course observed during our studies of CTL responses against autologous tumour cells.

In the AV melanoma system, we detected stable antigen expression only. With CTL generated in MLTC from patient MZ-2, Hérin *et al* (1987) described three different antigenic phenotypes of tumour cell clones. They defined an antigen A, which is found on all clones and subcultures of MZ-2 melanoma, and an antigen B, which can be lost upon long term culture. A third antigen, C, was first defined on melanoma clone 43 after exposure to a mutagen, MNNG (Boon and Kellerman, 1977). Further analysis showed that 5% of melanoma clones derived from the original culture and not exposed to MNNG were lysed by CTL reacting with antigen C. It is therefore unlikely that the detection of antigen C is the consequence of mutagen treatment. By direct testing of melanoma reactive CTL clones, Anichini *et al* (1986) reported a quantitative heterogeneity in antigens recognized by autologous CTL on melanoma subclones. Unstable antigens have also been described in another melanoma system (Degiovanni *et al*, 1988).

Immunoselection with CTL Clones

In methylcholanthrene induced mouse mastocytoma P815, multiple simultaneously expressed tumour antigens were detected with stable CTL clones used for immunoselection of antigen loss variants (Maryanski and Boon, 1982; Maryanski *et al*, 1982). With stable CTL clones available in the melanoma system AV/SK-MEL-29, we applied this approach of immunoselection to the study of antigens in melanoma (Knuth *et al*, 1989). With two different CTL clones directed against autologous tumour cells, target cell clones were incubated in 12- or 16-fold excess for 6 hours. To increase the chances of obtaining variants, target cells were subjected to irradiation with 10 Gy before selection. Two stable tumour cell variants were obtained, which were resistant to lysis by the respective CTL clone used for immunoselection. Other CTL clones, however, were still lytic for the selected variants. This indicated, firstly, that at least three stable CTL defined antigens are simultaneously expressed on AV melanoma cells and, secondly, that immunoselected variants did not acquire a general resistance to lysis by CTL.

Van den Eynde *et al* (1989) extended this approach in the MZ-2 melanoma system described above. In addition to the previously mentioned antigens discovered in this melanoma system by direct tests of CTL against autologous tumour cell clones, three other stable antigens were detected on tumour cell variants obtained by immunoselection. Again, only target cell variants, immunoselected with a particular CTL clone, were not lysed by this particular CTL clone, whereas other autologous CTL still lysed the immunoselected tumour cell variant. This analysis was extended with other CTL clones aimed at an estimation of the number of stable antigens recognized on this tumour by autologous CTL. All 13 additional CTL clones tested against these three stable antigens on immunoselected variants were directed against one of the three antigens that could be eliminated by immunoselection. This suggested that only a very limited number of antigens are recognized on this tumour by autologous CTL. In this issue, Boon *et al* outline a genetic approach aimed at cloning the gene coding for MZ-2E, one of the antigens defined by means of CTL immunoselection, as described above.

MHC Restricted Recognition of Tumour Cell Antigens by CTL

The importance of MHC restriction elements both for recognition by CTL in vitro and for tumour progression in vivo is well documented in several experimental tumour models (Tanaka *et al*, 1988). In several human cancers, alterations in HLA class I antigen expression have been described (Lampson *et al*, 1983; Doyle *et al*, 1985; Smith *et al*, 1988, 1989; Momburg *et al*, 1989; Natali *et al*, 1989). In some instances, a correlation between low HLA class I expression and histological criteria of malignancy was found (Momburg *et al*, 1986; Möller *et al*, 1987). The influence of interferons on MHC class I and class II antigen expression has been studied by several groups in various tumour systems. Nistico *et al* (1990) noted a general upregulation of both MHC class I and class II antigen expression at the cell surface of human melanoma by interferons.

In our study of immunoselection of melanoma clones in the AV/SK-MEL-29 system, recognition of an HLA class I restricted antigen on tumour target cells could be clearly demonstrated with autologous CTL clones. In the AV system, typing positive for HLA-A2, inhibition experiments with monospecific anti-HLA-A2 sera from pregnant women and with a monoclonal antibody to HLA-A2 showed that the HLA-A2 antigen is a restriction element for the recognition of AV melanoma cells by autologous CTL. The immunoselected tumour cell variants still typed positive for HLA-A2. Since no other HLA-A2 positive allogeneic melanoma tested with HLA-A2 restricted AV CTL clones was lysed in our specificity analysis, it seems very unlikely that the antigens found in this tumour system are common in other human melanomas.

In the course of our immunoselection experiments, we found tumour cell variants that could not be lysed by any autologous CTL clone tested. Further analysis revealed that these variants had lost the expression of the HLA restriction element, HLA-A2. Fluorescence activated cell sorter analysis of HLA-A2 negative variants after treatment with interferon-γ (IFN-γ) showed induction of HLA class II molecules on AV melanoma clones and an overall increase in the HLA class I expression on all clones. However, HLA-A2 expression could not be induced on the loss variant. Isoelectric focusing analysis of HLA class I antigens immunoprecipitated with W6/32 antibody directed against a framework determinant of HLA class I molecules confirmed the loss of HLA-A2 expression.

MLTC experiments with the HLA-A2 loss variant as stimulator cells generated CTL clones weakly cytolytic against the loss variant. Pretreatment of these target cells with IFN-γ restored the lysis in an interferon dose dependent fashion. HLA-A2 positive melanoma clones were also effectively lysed only after pretreatment with IFN-γ. Antibody blocking with antibodies to HLA-A2, common determinants of class I and class II antigens and antibodies against a common determinant of HLA-B antigens revealed that only the HLA-B antibody blocked the lysis of SK-MEL-29 cells by AV-CTL raised against HLA-A2 negative variants. This indicates the involvement of another restriction element in CTL recognition of this melanoma. A tumour cell variant, on which one of the stable antigens was defined by immunoselection, was found to be resistant to lysis by CTL raised against the HLA-A2 negative variant as well as by CTL of the first MLTC generation, even after pretreatment with IFN-γ. Preliminary data indicate that the antigen lost on this variant after immunoselection can be presented by two different HLA class I molecules, HLA-A2 and Bw6 (Wölfel et al, 1989).

In contrast to our findings, Slovin et al (1986) reported a common antigen recognized by CTL in association with HLA-A2 on human sarcomas. Other groups have derived, from melanoma patients, CTL clones that recognize autologous melanoma cells in an HLA class I antigen restricted fashion (Darrow et al, 1989; Crowley et al, 1990, 1991). These authors identified in their system HLA-A2 as a dominant restriction element for CTL recognition of autologous tumour cells when patients' lymphocytes were heterozygous at the HLA-A region, expressing both A1 and A2. In other patients, it was shown that HLA-A1 can be a restriction element as well, and A1 matched allogeneic melanoma cells also could substitute for autologous melanoma in inducing a proliferative response of CTL. Since only autologous HLA-A1 or HLA-A2 positive melanoma cells and HLA-A1 or HLA-A2 matched allogeneic melanoma cells, but not HLA-matched non-melanoma tumour target cells, stimulated CTL in this setting, it is speculated that these melanoma cells carry common melanoma associated tumour antigens that are recognized by CTL in the context of different HLA class I antigens. Once dominant restricting alleles are defined for a patient, appropriately matched allogeneic melanoma cells might become a source of vaccine for clinical use.

In Vivo Relevance of CTL Responses to Tumour Antigens

The in vivo relevance of in vitro findings with CTL on cultured autologous tumour target cells will be supported if these CTL can be shown to lyse fresh tumour cells or if fresh tumour samples can be shown to induce a specific proliferative response in CTL. Fresh tumour samples often contain debris and non-tumour cells, which are difficult to separate from tumour cell suspensions. This might interfere with cytolytic tests. Some authors, however, have been able to demonstrate lysis of freshly collected tumour target cells with CTL generated in vitro (Slovin *et al*, 1986). In other studies, it has been shown, for example, that freshly collected melanoma cells are lysed by TIL derived CTL. A very convincing demonstration of the in vivo relevance of in vitro findings with autologous CTL clones against melanoma was given by Degiovanni *et al* (1990). Freshly collected melanoma cells from a surgically removed tumour recurrence in a melanoma patient induced a strong proliferative response in CTL clones raised against the melanoma cell line in vitro from the same patient. Analysis of precursor frequencies against target antigens carried out at different times in the course of a patients medical history or in different stages of disease will further clarify this issue.

CTL IN OTHER MALIGNANT DISEASES

A wide variety of malignant diseases have been tested in vitro for the activity of CTL directed against autologous tumour target cells (Yssel *et al*, 1984; Ferrini *et al*, 1985; Sato *et al*, 1986; Slovin *et al*, 1986; Anichini *et al*, 1987; Fisch *et al*, 1989). Effector lymphocytes were mostly derived from mononuclear cell infiltrates of tumour specimens or malignant effusions. A systematic analysis in these settings often is hampered by the fact that preferentially cloned tumour target cell lines are rarely available, mainly because cancer cells other than melanoma are difficult to establish in permanent tissue culture. However, CTL clones with varying degrees of tumour restricted reactivity, mostly "natural killer" like activity, have been described (Belldegrun *et al*, 1988). Barnd *et al* (1989) reported on human cytotoxic T cells from patients with pancreatic cancer. These CTL showed preferential lysis of pancreatic cancer cells, breast cancer cells and some ovarian cancer cells. The CTL recognition in this case apparently is non-MHC restricted and is directed to tumour associated mucins.

REGULATORY T CELLS IN HUMAN CANCERS

The most straightforward approach to CTL in cancer is to investigate how these effectors attack the targets that otherwise kill the host. Not all CTL are lytic for autologous tumour, however. And in MLTC, not only CTL but also proliferative T cell progeny are generated (Mukherji *et al*, 1989; Chakraborty *et al*, 1990). The majority of these regulatory T cell cultures were of CD3+/

CD4+/CD8– phenotype. Some had helper function in the induction of CTL from PBMC, others suppressed cytotoxic responses. Upon removal of regulatory T cell subsets in systems derived from patients with urinary bladder cancer and laryngeal cancer, Cozzolino et al (1987) could show a restored proliferative response to autologous tumour cells.

TUMOUR ESCAPE FROM T CELL RECOGNITION

Findings in experimental tumour systems in rodents (Uyttenhove et al, 1983) and in studies of human cancers (Knuth et al, 1989; Van den Eynde et al, 1989; Wölfel et al, 1989) suggest that tumour cells might escape immune recognition in vivo through reduced or lost expression of (a) immunogenic peptides, (b) presenting HLA molecules (Momburg et al, 1986, 1989; Möller et al, 1987; Hämmerling et al, 1989) or (c) accessory molecules involved in cell adhesion, for example ICAM-1. In melanoma, in particular, increased or de novo expression of MHC class II or adhesion molecules is correlated with tumour progression, metastasis and poor prognosis (Bröcker et al, 1985; Holzmann et al, 1987, 1988; Johnson et al, 1989). Every one of these events is likely to occur, separately or in combination, in cancer progression and metastasis.

CLINICAL PERSPECTIVES AND APPROACHES TO A SPECIFIC IMMUNOTHERAPY

Anecdotal evidence for "spontaneous" regression of cancer has been accumulating for almost 100 years. There are numerous reports of immune manipulations in human cancers, specific and non-specific, sometimes with striking clinical results. As outlined above, some progress has been made in understanding the mechanisms involved in the recognition of cancer cells by the immune system. We have seen strikingly favourable, albeit anecdotal, clinical courses in melanomas and have made these targets of our research efforts. We are beginning to see how to choose a reasonable route for an approach to devise a scientifically sound and clinically effective immunotherapy. A better understanding of human cancer antigens is in prospect, as indicated by Boon et al in this issue; this also will be an essential step forward in finding rational ways to stimulate the immune system with clearly defined tumour cell vaccines. Comparatively little has been learned from approaches with less well defined "adoptive" or "active" immunotherapies, not even offering a chance for a more thorough understanding of the molecular basis underlying these "therapies", but exposing the patient to potentially enormous and sometimes life-threatening side effects. The cloning and sequencing of the first human cancer antigen eliciting a cellular immune response will be a major step forward defining new strategies in the immunotherapy of human cancers.

SUMMARY

The immunological and molecular mechanisms that govern T cell responses to human malignant tumours are just starting to be understood within a more complex framework of humoral, cellular and molecular interactions. The definition of multiple antigens simultaneously expressed on human melanoma, as detected with cytolytic T cells in immunoselection experiments, is a first step towards the molecular characterization of these antigens. Observations on the influence of expression of restriction elements of the major histocompatibility complex on the recognition of these tumour associated antigens have advanced our understanding of how the immune system responds to cancer cells in vivo. It is specificity that is tuning the immune system, not only in cancer. The molecular characterization of the first human cancer antigen recognized by CTL is now under way as outlined by Boon *et al* in this issue.

Acknowledgements

The work was supported by grants from Deutsche Forschungsgemeinschaft DFG-Kn180/3-4 to AK and DFG-Wo339/2-2 to TW and an investigator award from Cancer Research Institute, New York, to AK. We thank Prof B Fleischer for critical reading of the manuscript.

References

Anichini A, Fossati G and Parmiani G (1986) Heterogeneity of clones from a human metastatic melanoma detected by autologous cytotoxic T lymphocyte clones. *Journal of Experimental Medicine* **163** 215–220

Anichini A, Fossati G and Parmiani G (1987) Clonal analysis of the cytolytic T-cell response to human tumors. *Immunology Today* **8** 385–389

Anichini A, Mazzocchi A, Fossati G and Parmiani G (1989) Cytotoxic T lymphocyte clones from peripheral blood and from tumor site detect intratumor heterogeneity of melanoma cells: analysis of specificity and mechanisms of interaction. *Journal of Immunology* **142** 3692–3701

Barnd DL, Lan MS, Metzgar RS and Finn OJ (1989) Specific, major histocompatibility complex-unrestricted recognition of tumor-associated mucins by human cytotoxic T cells. *Proceedings of the National Academy of Sciences of the USA* **86** 7159–7163

Bean MA, Pees H, Rosen G and Oettgen HF (1973) Prelabelling target cells with ^{3}H-proline as a method for studying lymphocyte cytotoxicity. *National Cancer Institute Monographs* **37** 41–48

Belldegrun A, Muul LM and Rosenberg SA (1988) Interleukin 2 expanded tumor-infiltrating lymphocytes in human renal cell cancer: isolation, characterization, and antitumor activity. *Cancer Research* **48** 206–214

Bjorkman PJ, Saper MA, Samraoui B, Bennett WS, Strominger JL and Wiley DC (1987) The foreign antigen binding site and T cell recognition regions of class I histocompatibility antigens. *Nature* **329** 512–518

Boon T and Kellermann O (1977) Rejection by syngeneic mice of cell variants obtained by mutagenesis of a malignant teratocarcinoma cell line. *Proceedings of the National Academy of Sciences of the USA* **74** 272–275

Bröcker EB, Suter L, Brüggen J, Ruiter DJ, Macher E and Sorg C (1985) Phenotypic dynamics of tumor progression in human malignant melanoma. *International Journal of Cancer* **36**

29–35

Carey TE, Takahashi T, Resnick LA, Oettgen HF and Old LJ (1976) Cell surface antigens of human malignant melanoma I Mixed hemadsorption assays for humoral immunity to cultured autologous melanoma cells. *Proceedings of the National Academy of Sciences of the USA* **73** 3278–3282

Chakraborty NG, Twardzik DR, Sivanandham M, Ergin MT, Hellstrom KE and Mukherji B (1990) Autologous melanoma-induced activation of regulatory T cells that suppress cytotoxic response. *Journal of Immunology* **145** 2359–2364

Clark Jr WH, Mastrangelo MJ, Ainsworth AM, Berd D, Bellet RE and Bernardino EA (1977) Current concepts of the biology of human cutaneous malignant melanoma. *Advances in Cancer Research* **24** 267–338

Cozzolino F, Torcia M, Carossino AM *et al* (1987) Characterization of cells from invaded lymph nodes in patients with solid tumors: lymphokine requirement for tumor-specific lymphoproliferative response. *Journal of Experimental Medicine* **166** 303–318

Crowley NJ, Slingluff CL, Darrow TL and Seigler HF (1990) Generation of human autologous melanoma-specific cytotoxic T-cells using HLA-A2-matched allogeneic melanomas. *Cancer Research* **50** 492–498

Crowley NJ, Darrow TL, Quinn-Allen MA and Seigler HF (1991) MHC-restricted recognition of autologous melanoma by tumor-specific cytotoxic T cells: evidence for restriction by a dominant HLA-A allele. *Journal of Immunology* **146** 1692–1699

Darrow TL, Slingluff CL and Seigler HF (1989) The role of HLA class I antigens in recognition of melanoma cells by tumor-specific cytotoxic T lymphocytes: evidence for shared tumor antigens. *Journal of Immunology* **142** 3329–3335

Degiovanni G, Lahaye T, Hérin M, Hainaut P and Boon T (1988) Antigenic heterogeneity of human melanoma tumor detected by autologous CTL clones. *European Journal of Immunology* **18** 671–676

Degiovanni G, Hainaut P, Lahaye T, Weynants P and Boon T (1990) Antigens recognized on a melanoma cell line by autologous cytolytic T lymphocytes are also expressed on freshly collected tumor cells. *European Journal of Immunology* **20** 1865–1868

Doyle A, Martin WJ, Funa K *et al* (1985) Markedly decreased expression of class I histocompatibility antigens, proteins and mRNA in small cell lung cancer. *Journal of Experimental Medicine* **161** 1135–1151

Falk K, Rötzschke O, Stevanovic S, Jung G and Rammensee H-G (1991) Allele-specific motifs revealed by sequencing of self-peptides eluted from MHC molecules. *Nature* **351** 290–296

Ferrini S, Biassoni R, Moretta A, Bruzzone M, Nicolin A and Moretta L (1985) Clonal analysis of T lymphocytes isolated from ovarian carcinoma ascitic fluid: phenotype and functional characterization of T-cell clones capable of lysing autologous carcinoma cells. *International Journal of Cancer* **36** 337–343

Fisch P, Weil-Hillman G, Uppenkamp M *et al* (1989) Antigen-specific recognition of autologous leukemia cells and allogeneic class-I MHC antigens by IL-2-activated cytotoxic T cells from a patient with acute T-cell leukemia. *Blood* **74** 343–353

Furukawa KS, Furukawa K, Real FX, Old LJ and Lloyd KO (1989) A unique antigenic epitope of human melanoma is carried on the common melanoma glycoprotein gp95/p97. *Journal of Experimental Medicine* **169** 585–590

Garrett TPJ, Saper MA, Bjorkman PJ, Strominger JL and Wiley DC (1989) Specificity pockets for the side chains of peptide antigens in HLA-Aw68. *Nature* **342** 692–696

Grimm EA, Mazumder A, Zhang HZ and Rosenberg SA (1982) Lymphokine-activated killer cell phenomenon: lysis of natural killer-resistant fresh solid tumor cells by interleukin 2-activated autologous human peripheral blood lymphocytes. *Journal of Experimental Medicine* **155** 1823–1841

Hämmerling GJ, Maschek U, Sturmhöfel K and Momburg F (1989) Regulation and functional role of MHC expression on tumors, In: Melchers F *et al* (eds). *Progress in Immunology VII*, pp 1071–1078, Springer Verlag, Berlin

Hellström KE and Hellström I (1974) Lymphocyte-mediated cytotoxicity and blocking serum activity to tumor antigens. *Advances in Immunology* 18 209–277

Hérin M, Lemoine C, Weynants P *et al* (1987) Production of stable cytolytic T-cell clones directed against autologous human melanoma. *International Journal of Cancer* 39 390–396

Holzmann B, Bröcker EB, Lehmann JM *et al* (1987) Tumor progression in human malignant melanoma: five stages defined by their antigenic phenotypes. *International Journal of Cancer* 39 466–471

Holzmann B, Lehmann JM, Ziegler-Heitbrock HWL, Funke I, Riethmüller G and Johnson J (1988) Glycoprotein P3.58, associated with tumor progression in malignant melanoma, is a novel leukocyte activation antigen. *International Journal of Cancer* 41 542–547

Itoh K, Platsoucas CD and Balch CM (1988) Autologous tumor-specific cytotoxic T lymphocytes in the infiltrate of human metastatic melanomas: activation by interleukin 2 and autologous tumor cells and involvement of the T cell receptor. *Journal of Experimental Medicine* 168 1419–1441

Johnson JP, Stade BG, Holzmann B, Schwäble W and Riethmüller G (1989) De novo expression of intercellular-adhesion molecule 1 in melanoma correlates with increased risk of metastasis. *Proceedings of the National Academy of Sciences of the USA* 86 641–644

Knuth A, Danowski B, Oettgen HF and Old LJ (1984) T-cell-mediated cytotoxicity against autologous malignant melanoma: analysis with interleukin 2-dependent T-cell cultures. *Proceedings of the National Academy of Sciences of the USA* 81 3511–3515

Knuth A, Wölfel T, Klehmann E, Boon T and Meyer zum Büschenfelde K-H (1989) Cytolytic T-cell clones against an autologous human melanoma: specificity study and definition of three antigens by immunoselection. *Proceedings of the National Academy of Sciences of the USA* 86 2804–2808

Lampson LA, Fisher CA and Whelan JP (1983) Striking paucity of HLA-A,B,C and β2-microglobulin on human neuroblastoma cell lines. *Journal of Immunology* 130 2471–2478

Livingston PO, Shiku H, Bean MA, Pinsky CM, Oettgen HF and Old LJ (1979) Cell-mediated cytotoxicity for cultured autologous melanoma cells. *International Journal of Cancer* 24 34–44

Maryanski JL and Boon T (1982) Immunogenic variants obtained by mutagenesis of mouse mactocytoma P815 IV Analysis of variant-specific antigens by selection of antigen-loss variants with cytolytic T cell clones. *European Journal of Immunology* 12 406–412

Maryanski JL, Van Snick J, Cerottini J-C and Boon T (1982) Immunogenic variants obtained by mutagenesis of mouse mastocytoma P815 III Clonal analysis of the syngeneic cytolytic T lymphocyte response. *European Journal of Immunology* 12 401–406

Miescher S, Whiteside TL, Carrel S and von Fliedner V (1986) Functional properties of tumor-infiltrating and blood lymphocytes in patients with solid tumors: effects of tumor cells and their supernatants on proliferative responses of lymphocytes. *Journal of Immunology* 136 1899–1907

Möller P, Hermann B, Moldenhauer G and Momburg F (1987) Defective expression of MHC class I antigens is frequent in B cell lymphomas of high grade malignancy. *International Journal of Cancer* 40 32–39

Momburg F, Degener T, Bacchus E, Moldenhauer G, Hämmerling GJ and Möller P (1986) Loss of HLA-A,B,C and de novo expression of HLA-D in colorectal cancer. *International Journal of Cancer* 37 179–184

Momburg F, Ziegler A, Harpprecht J, Möller P, Moldenhauer G and Hämmerling GJ (1989) Selective loss of HLA-A or HLA-B antigen expression in colon carcinoma. *Journal of Immunology* 142 352–358

Mukherji B and MacAlister TJ (1983) Clonal analysis of cytotoxic T cell response against human melanoma. *Journal of Experimental Medicine* 158 240–245

Mukherji B, Guha A, Chakraborty NG *et al* (1989) Clonal analysis of cytotoxic and regulatory T cell responses against human melanoma. *Journal of Experimental Medicine* 169 1961–1976

Natali PG, Nicotra MR, Bigotti A *et al* (1989) Selective changes in expression of HLA class I polymorphic determinants in human solid tumors. *Proceedings of the National Academy of Sciences of the USA* **86** 6719–6723

Nistico P, Tecce R, Giacomini P *et al* (1990) Effect of recombinant human leukocyte, fibroblast and immune interferons on expression of class I and II major histocompatibility complex and invariant chain in early passage human melanoma cells. *Cancer Research* **50** 7422–7429

Old LJ (1981) Cancer immunology: the search for specificity–GHA Clowes Memorial Lecture. *Cancer Research* **41** 361–375

Parmiani G, Sensi M and Fossati G (1985) Allostimulation-induced tumor cytotoxic cells: from mouse to man. *Immunology Today* **6** 215–218

Sato T, Sato N, Takahashi S, Koshiba H and Kikuchi K (1986) Specific cytotoxicity of a long-term cultured T-cell clone on human autologous mammary cancer cells. *Cancer Research* **46** 4384–4389

Slovin SF, Lackman RD, Ferrone S, Kiely PE and Mastrangelo MJ (1986) Cellular immune response to human sarcomas: cytotoxic T cell clones reactive with autologous sarcomas I Development, phenotype and specificity. *Journal of Immunology* **137** 3042–3048

Smith MEF, Bodmer WF and Bodmer JG (1988) Selective loss of HLA-A,B,C locus products in colorectal adenocarcinoma. *Lancet* **i** 823–824

Smith ME, Marsh SGE, Bodmer JG, Gelsthorpe K and Bodmer WF (1989) Loss of HLA-A,B,C allele products and lymphocyte function-associated antigen 3 in colorectal neoplasia. *Proceedings of the National Academy of Sciences of the USA* **86** 5557–5561

Tanaka K, Yoshioka T, Bieberich C and Jay G (1988) Role of the major histocompatibility complex class I antigens in tumor growth and metastasis. *Annual Review of Immunology* **6** 359–380

Topalian SL, Solomon D and Rosenberg SA (1989) Tumor-specific cytolysis by lymphocytes infiltrating human melanomas. *Journal of Immunology* **142** 3714–3725

Townsend A and Bodmer H (1989) Antigen recognition by class I-restricted T lymphocytes. *Annual Review of Immunology* **7** 601–624

Townsend A, Rothbard J, Gotch F, Bahadur G, Wraith D and McMichael A (1986) The epitopes of influenza nucleoprotein recognized by cytotoxic T lymphocytes can be defined with short synthetic peptides. *Cell* **44** 959–968

Uyttenhove C, Maryanski J and Boon T (1983) Escape of mouse mastocytoma P815 after nearly complete rejection is due to antigen-loss variants rather than immunosuppression. *Journal of Experimental Medicine* **157** 1040–1052

Van den Eynde B, Hainaut P, Hérin M *et al* (1989) Presence on a human melanoma of multiple antigens recognized by autologous CTL. *International Journal of Cancer* **44** 634–640

Vose BM and Bonnard GD (1982) Specific cytotoxicity against autologous tumour and proliferative responses of human lymphocytes grown in interleukin 2. *International Journal of Cancer* **29** 33–39

Wölfel T, Klehmann E, Müller C, Schütt K-H, Meyer zum Büschenfelde K-H and Knuth A (1989) Lysis of human melanoma cells by autologous cytolytic T cell clones: identification of human histocompatibility leukocyte antigen A2 as a restriction element for three different antigens. *Journal of Experimental Medicine* **170** 797–810

Yssel H, Spits H and de Vries J (1984) A cloned human T line cytotoxic for autologous and allogeneic B lymphoma cells. *Journal of Experimental Medicine* **160** 239–254

Zarling JM, Robins HI, Raich PC, Bach FH and Bach ML (1978) Generation of cytotoxic T lymphocytes to autologous human leukemia cells by sensitisation to pooled allogeneic normal cells. *Nature* **274** 269–271

Zinkernagel RM and Doherty PC (1979) MHC-restricted cytotoxic T cells: studies on the biological role of polymorphic major transplantation antigens determining T-cell restriction specificity, function and responsiveness. *Advances in Immunology* **27** 51–177

The authors are responsible for the accuracy of the references.

T Cell Recognition of Epstein-Barr Virus Associated Lymphomas

A B RICKINSON[1] • R J MURRAY[1] • J BROOKS[1] • H GRIFFIN[1]
D J MOSS[2] • M G MASUCCI[1,3]

[1]Department of Cancer Studies, CRC Laboratories, University of Birmingham, Birmingham B15 2TJ; [2]Queensland Institute of Medical Research, The Bancroft Centre, Herston, Brisbane, 4029; [3]Department of Tumor Biology, Karolinska Institute, Box 60400, S-104 01 Stockholm

INTRODUCTION

Epstein-Barr virus (EBV), a herpesvirus widespread in human populations, has two major target tissues in vivo, B lymphocytes and squamous pharyngeal epithelium. In B cells, the infection is predominantly non-productive or "latent", although clearly there are situations where latently infected B cells can be triggered into the virus productive or "lytic" cycle (Miller, 1990). In epithelium, the infection is predominantly lytic, with complete replication of the virus linked to ordered squamous epithelial differentiation (Greenspan et al, 1985; Niedobitek et al, 1991). We have at least a partial understanding of the cytotoxic T lymphocyte (CTL) controls that are exercised over latently infected B cells in vivo and that are a potential defence against virus associated lymphomas (see below). By contrast, we have virtually no information on T cell responses directed towards productively infected epithelium. This is not to say that such responses do not exist, rather that the experimental protocols that might uncover them are not yet in place—a situation that reflects the absence of an in vitro system for reproducing the naturally infectious cycle in epithelium.

T CELL SURVEILLANCE OF EBV INFECTED B CELLS

Epstein-Barr virus readily infects B lymphocytes in vitro, inducing their growth transformation to permanent lymphoblastoid cell lines (LCL); most LCL carry the virus as a latent infection with limited expression of the episomally maintained viral genome (Kieff and Liebowitz, 1990). This has provided an accessible cell culture system with which to search for evidence of virus specific T cell mediated immunity in humans. The first inroad in this area came from the study of infectious mononucleosis (IM), a self-limiting lymphoproliferative disease of adolescence caused by delayed primary infection with the virus (Henle and Henle, 1979). The majority of those atypical mononuclear cells whose presence in the blood is diagnostic of IM were found to be not virus infected B lymphoblasts but T cells activated in response to the virus infection. Indeed, when freshly isolated preparations of such IM T cells (depleted of conventional natural killer activity) were tested on LCL targets in vitro, they appeared to display an EBV specific cytotoxicity, which transgressed the emerging rules of MHC restricted T cell function (Svedmyr and Jondal, 1975). Only much later was the truly EBV specific component of this polyclonal CTL response identified and shown to be HLA class I antigen restricted; this component can easily be masked by other CTL of unknown specificity that are coincidentally activated during IM and show cross reactive recognition of certain HLA mismatched LCL in in vitro assays (Strang and Rickinson, 1987). Coincidental activation of T cells on the scale seen in IM raises the possibility that one or more EBV coded proteins may function as "super-antigens" in a manner similar to that of certain bacterial proteins (White *et al*, 1989).

Following this early work on the primary T cell response to EBV infection, studies of virus induced lymphocyte transformation in vitro revealed the existence of long term T cell surveillance against the virus in all healthy previously infected individuals (Rickinson *et al*, 1981). Thus, experimentally infected cultures of blood mononuclear cells from virus immune individuals frequently showed regression of B cell outgrowth, an effect mediated predominantly through the in situ reactivation of a CTL response. Expansion and subsequent cloning of the reactive T cells in medium containing interleukin-2 (IL-2) demonstrated their operational specificity for EBV (ie recognition of LCL targets but not mitogen-activated B lymphoblasts) and restriction through HLA class I, or occasionally through HLA class II, antigens (Moss *et al*, 1981, 1988; Wallace *et al*, 1982; Misko *et al*, 1984). The above regression assay provided a simple limiting dilution protocol with which to monitor the frequency of EBV specific cytotoxic precursors (memory cells) in the circulating T cell pool of immune individuals. It showed that this frequency was unusually high (at least 1 per 10^3 to 10^4 circulating T cells) and also remarkably stable in healthy individuals monitored over several years (Rickinson *et al*, 1981). These immune variables reflect the persistent nature of EBV infection. Thus, the virus establishes a lifelong carrier state, with the original infecting strain remaining the dominant isolate in the B cell pool of each individual virus carrier (Yao *et al*, 1991). This provides an interesting contrast to the situation with a non-persistent virus such as influenza, where levels of virus specific CTL memory fall throughout the interval between successive acute infections (McMichael *et al*, 1983). Furthermore, the stability of EBV specific T cell memory strongly suggests that immunogenic virus infected B lymphoblasts (ie the in vivo equivalents of in vitro LCL) are continually being generated in symptom free virus carrying individuals as a chronic stimulus to the T cell system. In this context, it is interesting to compare EBV with the neurotropic herpesviruses, such as herpes simplex and varicella zoster, which persist as latent infections of the nervous system rather than of lymphoid tissues (Stevens, 1989). Such agents show no detectable viral antigen synthesis in latently infected neurons, and although reactivations from latency are probably a continuous feature of the neurotropic herpesvirus carrier state, the reactivating cells appear to pose less of an immunogenic challenge to the T cell system. For such viruses, the frequency of detectable CTL precursors, directed against antigens of the lytic cycle, is at least an order of magnitude below that of EBV specific CTL precursors (Hickling *et al*, 1987).

EBV TARGET ANTIGENS FOR VIRUS SPECIFIC CTL RECOGNITION OF LCL

The operational specificity of EBV induced CTL responses for virus transformed B lymphoblastoid cells was appreciated long before the complexity of EBV latent gene expression in such target LCL was understood. Only relatively recently has the spectrum of viral genes that are constitutively expressed in LCL been defined and their products, the EBV latent proteins, identified (Kieff and Liebowitz, 1990). These are illustrated diagrammatically in Fig. 1 above a *Bam*HI restriction map of the EBV genome (here shown in linear form rather than the covalently closed circular form present in LCL). The latent gene products include six EBV nuclear antigens, EBNA 1, 2, 3A, 3B, 3C and LP, encoded by individual messenger RNAs (mRNAs), all generated by alternative splicing of the same rightward running transcripts initiated in the *Bam*HI C and/or W region of the genome, and two latent membrane proteins, LMP 1 and 2, encoded by multiple spliced transcripts from promoters in the *Bam*HI N region. Note that LMP 2, whose expression requires circularization of the genome and transcription across the fused termini, is encoded in full length and in truncated forms by independent transcripts in LCL; however, in

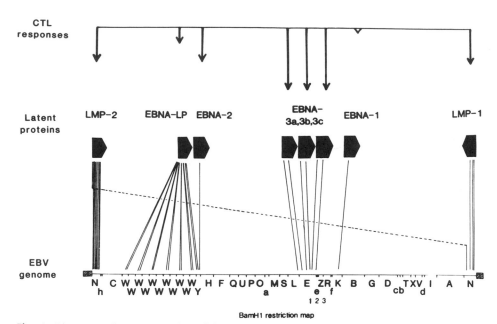

Fig. 1. Diagrammatic representation of the known spectrum of EBV latent proteins expressed in LCL cells, illustrating their individual coding sequences within the EBV genome and their relative immunogenicity for the human CTL response. The viral genome is shown in linear form as a *Bam*HI restriction map. The six EBNA are encoded by alternatively spliced mRNAs generated from the same long primary transcripts initiated in *Bam*HI C or W; the multiply spliced LMP mRNAs map within the *Bam*HI N region, expression of LMP 2 mRNA transcripts being dependent on circularization of the genome via fusion of the terminal repeats. Lines joining the genomic map and the individual latent proteins in each case indicate the number and position of the protein coding exons. The upper part of the figure summarizes current information on the relative immunogenicity of the latent proteins for CTL responses. Thus, EBNAs 3A, 3B and 3C appear to be preferred targets in many cases, whereas responses against target epitopes from EBNA 1 have not been detected in any of the donors examined thus far

the present context, we can confine attention to the full length form since this includes the whole primary sequence of the truncated protein.

Given what we now know about processing of endogenously synthesized proteins to small peptide fragments and their presentation on the cell surface as a complex with HLA class I antigens (Townsend *et al*, 1986; Silver *et al*, 1991), it is clear (a) that there are at least eight independent virus coded proteins with the potential to provide target epitopes for the EBV specific T cell response and (b) that epitope choice will in each case be critically dependent on the identity of the HLA restricting molecule. Analysis of CTL responses in this complex viral system has been made possible through collaboration with Dr M Kurilla and Dr E Kieff (Harvard Medical School, Boston, USA), who constructed a complete set of vaccinia recombinants expressing the individual latent proteins from relevant complementary DNA sequences of the standard type 1 EBV strain, B95.8. Such recombinants were first used to analyse the target antigen specificity of CTL preparations from rare donors showing selective reactivity against type 1 and not against type 2 virus strains. These two types of EBV are distinguished by a degree of sequence divergence in their EBNA 2, 3A, 3B, 3C and LP genes (Dambaugh *et al*, 1984; Sample *et al*, 1990). Thus, the experiments were conducted by expressing the type 1 versions of these genes from the recombinant vaccinia virus vectors in autologous type 2 virus transformed LCL. In this way, we were able to show examples of type 1 selective CTL that recognized in one case an epitope within the type 1 EBNA 2 protein and in another case an epitope within type 1 EBNA 3A (Murray *et al*, 1990).

Most polyclonal EBV specific CTL preparations, however, show cross reactive recognition of both type 1 and type 2 virus strains, and the analysis of these responses has required the introduction of vaccinia virus recombinants into autologous EBV negative target cells such as fibroblasts (Murray R, unpublished; Gavioli R, unpublished) or B cells activated to the lymphoblastoid state by ligation of surface IgM and costimulation with IL-2 and IL-4 (Khanna *et al*, 1991). Using these approaches, we have recently completed systematic surveys of EBV target antigen choice in a total of 30 healthy virus immune donors, representing a variety of different HLA backgrounds, from whom CTL were generated by stimulation with the autologous B95.8 virus transformed LCL. The overall conclusions from this work, analysing both polyclonal CTL preparations and derived clones (Murray R, Brooks J and Rickinson A, unpublished; Khanna R and Moss D, unpublished), can be summarized as follows: (a) there are clear differences in target antigen choice between different individuals, responses from any one individual often being a composite of reactivities against different virus antigens; (b) more than half of the component responses that have been mapped to date in these donors are directed towards one or other of the EBNA 3A, 3B and 3C family of high molecular weight nuclear antigens, whereas other components have been identified against EBNA 2, EBNA-LP, LMP 1 or LMP 2; (c) in a number of cases, it is possible to correlate dominance of antigen choice with a particular restricting determinant (eg HLA-B8 molecules frequently present an epitope from EBNA 3A; HLA-A11 molecules present an epitope from EBNA 3B; HLA-B44 and HLA-B27.05 present epitopes from EBNA 3C; and HLA-A2.1 presents an epitope from LMP 2).

To illustrate the type of results from which these overall conclusions are drawn, Fig. 2 presents the data obtained when polyclonal CTL preparations from two virus immune donors, CM_c (HLA type A2.1, A11, B8, B44) and WT (HLA type A2.1, A2.1, B14, B15), were raised and tested against the autologous LCL, an HLA mismatched LCL and autologous fibroblasts after acute infection with individual vaccinia virus recombinants from the panel. In both cases, responses were directed against more than one target antigen; thus, donor CM_c CTL preparations contain components reactive against EBNA 3A, EBNA 3B and EBNA 3C (Fig. 2a), whereas donor WT CTL contain components reactive against EBNA 3C and LMP 2 (Fig. 2b). Subsequently, either by retesting these same polyclonal effectors on appropriately HLA

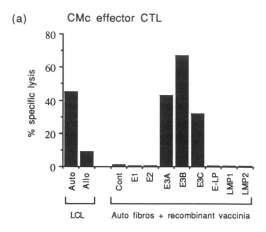

(a)   CMc effector CTL

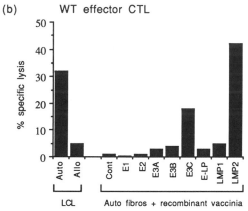

(b)   WT effector CTL

Fig. 2. Analysis of EBV target antigen choice in polyclonal CTL populations raised from EBV immune donors of different HLA antigen types. Results of representative 5 hr cytotoxicity assays are shown in which CTL from donors a) CMc (HLA-A2.1, A11, B8, B44) and b) WT (HLA-A2.1, A2.1, B14, B15) were assayed against the autologous LCL, an HLA class I antigen mismatched allogeneic LCL, and autologous fibroblasts acutely infected with recombinant vaccinia viruses expressing the individual EBV latent proteins. The CTL were generated by in vitro stimulation of peripheral blood mononuclear cells with the autologous B95.8 virus transformed LCL followed by expansion in IL-2, and were assayed at an effector:target ratio of 10:1

matched allogeneic fibroblast targets or by establishing T cell clones, it was possible to dissect such responses into their component reactivities. Thus, donor CM_c responses include a HLA-B8 restricted component recognizing an epitope from EBNA 3A, an HLA-A11 restricted component recognizing an epitope from EBNA 3B and a HLA-B44 restricted component recognizing an epitope from EBNA 3C; by contrast, the major component of the donor WT response is HLA-A2.1 restricted and recognizes an epitope from LMP 2.

More work will be required to determine the generality of these overall conclusions for EBV specific CTL responses in the population at large. However, we are confident that the specific combinations of HLA restricting determinant and EBV target antigen revealed in the studies to date are indeed meaningful, since in a number of cases, reconstitution experiments with synthetic peptides have formally identified the location of the CTL epitope within the primary sequence of the relevant viral antigen (Burrows *et al*, 1990a,b). Although the analysis of these 30 immune individuals has indicated that the source of EBV target antigens is quite diverse, we have never detected any cytotoxic response either at the polyclonal or at the clonal level directed towards the EBNA 1 antigen, despite the fact that this is a relatively large protein of 70 kDa, which (even allowing for its internal gly-ala repeat sequence) should represent a potentially rich source of T cell epitopes. A picture is therefore emerging of a hierarchy among the EBV latent proteins in terms of their immunogenicity for human CTL responses, and this ranking order is illustrated diagrammatically in Fig. 1. It is worth noting here that virus infection of resting B cells is associated with an ordered sequence of viral antigen expression, with abundant expression of EBNA 2 and EBNA-LP preceding the appearance of the other EBNA and subsequently of the LMP (Moss *et al*, 1986; Alfieri *et al*, 1991). Hence, CTL responses are not preferentially directed towards the two viral proteins (EBNA 2, EBNA-LP) expressed first post-infection, and this probably reflects the fact that virus infected B cells are efficient immunogens only after full activation to the lymphoblastoid state (see below). Such activation is almost certainly not achieved until all the latent proteins are expressed, because LMP 1, one of the last antigens to appear in the temporal sequence, is a key effector of virus induced cellular change (Wang *et al*, 1990).

Finally, in the context of target antigen choice, it should be noted that there are some donors whose EBV induced CTL response, analysed either as a polyclonal population or as derived clones, recognizes the autologous LCL efficiently and appears to be operationally EBV specific, yet does not map to any of the latent proteins included in the present panel. One possible explanation of such a result is that the list of viral proteins constitutively expressed in LCL is not yet complete; if true, this has important implications for the study of virus induced cell transformation. Another possibility is that, for reasons we do not understand, infection with the relevant recombinant vaccinia under some circumstances cannot generate the cognate HLA-peptide complex, thereby leading to false negative results. Further work is needed to resolve these uncertainties.

IMMUNOGENICITY OF THE LATENTLY INFECTED LCL CELL

Outside the EBV field, many in vitro studies of human T cell function have exploited EBV transformed LCL either as potent stimulator cells, for instance of

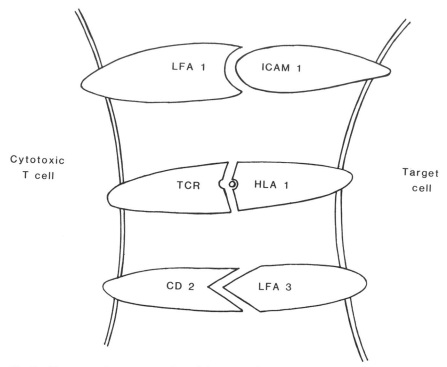

Fig. 3. Diagrammatic representation of the two adhesion pathways that can mediate CTL-target cell conjugation and thereby facilitate immunologically specific recognition via the T cell receptor/HLA-peptide complex. Adhesion can occur via interaction of LFA 1 on the CTL surface with ICAM 1 on the target, and via interaction of CD2 on the CTL with LFA 3 in the target; these interactions are independent of immunologically specific recognition but may be enhanced by it

allospecific responses in mixed lymphocyte culture (Reiss *et al*, 1980), or as efficient antigen presenting cells, whether the antigens in question are expressed endogenously from introduced vectors (Gotch *et al*, 1987) or are delivered as exogenous proteins into the endocytic pathway (Lanzavecchia, 1985). In these various situations, the high surface levels of HLA class I and class II antigens on LCL is one factor contributing to the efficiency of immunological recognition; however, another factor, perhaps equally important, is the strong expression of cellular adhesion molecules (Springer, 1990). Functionally, the best characterized of these molecules are the leukocyte function-associated antigens LFA 1 and LFA 3 and the intracellular adhesion molecule ICAM 1, all of which are present at high levels on the LCL surface. Indeed, the importance of these structures in facilitating cell adhesion was first recognized in in vitro studies using LCL as a model (Shaw *et al*, 1986). Thus, mutual interactions between LFA 1 and ICAM 1 underlie the ability of LCL to form homotypic adhesions (hence, the growth of these cells in large clumps), whereas ICAM 1 and LFA 3 expression determines the accessibility of LCL cells to conjugate formation with immune T cells (Shaw *et al*, 1986; Gregory *et al*, 1988). As shown diagrammatically in Fig. 3, ICAM 1 on the LCL surface interacts with LFA 1 on the T cell, and similarly, LFA 3 on the LCL interacts with the T cell specific surface molecule CD2 (LFA 2). These interactions constitute two separate adhesion pathways, which can occur independently of (but may be enhanced following) immunologically specific recognition of the HLA-peptide complex by the T cell receptor (Springer, 1990).

As a target for EBV specific T cell responses therefore, the LCL expresses not just the complete array of EBV latent proteins as potential target antigens but also the adhesion molecules that enhance target cell accessibility to effector T cells. Furthermore, LCL express a range of lymphocyte activation antigens such as CD23, CD30 and CD39 at high levels on the cell surface (Rowe *et al*, 1985) and secrete a variety of lymphokines (Gordon *et al*, 1984; Wakasugi *et al*, 1987); either of these additional features might also enhance LCL immunogenicity by facilitating immune T cell activation from the resting state. Finally, the natural location of EBV infected LCL like cells arising in vivo that is in lymphoid tissues would be expected to optimize the exposure of these cells to the T cell repertoire.

EBV ASSOCIATED LYMPHOMAS IN HUMANS

There are two forms of B cell lymphomas that are consistently EBV genome positive, but otherwise quite distinct in terms of their presentation, their histological classification and their pathogenesis. These are the "immunoblastic lymphomas" and the endemic form of Burkitt's lymphoma. To these well documented examples of EBV genome positive B cell lymphomas, we can now add Hodgkin's disease (HD), a third virus associated tumour thought to be of immature lymphoid origin.

Immunoblastic Lymphomas

The immunoblastic lymphomas arise in individuals whose T cell responses are impaired. Most susceptible in this regard are allograft recipients receiving long term immunosuppressive therapy for maintenance of their graft (Cleary *et al*, 1986) and patients infected with human immunodeficiency virus (HIV) who have become severely immunologically compromised (Kalter *et al*, 1985; Beral *et al*, 1991; MacMahon *et al*, 1991). The above tumours frequently present as multifocal lesions within lymphoid tissues and/or in the central nervous system and are classified histologically as immunoblastic or polymorphic B cell lymphomas, often with some plasmacytoid features. Analysis of immunoglobulin gene rearrangement or isotype expression indicates that even within a single patient, individual tumour foci tend to be distinct, each being composed of one or a small number of unique B cell clones (Cleary and Sklar, 1984; Martin *et al*, 1984; Starzl *et al*, 1984; Cleary *et al*, 1986; Shapiro *et al*, 1988).

Endemic Burkitt's Lymphoma

The endemic (high incidence) form of Burkitt's lymphoma (BL) is classically observed in equatorial regions of Africa and New Guinea, where it is the commonest malignancy of childhood (Magrath, 1990). These tumours tend to present at unusual anatomical sites outside lymphoid tissues, yet the lymphoma cells appear morphologically and from their surface markers to be of germinal centre origin (Gregory *et al*, 1987). The monoclonal nature of BL is clear not just from analysis of the productively rearranged immunoglobulin locus but also from the presence in each tumour of a unique chromosomal translocation that places the c-*myc* oncogene (on chromosome 8) in the vicinity either of the second immunoglobulin heavy chain locus (on chromosome 14) or of one of the light chain loci (on chromosomes 2 and 22). Although almost all cases of endemic BL are EBV genome positive, there is a much rarer sporadic form of the tumour that occurs worldwide, which has a similar translocation involving c-*myc* and is associated with EBV in only a minority (15–20%) of cases (Magrath, 1990). Individuals infected with HIV are themselves at increased risk of translocation positive BL but, unlike the immunoblastic lymphomas that are a feature of full blown acquired immunodeficiency syndrome, these Burkitt tumours tend to appear before any obvious impairment of immune function (Kalter *et al*, 1985) and resemble sporadic BL in their irregular association with EBV (Subar *et al*, 1988).

Hodgkin's Disease

Hodgkin's disease is an unusual tumour, observed worldwide, in which the malignant population of Reed-Sternberg and Hodgkin's cells constitutes only a small fraction of total cells in the biopsy specimen; subtyping of HD into lymphocyte predominant, nodular sclerosing, mixed cellularity and lymphocyte depleted forms reflects the different histological backgrounds of infiltrating normal cells in which the tumour cells are found. It is now clear that in 40–50% cases of HD, the malignant cell clone is EBV genome positive, the frequency of EBV association being particularly high in the clinically more aggressive mixed cellularity and lymphocyte depleted subtypes (Anagnostopoulos *et al*, 1989; Weiss *et al*, 1989; Herbst *et al*, 1991; Pallesen *et al*, 1991). This is a relatively new observation, and many of the fundamental questions concerning a possible role for EBV in the pathogenesis of HD remain to be formally addressed, as does the question of HD susceptibility to EBV specific T cell surveillance.

T CELL SURVEILLANCE AND IMMUNOBLASTIC B CELL LYMPHOMAS

There are now a number of independent reports indicating that immunoblastic lymphomas of the immunosuppressed display a pattern of EBV gene expression essentially similar to that seen in in vitro transformed LCL, that is expression of all six EBNA and of the LMP (Young *et al*, 1989a; Thomas *et al*, 1990; Gratama *et al*, 1991). The situation is best documented with respect to the viral antigens EBNA 2 and LMP 1, both of which have been consistently detected in the cells of these lesions when frozen tissue sections have been stained with the relevant antigen specific monoclonal antibodies (MAbs). Moreover, the cellular phenotype of these lymphoma cells mirrors that of LCL, with high surface expression of cellular adhesion molecules such as ICAM 1 and LFA 3 as well as of cellular activation antigens such as CD23.

Such evidence strongly suggests that these B cell lymphomas of the immunosuppressed, usually presenting as oligoclonal proliferations, are the in vivo counterparts of in vitro transformed LCL and as such are primarily EBV driven. However, the lesions can progress from oligo- to monoclonality and, in light of the situation in BL (see below), it would be interesting to know whether this reflects the acquisition by a rare cell within the EBV transformed population of a second genetic change, which either partially or fully liberates cell growth from its initial dependence on the virus. Two points can be made in this context. Firstly, there is as yet no genetic or cytogenetic evidence for any specific second event in the evolution of these tumours. Secondly, and more importantly, the same characteristic pattern of EBV latent gene expression and the same cellular phenotype have been consistently observed in immunoblastic lymphomas whether the lesions analysed were oligoclonal or monoclonal (Young et al, 1989a; Thomas et al, 1990; Gratama et al, 1991). The simplest interpretation of these findings is that evolution to monoclonality in vivo exactly mirrors a phenomenon already recognized in vitro, where experimental infection of resting B cells gives rise to an LCL that is at first polyclonal but on serial passage often becomes dominated by the fastest growing clone; however, continued growth of this dominant clone remains absolutely dependent on EBV. If this is also true in vivo, it implies a continuing role for the virus in driving lymphoma cell growth, irrespective of the clonality of the lesions; parallel studies on EBV induced B cell lymphomas in animal model systems (Cleary et al, 1985; Young et al, 1989b; Rowe et al, 1991) have led to a similar conclusion.

The sensitivity of immunoblastic lymphomas to EBV specific CTL has not been directly tested (a logistically difficult experiment), but the fact that the tumour cells both express the full spectrum of virus latent proteins and display a high adhesion molecule profile at the surface strongly implies that they will remain susceptible to immune recognition. Indeed, it is well established that in allograft recipients, relaxation of immunosuppressive therapy can lead to regression of the lymphomas whether the lesions are oligoclonal or monoclonal (Starzl et al, 1984), just as would be expected if the recovering virus specific T cell surveillance can still recognize and eliminate the tumour cells.

T CELL SURVEILLANCE AND BURKITT'S LYMPHOMA

Endemic BL is the classical example of a virus associated human tumour, and, once the existence of an EBV specific CTL surveillance system in healthy virus carrying individuals had been firmly established, it became important to determine whether BL itself was susceptible to such surveillance. The fact that BL patients often showed normal levels of virus specific CTL in the in vitro regression assay and yet gave no evidence of CTL control of the tumour in vivo implied that some form of immune evasion was at work (Rooney *et al*, 1985a). To address this question directly, paired cell lines were established from individual Burkitt patients, one the tumour derived BL cell line and the other the LCL generated from normal B cells by in vitro transformation either with a laboratory strain of EBV or preferably with the virus strain rescued from the tumour. Early passage BL cells displayed the group I surface phenotype of the original tumour and grew as single cells (Rooney *et al*, 1986b), whereas the LCL displayed the typical group III phenotype and grew in clumps. Group I BL lines were not recognized by EBV specific, HLA matched CTL in assays where the LCL derived from the same individual patients were efficiently killed (Rooney *et al*, 1985b). This represented the first clear demonstration of tumour cell escape from an appropriate CTL surveillance system in humans and prompted a series of investigations into the mechanisms underlying such immune evasion.

Clearly, this could not be ascribed to any inherent resistance of the group I BL cells to cell mediated cytolysis per se, since such lines were killed by some allospecific CTL clones (Torsteindottir *et al*, 1986) and were reproducibly more sensitive than their LCL counterparts to lysis by non-HLA restricted lymphokine activated T cell preparations (Misko *et al*, 1990). Subsequent studies have exploited the fact that many EBV positive BL cell lines are themselves phenotypically unstable and on serial passage can switch to a group III LCL like phenotype quite unlike that of the original tumour (Rooney *et al*, 1986b); these cells then become sensitive to EBV specific CTL recognition in the same way as LCL (Rooney *et al*, 1985b; Rowe DT *et al*, 1986). Comparisons can therefore be made between early and late passage cultures of the same BL cell line, or better still between phenotypically distinct group I and group III subclones established from the same tumour (Gregory *et al*, 1990). Below, we use this subclone analysis to illustrate three fundamental differences between group I and group III cells, any one of which could contribute to the different sensitivities of these cells to immune recognition.

HLA Class I Antigen Expression

It has been clear for many years that BL biopsy cells and derived BL cell lines do express HLA class I antigens on the cell membrane (the Daudi cell line is a celebrated exception to this rule and carries a functional deletion of the β_2-microglobulin [β_2m] gene [Quillet *et al*, 1988]). Furthermore, the levels of HLA antigens expressed on the group I BL cell surface are sufficient to sensitize these cells to lysis by appropriate allospecific CTL preparations (Torsteindottir *et al*, 1986; Griffin H and Rickinson A, unpublished), even though the lines themselves are much poorer stimulators of alloresponses in vitro than the corresponding LCL (Rooney *et al*, 1986a). However, studies with mono-

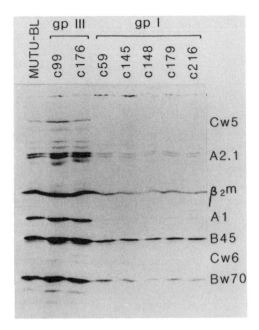

Fig. 4. HLA class I antigen expression in group I versus group III clones of the Mutu-BL cell line (HLA type A1, A2.1; B45, Bw70; Cw5, Cw6). Each of the clones was metabolically labelled with [^{35}S]methionine in exponential growth phase, and then protein extracts were made using NP-40. HLA class I antigens were immunoprecipitated from NP-40 extracts containing equal amounts of TCA precipitable radioactivity using the MAb W632; note that this MAb recognizes a monomorphic determinant on all mature HLA heavy chain/β_2 microglobulin complexes. The immunoprecipitated material was then separated in a one dimensional isoelectric focusing gel to reveal the individual allele specific heavy chains. Group I clones show reduced labelling of all HLA class I antigens compared with group III clones (and with the group III parental Mutu-BL cell line in late passage), and in addition, an allele selective downregulation of HLA-A1; note that longer exposures of the gel are required to show effects on HLA-C alleles

clonal antibodies to polymorphic rather than monomorphic determinants on class I antigens first raised the possibility of allele selective HLA downregulation in BL cells compared to the corresponding LCL (Masucci *et al*, 1987; Torsteindottir *et al*, 1988), and particular examples of this have subsequently been confirmed by immunoprecipitation and isoelectric focusing (Masucci *et al*, 1989; Masucci, 1990).

Figure 4 illustrates this phenomenon by comparing isogenic subclones of the Mutu-BL cell line, as well as the parental line itself after its switching to group III phenotype in late passage. Using the MAb W6/32, HLA class I molecules were immunoprecipitated from Nonidet P-40 (NP-40) extracts of metabolically labelled group I and group III clones containing equal amounts of TCA precipitable radioactivity. The immunoprecipitated material was then separated by one dimensional isoelectric focusing to allow identification of each allelic heavy chain as well as the invariant β_2m light chain. It is clear from the intensities of the β_2m bands that overall incorporation into HLA class I antigens is relatively low in group I clones, even though the cells are at least as metabolically active as their group III counterparts. In addition, however, there is an allele selective downregulation of HLA-A1 expression that is not observed for the HLA-A2.1, B45 and Bw70 antigens. These effects, and also effects on HLA C antigen expression, can be quantitated by excising the relevant regions of the gel and counting incorporated label. Clones that have progressed to a group III phenotype show "correction" of the allele selective effect on HLA-A1 and also a general increase in synthesis of all HLA class I antigens to LCL like levels. In other experiments (data not shown), these differences between group I and group III Mutu-BL clones apparent from metabolic labelling experiments have been confirmed when steady state levels of the individual HLA-A1, A2.1 and B45 antigens at the cell surface were measured in binding assays with allele specific monoclonal antibodies (Masucci M, unpublished).

There are a number of general points to be made with respect to HLA class I allele selective downregulation in BL. Firstly, the phenomenon has been observed in the majority of group I BL cell lines examined to date and usually involves either reduced expression or total absence of an HLA-A and/or HLA C antigen (Andersson *et al*, 1990). Secondly, downregulation appears to be imposed at the level of gene transcription rather than at the stage of protein assembly/transport to the membrane; indeed, where there is only partial downregulation, full expression of the allele can often be induced by interferon treatment (Andersson *et al*, 1990), presumably indicating that the affected class I gene retains functional interferon responsive elements in the promoter region (David-Watine *et al*, 1990). Thirdly, certain HLA alleles are affected much more often than others, the most striking example of consistent downregulation in BL involving HLA-A11. Finally, this phenomenon is not a direct consequence of selection pressure exerted by EBV specific CTL surveillance in vivo, since it is seen both in EBV positive and in (sporadic) EBV negative Burkitt tumours. It may therefore be either a specific feature of BL per se, perhaps reflecting some consequence of the deregulated c-*myc* expression that is characteristic of both endemic and sporadic tumours, or a feature of the normal germinal centre cell population from which BL is thought to arise. This issue has not yet been resolved.

Adhesion Molecule Expression

A second important feature of the BL tumour cell surface, revealed from the study of phenotypically stable group I BL cell lines (Gregory *et al*, 1988), is the absence or very low expression of the cellular adhesion molecules LFA 1, ICAM 1 and LFA 3. This is illustrated in Table 1 by the results of a cytofluorimetric analysis of group I versus group III Mutu-BL clones after immunofluorescence staining with monoclonal antibodies specific for the individual adhesion molecules. All three structures are essentially undetectable on

TABLE 1. Adhesion molecule profile of group I and group III Mutu-BL clones

Mutu cells	Phenotype group	Growth phenotype	Fluorescence/volume ratio after staining[a] for		
			LFA 1	ICAM1	LFA3
BL c59	I	Single cells	0.2	0	0
BL c167	I	Single cells	0.1	0	0
BL c179	I	Single cells	1.3	0.2	0.2
BL c62	III	Large clumps	20.0	39.3	28.8
BL c99	III	Large clumps	15.1	41.4	32.4
BL c176	III	Large clumps	17.1	44.6	22.3
LCL	III	Large clumps	24.7	43.6	31.0

[a]Results of cytofluorimetric analysis after indirect immunofluorescence staining of cells with the LFA 1α chain specific MAb MHM24, the ICAM1-specific MAb RR1/1 or the LFA 3 specific MAb TS2/9

group I clones yet are activated to high levels, equivalent to those seen in LCL, in clones that have switched to a group III phenotype.

These differences are reflected in the differing growth patterns of group I and group III cells; thus, group I cells grow as a single cell suspension rather than in clumps because the molecules mediating homotypic adhesion, namely LFA 1 and ICAM 1, are not detectably expressed. More importantly, the absence of ICAM 1 and LFA 3 on the group I BL cell surface is reflected functionally by the inability of such cells to form conjugates with activated T cells in short term in vitro assays (Gregory *et al*, 1988). Again, these characteristics are not unique to EBV positive BL, since cell lines established from cases of EBV negative sporadic BL also show the same phenotype. Here, one can certainly argue that the low adhesion molecule profile is a phenotypic vestige of the normal cell compartment from which BL is thought to arise, since a proportion of normal germinal centroblasts also appear to express adhesion molecules weakly if at all (Gregory CD, unpublished).

EBV Latent Gene Expression

A third key difference between group I BL cell lines and LCL is in the resident form of EBV latency. Thus, EBNA 1, a molecule essential for maintenance and duplication of the episomal viral genome (Yates *et al*, 1984), is the only detectable latent protein in such BL cells, with all other EBNA and the LMP downregulated (Rowe *et al*, 1987; Gregory *et al*, 1990). Restriction over viral gene expression is imposed at the transcriptional level; the latent gene promoters used in LCL are silent and a novel EBNA 1 specific promoter in the *Bam*HI F region of the genome is activated (Sample *et al*, 1991). Switching of BL cell lines from a group I to a group III phenotype in vitro is

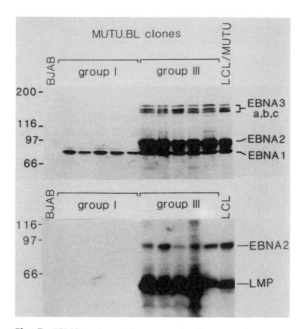

Fig. 5. EBV latent protein expression in group I versus group III clones of the Mutu-BL cell line. Protein extracts of each clone were separated by polyacrylamide gel electrophoresis, transferred and immunoblotted using either a polyclonal human serum with antibodies to EBNAs 1, 2, 3A, 3B and 3C (upper panel) or a mixture of MAbs PE2 and CS1-4 specific for EBNA 2 and LMP 1, respectively (lower panel). Control cell lines were the EBV negative BJAB line and an LCL (LCL/Mutu) established by in vitro transformation of normal B cells using the EBV strain rescued from Mutu-BL cells. Whereas group III Mutu-BL clones express all the relevant EBV latent proteins, only EBNA 1 is detectable in group I clones

associated with promoter switching and a concomitant broadening of EBV latent protein expression to that characteristic of LCL. Figure 5 illustrates the point by showing gels of protein extracts from group I and group III Mutu-BL clones that have been developed with a human serum containing high titre antibodies to the EBNA 1, 2, 3A, 3B and 3C proteins (upper panel) or with a pool of monoclonal antibodies against EBNA 2 and LMP 1 (lower panel). There is a dramatic difference in the pattern of expression of the same EBV genome in the two phenotypically distinct types of cells.

It is not hard to see the advantage that the highly restricted form of EBV latency offers group I BL cells in terms of immune evasion, since those viral antigens that constitute the dominant (perhaps the only) targets of virus specific CTL recognition are not expressed. However, one should be wary of the facile interpretation that this form of latency is forced upon the malignant cell clone by pressure from the immune surveillance mechanism in vivo, ie that downregulation of latent protein expression is a key selective step in the pathogenesis of BL. It may well be that EBV naturally adopts this form of infection in a variety of normal cells in vivo, particularly in naturally proliferative cell compartments (such as the germinal centre) where EBNA 1 mediated maintenance/replication of the viral genome would be all that is required to ensure that all progeny cells retain the virus infection. Highly restricted EBV latent gene expression may therefore be a regular feature of the target cell population from which BL arises, rather than a unique feature of a malignant cell clone selected for its ability to evade EBV specific CTL recognition.

PHENOTYPIC CHANGE AND THE RECONSTITUTION OF BL CELL IMMUNOGENICITY

It is clear from the work described above that BL cell progression from group I to group III is associated with dramatic changes both in cellular and in viral phenotypes. These are illustrated diagrammatically in Fig. 6. As to the relationship between these different sets of changes, it is the activation of viral latent gene expression that leads to the observed switch in cell phenotype and not vice versa. Thus, EBV negative sporadic BL cell lines almost all retain a group I like phenotype on serial passage (Rowe M *et al,* 1986), any changes

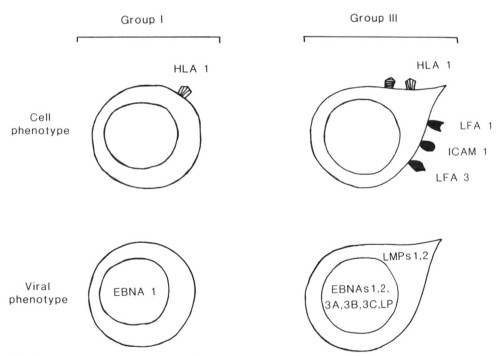

Fig. 6. Diagrammatic representation of group I versus group III BL cells illustrating differences both in cellular and in viral phenotypes that could influence the cells' immunogenicity for CTL responses. Group I cells display lower levels of all HLA class I alleles at the cell surface compared with group III cells and frequently show an additional downregulation selectively affecting certain alleles. Group I cells are essentially negative for, or show very weak expression of, the cellular adhesion molecules LFA 1, ICAM 1 and LFA 3, whereas all three proteins are highly expressed on the group III cell surface. Viral latent protein expression is restricted to EBNA 1 in group I cells compared with the full spectrum of eight latent proteins found in group III cells

that do occur being relatively minor, most often involving the appearance of low levels of ICAM 1 and/or LFA 1 on the cell surface. However, these lines can be switched towards the group III phenotype by experimental infection with EBV in vitro or by transfection with individual EBV latent genes (Rowe M *et al*, 1986; Torsteindottir *et al*, 1986; Wang *et al*, 1987, 1990). The most dramatic single gene effects in this context are mediated by LMP 1, which, if expressed in EBV negative BL cells, induces a dose dependent upregulation of all three adhesion molecules and of at least one activation antigen, CD23 (Wang *et al*, 1990). In the same situation, LMP 1 has not been seen to correct allele selective HLA class I downregulation (Cuomo *et al*, 1990).

As stated above, EBV positive BL cell lines that have switched to a group III phenotype and full pattern of latent gene expression were found to resemble LCL in their susceptibility to EBV specific cytolysis (Rooney *et al*, 1985b; Rowe D *et al*, 1986). In certain cases, it was even possible to follow the increasing susceptibility over time and show that this reflects the proportion of cells in the line that had switched to group III (Gregory *et al*, 1988). However, because all three immunologically relevant parameters (ie HLA antigens, adhesion molecules, viral antigens) tend to show coordinate upregulation in this system, it is very difficult to isolate any one variable and determine its individual importance. At this point, it is instructive to re-examine our published data (Gregory *et al*, 1988), here reproduced as Table 2, on the increasing susceptibility to virus specific cytolysis of an EBV positive BL cell line, BL72, with serial passage. These results, showing a correlation between levels of cytolysis and levels of adhesion molecule expression, were originally taken to indicate

TABLE 2. Sensitivity of BL72 and WW1-BL cells to EBV specific HLA-A11 restricted CTL: Data from Gregory et al (1988)

| Target cells[a] | Adhesion molecules[b] | | % Lysis with effector CTL[c] | | | | |
| | | | CM-T | | SW-T | KS-T | |
	ICAM 1	LFA 3	10:1	5:1	5:1	10:1	5:1
BL72 p25	4.1	0.7	0	0	0	0	2
BL72 p80	13.0	12.9	7	4	0	15	10
BL72 p140	24.1	21.5	23	18	11	34	26
72-LCL	34.4	58.9	37	27	18	47	44
WW1-BL	48.0	0.9	5	3	1	8	4
WW1-LCL	21.2	40.2	42	29	31	40	40
Allo-LCL	20.8	48.2	3	2	2	7	5

[a]Parallel cultures of BL72 at three passage numbers (p25, 80, 140) were tested simultaneously alongside the autologous LCL (72-LCL); WW1-BL was tested in late passage against the autologous LCL (WW1-LCL); an allogeneic HLA-A11 negative LCL (Allo-LCL) was included as a specificity control for the CTL assay

[b]Values measured as in Table 1

[c]Results of a 5 hr ^{51}Cr release assay using HLA-A11 restricted EBV specific effector T cell preparations from three donors, CM, SW and KS, at effector:target ratios shown

an important role for adhesion pathways in determining BL cell susceptibility to immune recognition. However, the dominant component in all three CTL preparations used in these assays was HLA-A11 restricted, and subsequent work has shown that BL72 actually displays an allele selective downregulation of HLA-A11 expression that is corrected on serial passage (Torsteindottir *et al*, 1988; Masucci M, unpublished). Changes in surface levels of HLA-A11, rather than changes in adhesion molecule profile, might therefore be sufficient to explain the increasing sensitivity of later passage BL72 cells to the CTL used in this particular work.

A more dramatic example of the same phenomenon, but one that opens up new experimental possibilities, involves the EBV positive BL cell line, WW1-BL, also originally derived from an HLA-A11 positive patient. This line switched to full virus latent gene expression at a very early passage (including expression of EBNA 3B, the protein usually associated with A11 restricted lysis) and assumed most features of an LCL like group III surface phenotype (Rowe *et al*, 1987). Despite this, the line was still not recognized by HLA-A11 restricted EBV specific CTL (Table 2) (Gregory *et al*, 1988). Subsequent work has shown that the WW1-BL cell line is unusual with respect to all three immunological variables relevant to A11 restricted recognition: (a) it shows complete allele selective suppression of HLA-A11 expression (Torsteindottir *et al*, 1988); (b) it has upregulated expression of the LFA 1 and ICAM 1 adhesion molecules but is unique among group III cell lines in remaining LFA 3 negative (Gregory *et al*, 1988); and (c) it carries a virus strain encoding a variant EBNA 3B protein, which apparently lacks the HLA-A11 restricted target epitope present within the standard B95.8 strain of EBNA 3B (Masucci M, unpublished).

TABLE 3. Reconstitution of WW1-BL cell sensitivity to EBV specific A11 restriction CTL[a]

	% Specific lysis with A11 restricted CTL	
Vaccinia infection of target cells[b]	WW1-BL	WW1-BL/A11[c]
None	6	6
Vacc-TK	4	5
Vacc-LFA3	6	5
Vacc-EBNA 3B	0	22
Vacc-LFA 3 + Vacc EBNA3B	8	20

[a]Results of a 5 hr ^{51}Cr release assay using EBV specific A11 restricted CTL at effector:target ratio of 10:1. In the same assay, lysis of the WW1-LCL was 20%

[b]Cells were infected with recombinant vaccinia viruses as described (Murray *et al*, 1990) prior to their inclusion as targets in the cytotoxicity assay. Vacc-TK⁻ is a control recombinant

[c]WW1-BL cells were transfected with a 5.1 kb HindIII genomic fragment containing the HLA-A11 gene cloned into the HindIII site of an EBV ori-p-based expression vector containing a hygromycin B drug resistance marker. Expression of HLA-A11 on the surface of the WW1-BL/A11 transfectant at levels equivalent to that seen on WW1-LCL cells was confirmed by immunofluorescence with the allele specific MAb AUF 5.13 and by isoelectric focusing as in Fig. 4

In our most recent experiments, we have reconstituted all three deficiencies in WW1-BL cells, either singly or together (a) by stable introduction of an A11-expressing plasmid, thereby completely restoring surface A11 expression; (b) by acute infection with a recombinant vaccinia virus expressing LFA 3, with proven restoration of LFA 3 dependent conjugate forming ability (Griffin H and Rickinson A, unpublished); and (c) by acute infection with a recombinant vaccinia virus expressing the standard EBNA 3B protein at levels in excess of those seen in LCL. We find that coexpression of A11 and EBNA 3B is both necessary and sufficient for recognition and lysis of WW1-BL cells by appropriate A11 restricted effectors, and that lysis under these conditions is not significantly increased by simultaneous expression of LFA 3. Illustrative results are shown from one such assay in Table 3. It is therefore clear that CTL function is not absolutely dependent on LFA 3 and that the LFA 3 pathway may have no auxiliary role in a situation where there is relative overexpression of the viral target protein (in this case EBNA 3B) and normal levels of the restricting antigen (in this case A11).

A similar conclusion, namely the redundancy of LFA 3 mediated adhesion for virus specific CTL function, has been reached in another study showing that group I BL cell lines with little or no LFA 3 can be sensitized to EBV specific CTL restricted through appropriate HLA antigens by exogenous addition of the defined EBV target epitope in synthetic peptide form (Khanna R and Moss D, unpublished). As shown in Fig. 7, the LFA 3 negative BL30 cell line (devoid of EBV sequences and derived from a sporadic Burkitt tumour) is sensitized to an HLA-B8 restricted EBNA 3A specific CTL clone c13 by addition of the relevant EBNA 3A derived peptide epitope. Similarly, the LFA 3 negative WW2-BL and BL29 cell lines (EBV positive but expressing only EBNA 1) are sensitized to an HLA-B18 restricted EBNA 2 specific CTL clone c27 by addition of the relevant EBNA 2 derived peptide epitope, whereas another LFA 3 negative EBV positive line BL36 can be sensitized to an HLA-B44 restricted EBNA 3C specific CTL clone c5 by addition of the relevant EBNA 3C derived epitope. Testing each effector:target combination with each of the three synthetic peptides ensures that the assay is internally controlled. A role for LFA 3 is therefore not apparent under these conditions. Furthermore, in the case of BL29, these cells appear to be completely negative not just for LFA 3 but also for ICAM 1 and LFA 1, thereby precluding involvement of either the LFA 3/CD2 or the ICAM 1/LFA 1 pathway in this particular peptide mediated cytolysis. Despite the clear-cut nature of the findings in these two particular experimental situations, it remains to be seen whether a facilitating role for adhesion pathways can be observed under limiting conditions, ie when the relevant EBV target protein is expressed at the low levels usually associated with latent EBV infection or when the exogenous peptide is titrated out to suboptimal concentrations.

Caution must be exercised in extrapolating from these highly artificial effector:target cell combinations in vitro to the reality of virus specific CTL surveillance in vivo. Nevertheless, our provisional conclusion is that downregula-

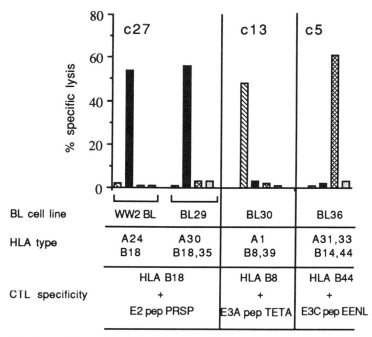

Fig. 7. Peptide mediated sensitization of LFA 3 negative group I BL cells to EBV specific cytolysis. Results of a 5 hr cytotoxicity assay using CTL clones c27 specific for the EBNA 2 derived peptide epitope PRSPTVFYNIPPMPL in the context of HLA-B18 (Moss DJ, unpublished), c13 specific for the EBNA 3A derived peptide epitope TETAQAWNAGFLRGRAYGIDLLRTE in the context of HLA-B8 (Burrows et al, 1990b) and c5 specific for the EBNA 3C derived peptide epitope EENLLDFVRFMGVMSSCNNP in the context of HLA-B44 (Burrows et al, 1990a). Targets included the EBV positive group I cell lines WW2-BL and BL29 both expressing HLA-B18, the EBV negative group I cell line BL30 expressing HLA-B8, and the EBV positive group I BL36 cell line expressing HLA-B44. Levels of lysis are shown for each of the effector:target combinations tested in medium alone (stippled) or in the presence of the c27 target peptide (closed), the c13 target peptide (hatched) or the c5 target peptide (crosshatched). Clearly, these LFA 3 negative target cells could be sensitized to the relevant EBV specific CTL clone on addition of optimal concentrations (1 µg/ml) of the appropriate peptide epitope; all three peptides were tested with all four effector:target combinations to provide internal controls

tion of EBV target antigens in BL cells represents the most effective and broad ranging mechanism underlying the escape of tumour cells from immune recognition. By comparison, the downregulation of HLA class I antigens should be less influential, since it is an allele selective phenomenon, and complete dominance of an individual's EBV specific CTL response by clones restricted through a single allele is rare. The very low expression/absence of adhesion molecules on BL cells seems unlikely to provide an absolute barrier to tumour cell recognition by CTL, although an important facilitating role for adhesion pathways under physiological conditions remains a possibility. It is worth remembering that all of the above CTL assays are carried out with already activated effector cells and reflect tumour cell antigenicity rather than immunogenicity. The reduced ability of group I compared with group III BL cells to stimulate CTL responses in vitro may well reflect the importance of adhesion pathways in this situation, since requirements for T cell activation from the resting state are known to be more stringent than for the effector function of already activated cells. In this context, group I BL cells are poor stimulators of responses in vitro (Rooney *et al*, 1986a), whereas derived LMP 1 transfectants, showing increased adhesion molecule expression but no change in surface levels of HLA antigens, have significantly improved stimulatory capacity (Cuomo *et al*, 1990). Prospects for immunotherapy against EBV positive BL using virus specific effectors are clearly limited. BL target cells should in principle be recognizable by EBNA 1 specific CTL, but our studies on healthy virus carriers suggest that CTL responses directed against EBNA 1 epitopes are rarely if ever detectable. Understanding why this is so remains an important future objective.

T Cell Surveillance and Hodgkin's Disease

The finding that a significant proportion of HD cases carry EBV specifically within the malignant cell population (Anagnostopoulos, 1989; Weiss *et al*, 1989) raises the question of immune surveillance against these tumours. A key issue in this context is the pattern of EBV gene expression in the tumour. Recent studies (Herbst *et al*, 1991); Pallesen *et al*, 1991), although still preliminary, suggest that HD cells sustain a third form of EBV latent infection, which is distinct from those seen in large cell lymphoma and in BL but much closer to that seen in the EBV associated epithelial malignancy, nasopharyngeal carcinoma. The latter is characterized by coexpression of EBNA 1, LMP 1 and LMP 2 in the absence of other EBNA (Brooks L, Yao QY, Rickinson AB, Young LS, unpublished).

Assuming, by analogy with BL, that the spectrum of available virus target proteins is the chief determinant of HD cell sensitivity to EBV specific surveillance, then this leads to an interesting prediction. Thus, although most virus specific CTL responses in healthy donors are directed towards EBNA (other than EBNA 1), there are certain HLA class I antigens that selectively present epitopes from the LMP. The most obvious example from our work to date is the presentation of an LMP 2 epitope (not yet defined at the peptide level) by the HLA-A2.1 antigen. Whereas an A2.1 restricted response is not usually the dominant component within a polyclonal CTL preparation from an A2.1 positive individual, T cells with the relevant LMP 2 reactivity are nevertheless detectable in many cases (Murray R, Brooks J and Rickinson A, unpublished). If such responses are mounted in vivo and are capable of recognizing LMP 2 as expressed in HD cells, then HLA-A2.1 could be protective against EBV positive HD but presumably not against the EBV negative form of the disease. Although there is still much to learn about EBV positive HD in terms of virus gene expression and of cellular immunogenicity, the possible role for EBV specific CTL responses in the control of this tumour provides an interesting focus for future work.

SUMMARY

Epstein-Barr virus, a lymphotropic herpesvirus of humans, has potent B cell growth transforming activity yet persists in the lymphoid tissues of most individuals as a lifelong asymptomatic infection. Virus induced B cell growth transformation in vitro is associated with the expression of a limited set of viral genes encoding six nuclear antigens (EBNA 1, 2, 3A, 3B, 3C and LP) and two latent membrane proteins (LMP 1, 2). Healthy virus carriers possess strong EBV specific CTL memory that can be reactivated in vitro. Here, we summarize experiments in which the antigenic specificities of these HLA class I restricted memory CTL responses have been mapped in a range of individuals with different HLA backgrounds. Of the known EBV latent proteins, EBNA 3A, 3B and 3C are frequently the dominant targets for such responses, but examples of responses directed against epitopes of EBNA 2, EBNA-LP or the LMP have been identified; by contrast, CTL responses against epitopes of EBNA 1 have not been observed. Epstein-Barr virus is associated with at least three malignancies of lymphoid origin—immunoblastic lymphomas of the immunosuppressed, endemic Burkitt's lymphoma and a subset of Hodgkin's disease. The immunoblastic lymphomas express the complete spectrum of EBV coded latent proteins and a cellular phenotype similar to that of in vitro transformed B lymphoblastoid cell lines; accordingly, they remain sensitive to EBV specific CTL recognition. Endemic BL cells are not recognized by such CTL, and at least three consistent features of this tumour could contribute to immune escape: (a) allele specific downregulation of HLA class I antigen expression, (b) absence/low expression of cellular adhesion molecules and (c) restriction of EBV latent protein expression to EBNA 1 only. The relative importance of these three features of the BL cell phenotype with regard to sensitivity to CTL recognition is re-interpreted in the light of recent results. Finally, the pattern of virus latent protein expression in EBV positive Hodgkin's disease is described, and the possibility of EBV specific CTL control against this tumour is discussed.

Acknowledgements

Our work is supported by the Cancer Research Campaign and Medical Research Council, UK (ABR), the National Health and Medical Research Council, Australia (DJM), and the Swedish Cancer Society (MGM). Currently, MGM is the recipient of a Wellcome-Swedish MRC Fellowship at the CRC Laboratories, Department of Cancer Studies, University of Birmingham, Birmingham, UK. We should like to acknowledge the valuable contributions to the CTL work that have come from our collaborators Dr M Kurilla and Dr E Kieff, Department of Microbiology and Molecular Genetics, Harvard Medical School, Boston, USA. Thanks are also due to our colleagues Dr CD Gregory and Dr M Rowe for permission to include data from their work in Table 1 and Fig. 5, and to Miss Deborah Williams for excellent secretarial assistance.

References

Alfieri C, Birkenbach M and Kieff E (1991) Early events in Epstein-Barr virus infection of human B lymphocytes. *Virology* **181** 595–608

Anagnostopoulos I, Herbst H, Niedobitek G and Stein H (1989) Demonstration of monoclonal EBV genomes in Hodgkin's disease and Ki-1 positive anaplastic large cell lymphoma by combined Southern blot and in situ hybridization. *Blood* **74** 810–816

Andersson ML, Stam N, Klein G, Ploegh H and Masucci MG (1990) Aberrations in the expression of HLA class I antigens in Burkitt's lymphoma cell lines. *International Journal of Cancer* **17** 544–550

Beral V, Peterman T, Berkelman R and Jaffe H (1991) AIDS-associated non-Hodgkin lymphoma. *Lancet* **337** 805–809

Burrows SR, Misko IS, Sculley TB, Schmidt C and Moss DJ (1990a) An Epstein-Barr virus-specific cytotoxic T cell epitope present on A- and B-type transformants. *Jounral of Virology* **64** 3974–3976

Burrows SR, Sculley TB, Misko IS, Schmidt C and Moss DJ (1990b) An Epstein-Barr virus-specific cytotoxic T cell epitope in EBNA 3. *Journal of Experimental Medicine* **171** 345–350

Cleary ML and Sklar J (1984) Lymphoproliferative disorders in cardiac transplant recipients are multiclonal lymphomas. *Lancet* **ii** 489–493

Cleary ML, Epstein MA, Finerty S *et al* (1985) Individual tumours of multifocal Epstein-Barr virus-induced malignant lymphomas in Tamarins arise from different B-cell clones. *Science* **228** 722–724

Cleary ML, Dorfman RF and Sklar J (1986) Failure in immunological control of the virus infection: post-transplant lymphomas, In: Epstein MA and Achong BG (eds). *The Epstein-Barr Virus: Recent Advances*, pp 163–181, Heinemann Medical Books, London

Cuomo L, Trivedi P, Wang F, Wimberg G, Klein G and Masucci MG (1990) Expression of the Epstein-Barr virus (EBV) latent membrane protein increases the stimulatory capacity of Burkitt's lymphoma cells in allogeneic mixed lymphocyte cultures. *European Journal of Immunology* **20** 2293–2299

Dambaugh T, Hennessy K, Chamnankit L and Kieff E (1984) U2 region of Epstein-Barr virus DNA may encode Epstein-Barr nuclear antigen 2. *Proceedings of the National Academy of Sciences of the USA* **81** 7632–7636

David-Watine B, Israel A and Kurilski P (1990) The regulation and expression of HLA class I genes. *Immunology Today* **11** 286–292

Gordon J, Ley SC, Melamed MD, English LS and Hughes-Jones NC (1984) Immortalized B lymphocytes produce B cell growth factor. *Nature* **310** 145–147

Gotch F, McMichael A, Smith G and Moss B (1987) Identification of viral molecules recognised by influenza-specific human cytotoxic T lymphocytes. *Journal of Experimental Medicine* **165** 408–416

Gratama JW, Zutter MM, Minarovits J *et al* (1991) Expression of Epstein-Barr virus-encoded growth-transformation-associated proteins in lymphoproliferations of bone marrow transplant recipients. *International Journal of Cancer* **47** 188–192

Greenspan JS, Greenspan D, Lennette ET *et al* (1985) Replication of Epstein-Barr virus within the epithelial cells of "hairy" leukoplakia, an AIDS-associated lesion. *New England Journal of Medicine* **313** 1564–1571

Gregory CD, Tursz T, Edwards CF *et al* (1987) Identification of a subset of normal B cells with a Burkitt's lymphoma (BL)-like phenotype. *Journal of Immunology* **139** 313–318

Gregory CD, Murray RJ, Edwards CF and Rickinson AB (1988) Down regulation of cell adhesion molecules LFA-3 and ICAM-1 in Epstein-Barr virus-positive Burkitt's lymphoma underlies tumour cell escape from virus-specific T cell surveillance. *Journal of Experimental Medicine* **167** 1811–1824

Gregory CD, Rowe M and Rickinson AB (1990) Different Epstein-Barr virus (EBV)-B cell interactions in phenotypically distinct clones of a Burkitt lymphoma cell line. *Journal of Gen-*

eral Virology **71** 1481–1495

Henle G and Henle W (1979) The virus as the etiologic agent of infectious mononucleosis, In: Epstein MA and Achong BG (eds). *The Epstein-Barr Virus,* pp 297–320, Springer-Verlag, Berlin

Herbst H, Dallenbach F, Hummel M *et al* (1991) Epstein-Barr virus latent membrane protein expression in Hodgkin and Reed-Sternberg cells. *Proceedings of the National Academy of Sciences of the USA* **88** 4766–4770

Hickling JK, Borysiewicz LK and Sissons JGP (1987) Varicella-zoster virus-specific cytotoxic T lymphocytes (TC): detection and frequency analysis of HLA class I-restricted TC in human peripheral blood. *Journal of Virology* **61** 3463–3469

Kalter SP, Riggs SA, Cabanillas F *et al* (1985) Aggressive non-Hodgkin's lymphomas in immunocompromised homosexual males. *Blood* **66** 655–659

Khanna R, Jacob CA, Burrows SR *et al* (1991) Expression of Epstein-Barr virus nuclear antigens in anti-IgM stimulated B cells following recombinant vaccinia infection and their recognition by human cytotoxic T cells. *Immunology* **74** 504–510

Kieff E and Leibowitz D (1990) Epstein-Barr virus and its replication, In: Fields BN, Knipe DM (ed). *Virology,* 2nd edition, pp 1889–1920, Raven Press, New York

Lanzavecchia A (1985) Antigen-specific interaction between T and B cells. *Nature* **314** 537–540

MacMahon E, Glass JD, Hayward SD *et al* (1991) EBV in AIDS primary CNS lymphoma. *Lancet* **338** 969–973

McMichael AJ, Gotch FM, Dongworth DW, Clark A and Potter CW (1983) Declining T cell immunity to influenza 1977-1982. *Lancet* **ii** 762–764

Magrath I (1990) The pathogenesis of Burkitt's lymphoma. *Advances in Cancer Research* **55** 133–270

Martin PJ, Shulman HM, Schubach WH *et al* (1984) Fatal EBV-associated proliferation of donor B cells after treatment of acute graft-versus-host disease with a murine monoclonal anti-T cell antibody. *Annals of Internal Medicine* **101** 310–315

Masucci MG (1990) Cell phenotype dependent down-regulation of MHC class I antigens in Burkitt's lymphoma cells. *Current Topics in Microbiology and Immunology* **166** 309–316

Masucci MG, Torsteindottir S, Colombani BJ, Brautbar C, Klein E and Klein G (1987) Down-regulation of class I HLA antigens and of the Epstein-Barr virus (EBV)-encoded latent membrane protein (LMP) in Burkitt lymphoma lines. *Proceedings of the National Academy of Sciences of the USA* **84** 4567–4571

Masucci MG, Stam N, Torsteinsdottir S, Neefjes J, Klein G and Ploegh H (1989) Allele specific down-regulation of MHC class I antigens in Burkitt's lymphoma lines. *Cellular Immunology* **120** 396–400

Miller G (1990) Epstein-Barr virus: biology, pathogenesis, and medical aspects, In: Fields BN, Knipe D M (ed). *Virology,* 2nd edition, pp 1921–1958, Raven Press, New York

Misko IS, Pope JH, Hutter P, Soszynski TD and Kane RG (1984) HLA-DR-antigen-associated restriction of EBV-specific cytotoxic T-cell colonies. *International Journal of Cancer* **33** 239–243

Misko, IS, Schmidt C, Martin N *et al* (1990) Lymphokine-activated killer (LAK) cells discriminate between Epstein-Barr virus (EBV)-positive Burkitt's lymphoma cells. *International Journal of Cancer* **46** 399–404

Moss DJ, Wallace LE, Rickinson AB and Epstein MA (1981) Cytotoxic T cell recognition of Epstein-Barr viurs-infected B cells. I. Specificity and HLA restriction of effector cells reactivated *in vitro. European Journal of Immunology* **11** 686–693

Moss DJ, Sculley TB and Pope JH (1986) Induction of Epstein-Barr virus nuclear antigens. *Journal of Virology* **58** 988–990

Moss DJ, Misko IS, Burrows SR, Burman K, McCarthy R and Sculley TB (1988) Cytotoxic T-cell clones discriminate between A- and B-type Epstein-Barr virus transformants. *Nature* **331** 719–721

Murray RJ, Kurilla MG, Griffin HM *et al* (1990) Human cytotoxic T cell responses against

Epstein-Barr virus nuclear antigens demonstrated using recombinant vaccinia viruses. *Proceedings of the National Academy of Sciences of the USA* **87** 2906–2910

Niedobitek G, Young LS, Lau R *et al* (1991) Epstein-Barr virus infection in oral hairy leukoplakia:virus replication in the absence of a detectable latent phase. *Journal of General Virology* **72** 3035–3046

Pallesen G, Hamilton-Dutoit SJ, Rowe M and Young LS (1991) Expression of Epstein-Barr virus latent gene products in tumour cells of Hodgkin's disease. *Lancet* **337** 320–322

Quillet A, Presse F, Marchiol-Fournigault C *et al* (1988) Increased resistance to non-MHC-restricted cytotoxicity related to HLA-A, B expression. *Journal of Immunology* **141** 17–20

Reiss CS, Hemler ME, Englehard VH, Mier JW, Strominger JL and Burakoff SJ (1980) Development and characterization of allospecific long-term human cytolytic T-cell lines. *Proceedings of the National Academy of Sciences of the USA* **77** 5432–5436

Rickinson AB, Moss DJ, Wallace LE *et al* (1981) Long-term T-cell-mediated immunity to Epstein-Barr virus. *Cancer Research* **41** 4216–4221

Rooney CM, Rickinson AB, Moss DJ, Lenoir GM and Epstein MA (1985a) Cell-mediated immunosurveillance mechanisms and the pathogenesis of Burkitt's lymphoma, In: Lenoir GM, O'Conor GT and Olweny CLM (eds). *Burkitt's Lymphoma: A Human Cancer Model*, pp 249–264, International Agency for Research on Cancer, Lyon

Rooney CM, Rowe M, Wallace LE and Rickinson AB (1985b) Epstein-Barr virus-positive Burkitt's lymphoma cells not recognized by virus-specific T-cell surveillance. *Nature* **317** 629–631

Rooney CM, Edwards CF, Lenoir GM, Rupani H and Rickinson AB (1986a) Differential activation of cytotoxic responses by Burkitt's lymphoma (BL)-cell lines: relationship to the BL-cell surface phenotype. *Cellular Immunology* **102** 99–112

Rooney CM, Gregory CD, Rowe M *et al* (1986b) Endemic Burkitt's lymphoma: Phenotypic analysis of tumour biopsy cells and of the derived tumour cell lines. *Journal of the National Cancer Institute* **77** 681–687

Rowe DT, Rowe M, Evan GI, Wallace LE, Farrell PJ and Rickinson AB (1986) Restricted expression of EBV latent genes and T-lymphocyte-detected membrane antigen in Burkitt's lymphoma cells. *EMBO Journal* **5** 2599–2607

Rowe M, Rooney CM, Rickinson AB *et al* (1985) Distinctions between endemic and sporadic forms of Epstein-Barr virus-positive Burkitt's lymphoma. *International Journal of Cancer* **35** 435–442

Rowe M, Rooney CM, Edwards CF, Lenoir GM and Rickinson AB (1986) Epstein-Barr virus status and tumour cell phenotype in sporadic Burkitt's lymphoma. *International Journal of Cancer* **37** 367–372

Rowe M, Rowe DT, Gregory CD *et al* (1987) Differences in B cell growth phenotype reflect novel patterns of Epstein-Barr virus latent gene expression in Burkitt's lymphoma cells. *EMBO Journal* **6** 2743–2751

Rowe M, Young LS, Crocker J, Stokes H, Henderson S and Rickinson AB (1991) Epstein-Barr virus (EBV)-associated lymphoproliferative disease in the SCID mouse model: implications for the pathogenesis of EBV-positive lymphomas in man. *Journal of Experimental Medicine* **173** 147–158

Sample J, Young L, Martin B *et al* (1990) Epstein-Barr virus type-1 (EBV-1) and 2 (EBV-2) differ in their EBNA 3A, EBNA 3B, and EBNA 3C genes. *Journal of Virology* **64** 4084–4092

Sample J, Brooks L, Sample C *et al* (1991) Restricted Epstein-Barr virus protein expression in Burkitt lymphoma is due to a different Epstein-Barr Nuclear Antigen-1 transcriptional initiation site. *Proceedings of the National Academy of Sciences of the USA* **88** 6343–6347

Shapiro RS, McClain K, Frizzera G *et al* (1988) Epstein-Barr virus-associated B cell lymphoproliferative disorders following bone marrow transplantation. *Blood* **71** 1234–1243

Shaw S, Luce GEG, Quinones R, Gress RE, Springer TA and Sanders ME (1986) Two antigen-independent adhesion pathways used by human cytotoxic T cell clones. *Nature* **323** 262–264

Silver ML, Parker KC and Wiley DC (1991) Reconstitution by MHC-restricted peptides of HLA-A2 heavy chain with β2-microglobulin, in vitro. *Nature* **350** 619–622

Springer TA (1990) Adhesion receptors of the immune system. *Nature* **364** 425–434

Starzl TE, Nalesnik MA, Porter KA *et al* (1984) Reversibility of lymphomas and lymphoproliferative lesions developing under cyclosporin A-steroid therapy. *Lancet* **i** 583–587

Stevens JG (1989) Human herpesviruses: a consideration of the latent state. *Microbiology Reviews* **53** 318–332

Strang G and Rickinson AB (1987) Multiple HLA class I-dependent cytotoxicities constitute the non-HLA-restricted response in infectious mononucleosis. *European Journal of Immunology* **17** 1007–1013

Subar M, Neri A, Inghirami G, Knowles DM and Dalla Favera R (1988) Frequent c-myc oncogene activation and infrequent presence of Epstein-Barr virus genome in AIDS-associated lymphoma. *Blood* **72** 667–671

Svedmyr E and Jondal M (1975) Cytotoxic effector cells specific for B cell lines transformed by Epstein-Barr virus are present in patients with infectious mononucleosis. *Proceedings of the National Academy of Sciences of the USA* **72** 1622–1626

Thomas JA, Hotchin NA, Allday MJ, Yacoub M and Crawford DH (1990) Immunohistology of Epstein-Barr virus-associated antigens in B cell disorders from immunocompromised individuals. *Transplantation* **49** 944–953

Torsteinsdottir S, Masucci MG, Ehlin-Henrikson B *et al* (1986) Differentiation-dependent sensitivity of human B cell derived lines to MHC-restricted T cell cytotoxicity. *Proceedings of the National Academy of Sciences of the USA* **83** 5620–5625

Torsteinsdottir S, Brautbar C, Klein E, Klein G and Masucci MG (1988) Differential expression of HLA antigens on human B cell lines of normal and malignant origin: a consequence of immune surveillance or a phenotypic vestige of the progenitor cells? *International Journal of Cancer* **41** 913–919

Townsend ARM, Rothbard J, Gotch FM, Bahadur G, Wraith D and McMichael AJ (1986) The epitopes of influenza nucleoprotein recognised by cytotoxic T lymphocytes can be defined with short synthetic peptides. *Cell* **44** 959–968

Wakasugi H, Rimsky L, Mahe Y *et al* (1987) Epstein-Barr virus-containing B-cell line produces an interleukin 1 that it uses as a growth factor. *Proceedings of the National Academy of Sciences of the USA* **84** 804–808

Wallace LE, Rickinson AB and Epstein MA (1982) Epstein-Barr virus-specific cytotoxic T cell clones restricted through a single HLA antigen. *Nature* **297** 413–415

Wang F, Gregory CD, Rowe M *et al* (1987) Epstein-Barr virus nuclear protein 2 specifically induces expression of the B cell activation antigen CD23. *Proceedings of the National Academy of Sciences of the USA* **84** 3452–3456

Wang F, Gregory CD, Sample C *et al* (1990) Epstein-Barr virus latent membrane protein (LMP-1) and nuclear proteins 2 and 3C are effectors of phenotypic changes in B lymphocytes: EBNA2 and LMP-1 cooperatively induce CD23. *Journal of Virology* **64** 2309–2318

Weiss LM, Mohared LA, Warnke RA and Sklar J (1989) Detection of Epstein-Barr virus genomes in Reed-Sternberg cells of Hodgkin's disease. *New England Journal of Medicine* **320** 502–506

White J, Herman A, Pullen AM, Kubo R, Kappler JW and Marrack P (1989) The Vb-specific superantigen staphylococcal enterotoxin B: stimulation of mature T cells and clonal deletion in neonatal mice. *Cell* **56** 27–35

Yao QY, Rowe M, Martin B, Young LS and Rickinson AB (1991) The Epstein-Barr virus carrier state: dominance of a single growth-transforming isolate in the blood and in the oropharynx of healthy virus carriers. *Journal of General Virology* **72** 1579–1590

Yates J, Warren N, Reisman D and Sugden B (1984) A *cis*-acting element from the Epstein-Barr viral genome that permits stable replication of recombinant plasmids in latently-infected cells. *Proceedings of the National Academy of Sciences of the USA* **81** 3806–3810

Young L, Alfieri C, Hennessy K *et al* (1989a) Expression of Epstein-Barr virus transformation-associated genes in tissues of patients with EBV lymphoproliferative disease. *New England Journal of Medicine* **321** 1080–1085

Young LS, Finerty S, Brooks L, Scullion F, Rickinson AB and Morgan AJ (1989b) Epstein-Barr virus gene expression in malignant lymphomas induced by experimental virus infection of cotton-top tamarins. *Journal of Virology* **63** 1967–1974

The authors are responsible for the accuracy of the references.

Lessons from T Cell Responses to Virus Induced Tumours for Cancer Eradication in General

C J M MELIEF • W M KAST

Department of Immunohematology and Blood Bank, University Hospital, PO Box 9600, 2300 RC Leiden, Netherlands

Introduction
Nature of T cell response against virus induced tumours
    Antigen processing for recognition by T helper cells and cytotoxic T lymphocytes
    Critical importance of peptide size for recognition by cytotoxic T lymphocytes
    MHC allele specific motifs in MHC binding peptides
Eradication of virus induced tumours by T cells
Mechanisms of tumour escape from T cell immunity
Immunogenicity of non-virus induced tumours
Strategies to raise T cells against poorly immunogenic tumours
Peptide vaccination to elicit protective T cell immunity
Prospects of peptide vaccination against human cancer
Summary

INTRODUCTION

The number of viruses found to cause cancer in humans is still rising. The list now includes Epstein-Barr virus (EBV), which is associated with Burkitt's lymphoma, notably in endemic areas (Klein 1975; Dalla Favera *et al*, 1982; Burkitt, 1983), and with lymphomas in immunocompromised individuals (Levine *et al*, 1984; Ziegler *et al*, 1984; Kalter *et al*, 1985).

Another culprit is human T lymphotropic virus I (HTLV-I), which is associated with adult T cell leukaemia lymphoma (ATLL), mainly in the Caribbean and in Japan (Poiesz *et al*, 1980; Hinuma *et al*, 1981; Gallo and Wong-Staal, 1984). A large and nasty family of viruses is that of the human papillomaviruses (HPV), more than 60 serotypes of which have now been described. Some types of HPV (including HPV types 1–4) cause innocent warts. Certain HPV types cause skin cancer, especially in immunocompromised patients (HPV types 5, 8, 14, 17 and 20). Yet other HPV types are associated with cancer of the uterine cervix, vulva, penis or anus (HPV types 16, 18, 31 and others). Finally, a fourth category of HPV can cause so-called condylomata acuminata, a peculiar wart like lesion in the genital area (HPV types 6, 11, 42) (Zur Hausen *et al,* 1984; Bennett, Jenson and Lancaster, 1990). An often neglected tumour virus should also be mentioned here: hepatitis B virus. World wide, about 250 million people carry this virus and have a 100-fold increased chance of liver cancer (Beasley *et al,* 1981; Chisari *et al,* 1989). Despite the identification of these tumour viruses in humans, most forms of human cancer are not thought to be associated with or caused by viruses (Bishop, 1991). In this review, we shall discuss how virus induced tumours can be recognized by T cells. It will be argued that T cell immunity against virus induced tumours does not, in essence, differ from anti-viral immunity in general. In some cases, tumour specific T cells can eradicate large tumour masses, but escape mechanisms are numerous. However, strategies to deal effectively with these escapes should lead to more precise delivery of immunotherapy.

In non-virus induced tumours, the current strategy is to concentrate on tumour infiltrating lymphocytes (TIL). Although this effort is rewarding, especially in malignant melanoma and renal cell carcinoma (Melief, 1991), we propose an alternative strategy (outlined later), based both on recent evidence that protective cytotoxic T cells can be induced in vivo by vaccination with immunodominant viral peptides binding to the major histocompatibility complex (MHC) class I molecules and on the recent insight that, in many cases, T cell tolerance is not based on clonal deletion but on clonal anergy of T cells. It is proposed that dormant anergic T cells can be directed against target molecules of choice in the tumour. This can be achieved by first seeking out target molecules of choice for T cells. In non-virus induced tumours, these can be differentiation antigens of restricted tissue distribution and overexpressed or mutated oncogene products. Peptide sequences that bind to the MHC class I molecules of the tumour bearing host can then be identified. Subsequently, the peptides that can induce cytotoxic T lymphocyte responses capable of lysing tumour cells can be isolated. For this to occur, the epitopes on the tumour associated antigens must be processed appropriately in tumour cells for presentation by MHC class I molecules.

NATURE OF T CELL RESPONSE AGAINST VIRUS INDUCED TUMOURS

The T cell response against virus induced tumours is subject to the rules of T cell immunity against viruses in general. Thus, both CD4+ helper T cell and CD8+ cytotoxic T lymphocyte (CTL) responses take place against antigenic peptides processed from longer tumour antigens and presented by MHC molecules at the tumour cell surface. If the tumour cells are MHC class II negative, the class II recognition pathway can only function indirectly by presentation of tumour antigen peptides that are processed by MHC class II positive cells of the immune system (macrophages and dendritic cells) that have taken up antigenic material from tumour cells.

Surprisingly, both at the induction level and at the effector level, destruction of MHC class II negative tumours by CD4+ cells, recognizing tumour derived peptides in the context of MHC class II molecules, can be an effective mechanism (Greenberg *et al*, 1988). In an experimental Friend murine leukaemia virus induced tumour model in mice, tumour destruction was mediated via macrophages that had become tumouricidal after activation by cytokines secreted by tumour specific CD4+ helper T cells (Greenberg *et al*, 1988). However, CD8+ CTL recognizing tumour derived peptides in the groove of MHC class I molecules are the most powerful mediators of tumour destruction (Melief, 1991; Melief and Kast, 1991a,b).

Antigen Processing for Recognition by T Helper Cells and Cytotoxic T Lymphocytes

Recently, our insights in the cellular events of antigen processing have dramatically increased (Townsend and Bodmer, 1989; Braciale and Braciale, 1991; Brodsky and Guagliardi, 1991; Melief, 1991). MHC class I molecules primarily present peptides that are loaded into the class I antigen presenting groove in the endoplasmic reticulum (ER). Peptide fragments are generated from proteins degraded within the cytoplasm (or perhaps even the ER itself). Peptide (or protein) pumps are necessary to get sufficient material into the ER for loading into the MHC class I groove and proper association of the trimolecular complex peptide/MHC class I heavy chain/β_2-microglobulin. If the peptide/protein pump mechanisms are defective, assembly of the complex is poor and the cell surface MHC class I expression is low, presumably resulting from either impaired transport to the surface, instability at the cell surface or both (Townsend *et al*, 1989, 1990; Ljunggren *et al*, 1990; Schumacher *et al*, 1990).

In cell lines with such an antigen processing defect, the unstable MHC class I molecules at the cell surface can be efficiently loaded with exogenous peptides of the right size, especially at reduced temperature (Ljunggren *et al*, 1990; Schumacher *et al*, 1991). Thus, such cell lines express "empty" MHC molecules at the cell surface that can be stabilized by reduction in temperature (approximately 22–26ºC) and peptide loading. In normal cells, only a minor proportion of MHC class I molecules at the cell surface are "empty". Nevertheless, sufficient binding of exogenously added peptide to MHC class I molecules can occur for target cell sensitization to take place (Townsend *et al*, 1986), presumably because even this small fraction is stabilized at 37ºC by exogenous peptide (Ljunggren *et al*, 1990; Schumacher *et al*, 1990).

Recently, four independent reports described candidate peptide transport molecules (peptide pumps) that are likely to be involved in the active transmembrane transport of peptides from the cytoplasm to the ER (Deverson *et al*, 1990; Monaco *et al*, 1990; Spies *et al*, 1990; Trowsdale *et al*, 1990). The genes encoding these transporter molecules are located in the MHC class II region in rat, mouse and humans. The processing defective murine cell line RMA-S (Townsend *et al*, 1989) and similar processing defective human cell lines (Salter and Cresswell 1986; Mellins *et al*, 1989; Cerundolo *et al*, 1990; Cotner *et al*, 1991; Elliott *et al*, 1991; Spies and De Mars, 1991) may have defects in these or other genes encoding transporter molecules. The processing defective cell lines are very useful for the identification of potential CTL epitopes and induction of CTL responses to these epitopes. Firstly, MHC binding peptides can be easily identified by their capacity to stabilize MHC class I expression at the surface of such cells. By immunofluorescence analysis, easy identification of CTL epitopes and of MHC/T cell receptor contact residues in each peptide is therefore possible (Kast and Melief, 1991). Secondly, loading of empty MHC molecules with a single peptide allows induction of primary in vitro CTL responses (De Bruijn *et al*, 1991).

In contrast to MHC class I molecules, MHC class II molecules are specialized in the presentation of exogenous protein antigens. This type of antigen processing involves endocytosis of protein antigens from outside the cells. Breakdown of these antigens occurs in the endosomal/lysosomal route, where loading of peptides into MHC class II molecules occurs. The so-called I invariant (Ii) chain is associated with MHC class II but not MHC class I, which probably accounts for most of the specialization of class II in exogenous antigen presentation. Firstly, the Ii chain is firmly bound to MHC class II in the ER, blocking access of peptides to the antigen presenting groove (Roche and Cresswell, 1990; Teyton *et al*, 1990). Secondly, the Ii chain contains a sorting signal for transport of the MHC class II molecule from the ER to the endosomal lysosomal compartment (Bakke and Dobberstein, 1990). Once in the acidic environment of late endosomal/lysosomal compartments, the Ii chain detaches, opening up the antigen binding groove to peptides generated by proteolytic digestion of endocytosed proteins.

The intersection of biosynthetic and endocytic routes required in this scenario was recently shown to occur for MHC class II but not class I molecules (Neefjes *et al*, 1990; Peters *et al*, 1991).

Critical Importance of Peptide Size for Recognition by Cytotoxic T Lymphocytes

The first indication of the stringent length requirement for peptides presented to CTL came from studies on the size of peptides eluted from MHC class I molecules on virus infected cells. In two different viral systems, vesicular stomatitis virus and influenza virus, the naturally processed peptides bound to MHC class I molecules turned out to be an octapeptide (Van Bleek and Nathenson, 1990) and nonapeptide (Rötzschke *et al*, 1990). These peptides were presented to CTL by the H-2K^b and H-2K^d MHC class I molecules, respectively. Similarly, in the case of a Sendai virus CTL epitope studied in our laboratory, the critical size of the biologically active peptide was nine aminoacids (Schumacher *et al*, 1991). It is likely that biological activity ascribed to longer peptides is due to truncated by-products of longer synthetic peptides (Rötzschke *et al*, 1990; Schumacher *et al*, 1990). These findings indicate that peptides recognized by CD8+ CTL fit precisely into the MHC class I groove and that an accurate proteolytic process is required to generate the proper peptide.

MHC Allele Specific Motifs in MHC Binding Peptides

Once the precise length of peptides involved in CTL recognition became known, and peptides of the proper length had been eluted from MHC molecules, it was discovered that even self peptides eluted from MHC molecules contain allele specific motifs (Falk *et al*, 1991). These motifs are characterized by the presence of two dominant anchor residues at fixed allele specific positions, for example L (or M) and V at positions 2 and 9, respectively, of HLA-A2.1 binding peptides and F (or Y) and L at positions 5 and 8, respectively, of H-2K^b binding peptides (Falk *et al*, 1991). In addition, "strong" and "weak" residues at each position in the peptide can be distinguished.

On the basis of these profiles, predictions can be made of sequences in proteins that are likely to bind to given MHC class I alleles. Known CTL epitopes of viruses, parasites and tumour antigens mostly follow these rules (Falk *et al*, 1991), but exceptions may occur. Of all algorithms reported to date, these allele specific motifs are most likely to allow an estimate of the number of potential CTL epitopes in a candidate target molecule, such as a tumour associated antigen.

ERADICATION OF VIRUS INDUCED TUMOURS BY T CELLS

Adoptive therapy of murine tumours with T cells has been reviewed recently (Greenberg *et al*, 1988; Melief *et al*, 1989; North *et al*, 1989; Melief, 1991; Melief and Kast, 1991a,b). In brief, murine tumours induced by either RNA or DNA tumour viruses can be successfully eradicated by cloned CD8+ or CD4+ T cells. CD8+ CTL clones are particularly effective, usually in combination with interleukin-2 (IL-2). Complete eradication of large established tumour masses has been achieved in the case of Friend virus induced leukaemia and human adenovirus type 5 (Ad5) early region one (E1) induced tumours in mice with cloned T cells and IL-2 (Greenberg *et al*, 1988; Kast *et al*, 1989; Melief *et al*, 1989; Melief and Kast, 1990, 1991a,b; Kast and Melief, 1991; Melief, 1991). In both models, the target antigens recognized by the curative T cell clones are viral structural proteins (Kast *et al*, 1989; Klarnet *et al*, 1989; Kast and Melief, 1991). A single immunodominant epitope is the target of

CD8+ CTL directed against Ad5 E1 induced tumour cells in the H-2^b haplotype. This epitope is the peptide SGPSNTPPEI encoded by the E1A viral nuclear oncogene and presented by the H-2D^b MHC class I molecule (Kast et al, 1989; Kast and Melief, 1991).

In this sequence, the residues SGPSN and I were found to be important for binding to the H-2D^b molecule, although the sequence TPPE was not (Kast and Melief, 1991). The involvement of the N residue at position 5 and the I residue at position 10 in binding to the D^b molecule agrees with the observation that N at 5 is a dominant anchor residue and I at 10 is a strong D^b interactive residue (Falk et al, 1991). In self peptides eluted from MHC molecules, the I is found at position 9. This difference in position of I could be related to the fact that the Ad5 E1A peptide sticks out of the groove at the carboxyterminal end (TPPE) with the exception of the I residue that lies deep in the groove, according to molecular modelling (Kast KM, Nieland J and Melief CJM, unpublished) based on the MHC class I crystal model (Bjorkman et al, 1987a,b). The SGPSN sequence at the aminoterminal end of the peptide is also deep in the H-2D^b groove in this model, a finding that is compatible with its D^b binding quality. Both from aminoacid deletion (Kast and Melief, 1991) and replacement studies (Kast KM, Meloen R, Drijfhout JW and Melief CJM, unpublished), all residues in the TPPE sequence are important for CTL recognition (Kast and Melief, 1991). We hypothesize that the TPPE sequence is important for CTL recognition because it sticks out of the groove and could contact the T cell receptor (TcR). The other residues in the decamer might be important, because they contribute to both MHC binding and TcR interaction or to general positioning within the groove and the TcR-interaction interface.

In the Ad5 E1 tumour model, the CTL have remarkable anti-tumour activity. Large subcutaneous tumour masses in T cell deficient mice were completely and permanently eradicated within 12 days of intravenous injection of 1.5×10^7 cloned CTL, combined with 10^5 units of IL-2 given as a single depot injection in incomplete Freund's adjuvant at a subcutaneous site distant from the tumour (Kast et al, 1989). The IL-2 is needed because these CD8+ CTL clones are IL-2 dependent both in vitro and in vivo (Kast et al, 1989). These results show that it is feasible to direct CTL therapy successfully at nuclear oncogene products and highlight the fact that CTL target proteins need not be expressed at the cell surface as long as processed peptides get to the cell surface bound in the antigen presenting groove of MHC class I molecules.

MECHANISMS OF TUMOUR ESCAPE FROM T CELL IMMUNITY

The following mechanisms can account for failure of tumour specific T cells to eradicate large tumour masses effectively: (a) immunoselection of tumour antigen negative variants; (b) downregulation of MHC class I expression; (c) "suppressive" T cells and (d) other T evasive activity exerted by tumour cells. These mechanisms have been discussed in two recent reviews (Melief, 1991;

Melief and Kast, 1991a). Downregulation of MHC class I expression is discussed in other recent papers (Smith *et al*, 1989; Ostrand-Rosenberg *et al*, 1991; Schrier *et al*, 1991; Wang *et al*, 1991; Möller and Hämmerling, this issue).

If so many different mechanisms can cause escape of tumour cells from the deadly embrace of CTL, how can CTL be effective at all in tumour eradication? Obviously, CTL can eradicate large tumour masses, as shown in the murine models discussed in the previous paragraph. In these models, a series of favourable factors contribute to successful tumour eradication by CTL. Ad5 E1 tumour eradication by CD8+ CTL and IL-2 is a case in point. Firstly, the therapeutically active T cells are directed against a product (E1A peptide) of one of the two genes (E1A and E1B) essential for the neoplastic state of these cells. Downregulation of E1A would inevitably lead to loss of the transformed state. Also, very little time is available for epitope deletion or mutation, because complete tumour eradication occurs within 2 weeks. Secondly, in Ad5 E1 transformed cells, there is no MHC class I downregulation. By contrast, in Ad12 E1 transformed cells, MHC class I is downregulated as a function of Ad12 E1A (Bernards *et al*, 1983; Schrier *et al*, 1983; Eager *et al*, 1985; Tanaka *et al*, 1985; Meijer *et al*, 1989), and these cells, in contrast to Ad5 E1 transformed tumour cells, grow out in immunocompetent hosts. Restoration of MHC class I expression by, for example, interferon-γ leads to loss of tumorigenicity of Ad12 E1 transformed cells (Hayashi *et al*, 1985). Thirdly, "suppressive" T cells that subvert the tumouricidal action of CTL in many models (North *et al*, 1989; Melief, 1991) have no role in the Ad5 E1 tumour adoptive T cell therapy model because the tumour bearing hosts are T cell deficient nu/nu mice that have very few immunoregulatory T cells. There is also no evidence that detrimental immunoregulatory cells abolish Ad5 E1 specific CTL activity in immunocompetent mice, because these animals are entirely resistant to Ad5 E1 tumour formation (Kast WM and Melief CJM, unpublished). Finally, Ad5 E1 transformed cells do not produce active transforming growth factor-β (TGF-β). This factor is one of the prime suspects of immunosuppressive cytokines liberated by a variety of tumour cells (Melief, 1991; Melief and Kast, 1991a).

All circumstances for Ad5 E1 tumour regression by CTL and IL-2 are thus favourable. Rather than become discouraged by the notion that such complete tumour eradication by CTL is unusual, we should try to mimic these conditions as much as possible in the therapy of human cancer. This is a formidable task, but many defined aims can be set. As already stated, one is to direct T cells to changes essential to the neoplastic state, such as overexpressed or mutated oncogene products. A second measure is to restore MHC expression whenever possible by, for example, interferon treatment. A third measure is to eliminate "suppressive" T cells by cyclophosphamide, irradiation, anti-CD4 treatment or other means (North *et al*, 1989; Melief, 1991). Finally, the production of factors such as TGF-β could be counteracted by tumour necrosis factor-α (Ranges *et al*, 1987) or TGF-β neutralizing antibodies.

IMMUNOGENICITY OF NON-VIRUS INDUCED TUMOURS

The prevalence and nature of tumour antigens in non-virus induced tumours have been reviewed recently (Melief, 1991; Melief and Kast, 1991a). A distinction must be made between tumours induced by exogenous insults, such as chemical carcinogens and ultraviolet light, and so-called "spontaneous" tumours.

Chemical carcinogens and ultraviolet light are both highly mutagenic. Therefore, random mutations in cellular genes are induced, some of which cause deregulated cell growth and some of which do not. Both types of mutations may generate immunogenic peptides recognizable by T cells. However, mutations in proto-oncogene products have so far not been proven to be naturally immunogenic, although a point mutated *ras* peptide can elicit a CD4+ T cell response (Jung and Schluesener, 1991; Peace *et al*, 1991). Indeed, most mutations in chemically and ultraviolet light induced tumours, which have caused immunogenicity, have occurred in random cellular genes. This explains the following characteristics of tumour antigens on chemically and ultraviolet light induced tumours: (a) their individually distinct nature, (b) their detection by T cells but not antibody and (c) their genetic stability (Melief, 1991; Melief and Kast, 1991a). Although the molecular nature of these antigens has not been elucidated with certainty (Melief, 1991), they are probably similar to the tumour-rejection antigen induced by mutagenic treatment in vitro of already existing tumours (Boon *et al*, 1989a,b; Melief, 1991; Melief and Kast, 1991a). The mutagenic tumour cells, selected for their failure to grow out in syngeneic mice are designated as tumour minus (tum⁻) variants. All genes encoding tum⁻ antigens cloned to date showed no homology with other known genes and all were distinct from each other (Boon *et al*, 1989a,b; Lurquin *et al*, 1989; Sibille *et al*, 1990; Szikora *et al*, 1990). In the cases investigated in detail, strongly immunogenic peptides were generated by point mutation. The mutation can cause the peptide to bind to an MHC class I molecule, in contrast to the peptide encoded by the normal gene, thereby making it immunogenic. Alternatively, both the native and mutant peptides bind to a class I molecule, but the mutant peptide is recognized by the T cell repertoire (Boon *et al*, 1989a,b; Lurquin *et al*, 1989; Sibille *et al*, 1990; Szikora *et al*, 1990). The T cell response against tum⁻ antigens can facilitate a T cell response against cryptic antigens of non-immunogenic spontaneous tumours (Van Pel *et al*, 1983). Whether or not such cryptic antigens can be autoantigens is open to debate.

Recently, it was shown conclusively that a non-mutated autoantigen can serve as a major rejection antigen on the chemically induced P815 DBA/2 mouse mastocytoma tumour line (Van Den Eynde *et al*, 1991). It is not known to what extent this antigen can elicit a CTL response on its own or can do so only in the wake of a response against other CTL epitopes caused by chemically induced mutation of P815 (Van Den Eynde *et al*, 1991). The normal gene encoding the P815 autoantigen serving as a tumour rejection antigen was silent or expressed at a very low level in adult mice, including normal mast cells, perhaps allowing abolition of immunological tolerance to the antigen.

High expression was found, however, in another tumorigenic mast cell line (Van Den Eynde *et al*, 1991). The expression of this antigen is reminiscent of oncofetal antigens. This study constitutes the first example of the tumour rejection potential of CTL directed against a molecularly defined autoantigen.

The immunogenicity of so-called "spontaneous" tumours, ie tumours not caused by clearly defined tumorigenic influences, is low to non-existent (Melief, 1991). Most human cancers belong to this category. It is now realized that these tumours are the result of subtle changes in proto-oncogenes leading to deregulated cell growth (Bishop, 1991). There is no evidence that these changes are immunogenic without additional immunotherapeutic measures. It will be argued, however, that immune responses to HLA binding peptides associated with these changes may be elicited by a deliberate vaccination strategy, as outlined later. Alternative strategies are summarized in the next section.

STRATEGIES TO RAISE T CELLS AGAINST POORLY IMMUNOGENIC TUMOURS

Vaccination against cancer in experimental models and in clinical disease has a long history (Old, 1989). Encouraging results were obtained with bacterial immunostimulants such as BCG (Zbar and Rapp, 1974; Bast *et al*, 1976) or *Corynebacterium parvum* (Shu *et al*, 1989). BCG instillation in the bladder is now used successfully in the adjuvant treatment of bladder carcinoma (De Jong *et al*, 1990).

A second way to vaccinate effectively against poorly immunogenic tumours is to immunize with an allogeneic virus induced tumour followed by challenge with a poorly immunogenic syngeneic tumour induced by the same virus (Azuma *et al*, 1987). Clearly, this method requires processing of allogeneic tumour proteins by host antigen presenting cells to generate memory T cells for the syngeneic tumour. Therefore, common tumour antigens shared between allogeneic and syngeneic tumours are necessary, a requirement only met by virus induced tumours. In the case of individually unique tumour antigens of weakly immunogenic, chemically or ultraviolet light induced tumours, the "allogeneic stimulus" principle can be used in a different way, namely by introduction of allogeneic MHC class I genes into the tumour (Gelber *et al*, 1989; Isobe *et al*, 1989; Ostrand-Rosenberg *et al*, 1991). Of course, this principle can also be used for virus induced tumours (Hui *et al*, 1989). Effective tumour immunity in one case was also induced by immunization with tumour cells transfected with syngeneic MHC class II genes (Ostrand-Rosenberg *et al*, 1991).

A third way to promote immunogenicity of tumours is to make tumour cells "foreign" in ways other than introduction of allogeneic MHC class I or autologous MHC class II molecules. This endpoint has been achieved by modification of tumour cells with Newcastle disease virus (Van Hoegen *et al*, 1988;

Schild *et al*, 1989) or by transfection of the haemagglutinin gene of influenza virus into tumour cells (Fearon *et al*, 1988).

A fourth way to overcome poor immunogenicity is by means of immunization with an immunogenic tum⁻ variant discussed in the preceding paragraph. The response against the strongly immunogenic tum⁻ antigens apparently has an adjuvant effect on the generation of an immune response against cryptic antigens also present on the original non-immunogenic tumour (Van Pel *et al*, 1983). Conceivably, as discussed in the preceding section, in certain instances, such tumour antigens could be autoantigens (Van Den Eynde *et al*, 1991).

A fifth method of raising T cells against poorly immunogenic tumour cells is high dose systemic IL-2. In one example, the immune cells mediating tumour immunity induced by this treatment were CD8+ CTL (Mulé *et al*, 1987). In this same study, however, no CD8+ T cell immunity was induced by high dose IL-2 treatment against non-immunogenic tumours. The IL-2 treatment had some therapeutic effect against these tumours, which was less pronounced and was mediated by IL-2 activated NK cells (Mulé *et al*, 1987). High dose systemic IL-2 has the disadvantage of activating large numbers of irrelevant T and NK cells with little or no tumour reducing capacity and at the cost of substantial toxicity. A more effective and less toxic mode of IL-2 delivery may be local IL-2 production after introduction of the IL-2 gene itself into poorly immunogenic tumour cells. This leads to local sustained IL-2 release by the same cell that presents antigen in the groove of MHC class I, bypassing the need for T helper cell activation in the complete absence of systemic toxicity (Fearon *et al*, 1990; Gansbacher *et al*, 1990b; Ley *et al*, 1990). Similar results have been obtained with the introduction of the interferon-γ gene into poorly immunogenic tumour cells and vaccination with such cells (Gansbacher *et al*, 1990a).

The common denominator in all these strategies is the abolition of defective helper T cell activation and associated cytokine release, which is required for induction of effective T cell immunity. This defect can be overcome by concomitant stimulation of other T cells (tumour cells with allogeneic MHC class I or autologous class II antigens, tumour cells with introduced viruses or viral antigen and mutagenized tumour cells with tum⁻ antigens) that substitute the defective helper T cell activation. Alternatively, the helper factors themselves, such as IL-2 and interferon-γ, can be provided directly, either systemically or (probably more efficiently) locally at the tumour site. Sustained production of these cytokines after gene transfer into tumour cells is preferred over locoregional injection of cytokine, because in the latter case, a very short biological half-life and less precise delivery are disadvantages. Vaccination with irradiated IL-2 producing tumour cells is efficient because irradiated tumour cells can produce large amounts of IL-2 for at least 3 days after irradiation (Visseren M and Melief CJM, unpublished). In all cases, once T cells are induced to react against the weakly immunogenic tumour antigens, such tumour specific T cells cross react against the original tumour. This illustrates the fact that initiation of a T cell response requires optimal conditions for antigen presentation, which are much more stringent than conditions of tumour antigen recognition by already activated T cells.

PEPTIDE VACCINATION TO ELICIT PROTECTIVE T CELL IMMUNITY

In two virus systems, it has now been possible to raise protective T cell immunity by vaccination with a single free short synthetic peptide. In each case, this peptide contained the immunodominant CTL epitope presented by an MHC class I molecule of the vaccinated mouse (Kast *et al*, 1991; Schulz *et al*, 1991). Thus, even though MHC class I molecules are specialized in the presentation of endogenously processed antigens, exogenously offered MHC class I binding immunodominant peptides can effectively elicit virus specific memory cells and vaccinate against lethal virus infection (Kast *et al*, 1991; Schulz *et al*, 1991). This finding corresponds with the widely observed phenomenon that target cell sensitization with exogenous peptides for CTL recognition is easy. Our own work indicates that the stringent length requirement for peptides in in vitro MHC class I binding and target cell recognition is not observed in in vivo peptide vaccination (Kast WM and Melief CJM, unpublished). A possible candidate cell functioning as peptide presenting cells is the lymphoid dendritic cell (DC). Peptide loaded DC are capable of initiating primary CTL responses in vitro, ie CTL responses in lymphocytes from non-immunized mice (Macatonia *et al*, 1989; De Bruijn MLH, Nieland JD, Kast WM and Melief CJM, unpublished).

Density of peptide-loaded MHC class I molecules is probably an important factor in response initiation, because processing of defective peptide loaded RMA-S cells, in contrast to parental RMA cells, can lead to initiation of primary H-2K^b and H-2D^b restricted CTL responses (De Bruijn *et al*, 1991). The MHC molecules on RMA-S cells are devoid of peptide, which causes MHC class I instability. On a per cell basis, RMA-S cells can bind more exogenous peptide to K^b or D^b molecules than RMA cells, especially at reduced peptide loading temperatures that counteract MHC class I degradation (De Bruijn *et al*, 1991). An additional factor explaining the difference in primary response induction between RMA and RMA-S cells is related to the CD8 dependence of these responses. MHC class I molecules occupied with irrelevant peptides (a majority present on RMA, largely absent on RMA-S) may interfere in the interaction of the CD8 molecule with relevant MHC/peptide complexes (Alexander *et al*, 1991; De Bruijn *et al*, 1991).

The concentration of peptide required for primary CTL response induction in vitro is much higher than required for target cell sensitization (De Bruijn *et al*, 1991), in agreement with the findings of Alexander *et al* (1991) for induction of H-2L^d positive peptide specific CTL responses. This raises the interesting prospect that responsiveness can be induced if antigen presenting cells are loaded with a sufficient number of MHC binding peptide molecules.

Under these conditions, CD8+ peptide specific CTL responses are CD4+ T helper cell independent (De Bruijn *et al*, 1991).

PROSPECTS OF PEPTIDE VACCINATION AGAINST HUMAN CANCER

The recent progress in understanding both peptide/MHC/T cell receptor interaction and antigen processing allows a novel strategy for induction of tumour derived T cells. Rather than concentrating on activation and expansion of TIL, we propose to intentionally direct T cells to respond to target antigens of choice in the neoplastic cells. Such antigens can be viral antigens in virus induced tumour cells, in addition to both differentiation antigens of restricted tissue distribution and overexpressed or mutated oncogene products in non-virus induced tumour cells. On the basis of work by Falk *et al* (1991), it is now possible to predict which aminoacid sequences of a given protein contain motifs involved in peptide binding to a given MHC class I molecule. So far, this has only been worked out for a single HLA class I antigen, HLA-A2.1 (Falk *et al*, 1991), but peptide motifs involved in binding of peptides to other HLA class I alleles and also HLA class II alleles are likely to follow soon. Once peptide sequences bearing HLA class I allele specific sequences are identified, it is possible to test which of these candidate peptides are capable of inducing primary CTL responses in vitro. For antigen presentation in such assays, one can consider using the human counterparts of the processing defective murine cell line RMA-S (Salter and Cresswell, 1986; Mellins *et al*, 1989; Cerundolo *et al*, 1990; Cotner *et al*, 1991; Elliott *et al*, 1991; Spies and DeMars, 1991; De Bruijn *et al*, in press) or human dendritic cells.

With this procedure, CTL epitopes can be identified in target molecules of choice, presented by specific HLA class I alleles. Even if such peptides contain exclusively autologous sequences, CTL response induction is not a priori impossible as shown by Van Den Eynde *et al* (1991). Factors that favour response induction are the possibility to overcome tolerance/anergy by high dose peptide presentation and the possibility to manipulate the response induction system in vitro. It is now realized that in many cases, immunological tolerance is not based on clonal deletion but on clonal anergy of T cells (Blackman *et al*, 1990; Ramsdell and Fowlkes, 1990; Sprent *et al*, 1990).

Subsequent to CTL epitope identification, deliberate vaccination with peptides of choice seems feasible in view of the successful results with immunodominant viral peptides (Kast *et al*, 1991; Schulz *et al*, 1991). Peptide vaccination can be tried both in virus associated tumours, such as cervical carcinoma and EBV positive Burkitt's lymphoma, and in non-virus induced tumours. In the latter instance, desirable targets for tumour specific CTL are the products of point mutated oncogenes (Bishop, 1991), including *ras* (Jung and Schluesener, 1991; Peace *et al*, 1991) and *p53* (Halevy *et al*, 1990; Rodriguez *et al*, 1990), provided the relevant peptides are naturally processed and bound to MHC class I molecules. Other potential targets are breakpoint peptides of translocated oncogene products such as *bcr/abl* (Van Denderen *et al*, 1990) or differentiation antigens such as the CD19 and CD20 antigens of B lymphoma cells (Hekman *et al*, 1991).

Although there is no guarantee of success, each step in this approach is well defined and has been proven to work in induction of protective immunity against viruses. Thus, instead of the wait-and-see-what-we-get strategy of TIL cultures, we propose to reverse the strategy and start with the target peptides of choice for CTLs and to overcome tolerance/anergy that precludes the induction of T cell responses to these peptides under normal circumstances. In the long run, we believe that this strategy will be more effective for the following reasons: (a) therapy will be directed against peptides common to the same type of tumour in hosts of the same HLA type; (b) in many instances, therapy will be directed at changes in oncogenes that lie at the base of the transformed phenotype: escapes from therapy are therefore more likely to lead to loss of neoplastic phenotype; (c) multiple target molecules in the same tumour may be targeted, reducing the escape possibilities and (d) the laborious, cumbersome and expensive adoptive T cell therapy can be replaced with convenient peptide vaccination procedures, preferably when residual disease is minimal.

SUMMARY

Immunotherapy of virus induced tumours by adoptive transfer of virus specific cytotoxic T cells (CTL) is now feasible in experimental murine systems. These CTL recognize viral peptide sequences of defined length presented in the groove of MHC class I molecules. Effective eradication of large tumour masses requires coadministration of IL-2. In essence, T cell immunity against virus induced tumours does not differ from anti-viral T cell immunity in general. Tumour escape strategies are numerous but, in various instances, can be counteracted by defined measures. Initiation of CTL responses against poorly immunogenic non-virus induced tumours (the majority of human cancer) requires novel strategies to overcome T cell inertia. Rather than waiting to see whether tumour specific CTL (against unknown antigens) can be cultured from TIL, we propose an alternative strategy in which CTL are raised against target molecules of choice, including differentiation antigens of restricted tissue distribution (autoantigens) or mutated/overexpressed oncogene products. The various steps proposed include: (a) identification of target molecules of choice; (b) identification in these target molecules of MHC allele specific peptide motifs involved in peptide binding to MHC molecules; (c) evaluation of actual binding of such peptides to specific MHC class I molecules; (d) in vitro CTL response induction by such peptides, presented either by highly efficient antigen presenting cells (such as processing defective cells, which carry empty MHC class I molecules) loaded with a single peptide or by dendritic cells, both cell types being capable of primary CTL response induction in vitro and (e) adoptive transfer of tumour specific CTL generated in vivo or, more conveniently, vaccination with immunodominant peptides. The latter possibility seems to be feasible because peptide vaccination with a single immuno-dominant viral peptide can install CTL memory and confer protection against lethal virus infection.

Acknowledgements

We thank René RP de Vries and Peter I Schrier for stimulating discussions and critical reading of the manuscript. WMK is a fellow of the Royal Dutch Academy of Sciences. Our work reported in this review was supported by the Dutch Cancer Society and by the Netherlands Organization of Scientific Research (NWO).

References

Alexander MA, Damico CA, Wieties KM, Hansen TH and Connolly JM (1991) Correlation between CD8 dependency and determinant density using peptide-induced, L^d-restricted cytotoxic T lymphocytes. *Journal of Experimental Medicine* **173** 849–858

Azuma H, Phillips JD and Green WR (1987) Clonal heterogeneity of anti-AKR/Gross leukemia virus cytotoxic T lymphocytes. *Journal of Immunology* **139** 2464–2473

Bakke O and Dobberstein B (1990) MHC class II associated invariant chain contains a sorting signal for endosomal compartments. *Cell* **63** 707–716

Bast RC, Bast BS and Rapp HJ (1976) Critical review of previously reported animal studies of tumour immunotherapy with nonspecific immunostimulants. *Annals of the New York Academy of Sciences* **277** 60–93

Beasley RP, Hwang L-Y, Lin C-C and Chien C-S (1981) Hepatocellular carcinoma and hepatitis B virus. *Lancet* **ii** 1129–1133

Bennett Jenson A and Lancaster WD (1990) Association of human papillomavirus with benign, premalignant and malignant anogenital lesions, In: Pfister H (ed). *Papillomaviruses and human cancer*, pp 11–43, CRC Press, Boca Raton, Forida

Bernards R, Schrier PI, Houweling A, Bos JL, Van der Eb AJ, Zijlstra M and Melief CJM (1983) Tumorigenicity of cells transformed by adenovirus type 12 by evasion of T cell immunity. *Nature* **305** 776–779

Bishop JM (1991) Molecular themes in oncogenesis. *Cell* **64** 235–248

Bjorkman P, Saper MA, Samraoui B, Bennett WS, Strominger JL and Wiley DC (1987) Structure of human class I histocompatibility antigen HLA-A2. *Nature* **329** 506–512

Bjorkman PJ, Saper MA, Samraoui B, Bennett WS, Strominger JL and Wiley DC (1987) The foreign antigen binding site and T cell recognition regions of class I histocompatibility antigens. *Nature* **329** 512–518

Blackman M, Kappler J and Marrack P (1990) The role of the T cell receptor in positive and negative selection of developing T cells. *Science* **248** 1335–1341

Boon T, Van Pel A, De Plaen E *et al* (1989) Genes coding cell defined tum⁻ transplantation antigens: point mutations, antigenic peptides, and subgenic expression. *Cold Spring Harbor Symposia on Quantitative Biology* **54** 587–596

Boon T, Van Pel A and De Plaen, E (1989) Tum⁻ transplantation antigens, point mutations, and antigenic peptides: a model for tumor - specific transplantation antigens. *Cancer Cells* **1** 25–28

Braciale TJ and Braciale VL (1991) Antigen presentation: structural themes and functional variations. *Immunology Today* **12** 124–129

Brodsky F and Guagliardi LE (1991) The cell biology of antigen processing and presentation. *Annual Reviews of Immunology* **9** 707–744

Burkitt DP (1983) The discovery of Burkitt's lymphoma. *Cancer* **51** 1777–1786

Cerundolo V, Alexander J, Anderson K *et al* (1990) Presentation of viral antigen controlled by a gene in the major histocompatibility complex. *Nature* **345** 449–452

Chisari FV, Klopchin K, Moriyama *et al* (1989) Molecular pathogenesis of hepatocellular carcinoma in hepatitis B virus transgenic mice. *Cell* **59** 1145–1156

Cotner T, Mellins E, Johnson AH and Pious D (1991) Mutations affecting antigen processing impair class II restricted allorecognition. *Journal of Immunology* **146** 414–417

Dalla-Favera R, Bregni R, Erickson J, Patterson D, Gallo RC and Croce CM (1982) Human c-myc onc gene is located on the region of chromosome 8 that is translocated in Burkitt lymphoma cells. *Proceedings of the National Academy of Sciences of the USA* **79** 7824–7827

De Bruijn MLH, Schumacher TNM, Nieland JD, Ploegh HL, Kast WM and Melief CJM (1991) Peptide loading of empty MHC molecules on RMA-S cells allows the induction of primary cytotoxic T lymphocyte responses. *European Journal of Immunology* **21** 2963–2970

De Jong WH, De Boer EC, Van Der Meijden *et al* (1990) Presence of interleukin-2 in urine of superficial bladder cancer patients after intravesical treatment with bacillus Calmette-Guérin. *Cancer Immunology and Immunotherapy* **31** 182–186

Deres K, Schild H, Wiesmer KH, Jung G and Rammensee HG (1989) In vivo priming of virus-specific cytotoxic T lymphocytes with synthetic lipopeptide vaccine. *Nature* **342** 561–564

Deverson EV, Gow IR, Coadwell WJ, Monaco JJ, Butcher GW and Howard JC (1990) MHC class II region encoding proteins related to the multidrug resistance family of trans-membrane transporters. *Nature* **348** 738–741

Eager KB, Williams J, Breiding D *et al* (1985) Expression of histocompatibility antigens H-2K, -D, and -L is reduced in adenovirus-12-transformed mouse cells and is restored by interferon gamma. *Proceedings of the National Academy of Sciences of the USA* **82** 5525–5529

Elliott T, Cerundolo V, Elvin J and Townsend A (1991) Peptide-induced conformational change of the class I heavy chain. *Nature* **351** 402–406

Falk K, Rötzschke O, Stevanovic S, Jung G and Rammensee HG (1991) Allele-specific motifs revealed by sequencing of self-peptides eluted from MHC molecules. *Nature* **351** 290–296

Fearon ER, Itaya T, Hunt B, Vogelstein B and Frost P (1988) Induction in a murine tumour of immunogenic tumour variants by transfection with a foreign gene. *Cancer Research* **48** 2975–2980

Fearon ER, Pardoll DM, Itaya T *et al* (1990) Interleukin-2 production by tumour cells bypasses T helper function in the generation of anti-tumour response. *Cell* **60** 397–403

Gallo RC and Wong-Staal F (1984) Current thoughts on the viral etiology of certain human cancers. *Cancer Research* **44** 2743–2749

Gansbacher B, Bannerji R, Daniels B, Zier K, Cronin K and Gilboa E (1990a) Retroviral vector-mediated γ-interferon gene transfer into tumour cells generates potent and long lasting antitumour immunity. *Cancer Research* **50** 7820–7825

Gansbacher B, Zier K, Daniels B, Cronin K, Bannerji R and Gilboa E (1990b) Interleukin-2 gene transfer into tumour cells abrogates tumorigenicity and induces protective immunity. *Journal of Experimental Medicine* **172** 1217–1224

Gelber C, Plaksin D, Vadai E, Feldman M and Eisenbach L (1989) Abolishment of metastasis formation by murine tumour cells transfected with foreign H-2K genes. *Cancer Research* **49** 2366–2373

Greenberg PD, Klarnet JP, Kern DE and Cheever MA (1988) Therapy of disseminated tumours by adoptive transfer of specifically immune T cells. *Progress in Experimental Tumour Research* **32** 104–127

Halevy O, Michalovitz D and Oren M (1990) Different tumour-derived p53 mutants exhibit distinct biological activities. *Science* **250** 113–116

Hayashi H, Tanaka K, Jay F, Khoury G and Jay G (1985) Modulation of the tumorigenicity of human adenovirus 12 transformed cells by interferon. *Cell* **43** 263–267

Hekman A, Honselaar A, Vuist WJM *et al* (1991) Initial experience with treatment of human B cell lymphoma with anti-CD19 monoclonal antibody. *Cancer Immunology and Immunotherapy* **32** 364–372

Hinuma Y, Nagato K, Hanaoka M *et al* (1981) Adult T cell leukemia: antigen in an ATL cell line and detection of antibodies to the antigen in human sera. *Proceedings of the National Academy of Sciences of the USA* **78** 6476–6480

Hui KM, Sim T, Foo TT and Oei AA (1989) Tumour rejection mediated by transfection with allogeneic class I histocompatibility gene. *Journal of Immunology* **143** 3835–3843

Isobe K-I, Hasegawa Y, Iwamoto T *et al* (1989) Induction of antitumour immunity in mice by allo-major histocompatibility complex class I gene transfectant with strong antigen expression. *Journal of the National Cancer Institute* **81** 1823–1828

Jung S and Schluesener J (1991) Human T lymphocytes recognize a peptide of single point-mutated, oncogenic ras proteins. *Journal of Experimental Medicine* **173** 273–276

Kalter SP, Riggs SA, Cabanillas F *et al* (1985) Aggressive non-Hodgkin's lymphomas in immunocompromised homosexual males. *Blood* **66** 655–659

Kast WM and Melief CJM (1991) Fine peptide specificity of cytotoxic T lymphocytes directed against adenovirus-induced tumours and peptide-MHC binding. *International Journal of Cancer* **6** (**Supplement**) 90–94

Kast WM, Offringa R, Peters PJ *et al* (1989) Eradication of adenovirus E1-induced tumours by E1A-specific cytotoxic T lymphocytes. *Cell* **59** 603–614

Kast WM, Roux L, Curren J *et al* (1991) Protection against lethal Sendai virus infection by in vivo priming of virus-specific cytotoxic T lymphocytes with a free synthetic peptide. *Proceedings of the National Academy of Sciences of the USA* **88** 2283–2287

Klarnet JP, Kern DE, Okuno K, Holt C, Lilly F and Greenberg PD (1989) FBL-reactive CD8+ cytotoxic and CD4+ helper T lymphocytes recognize distinct Friend murine leukemia virus-encoded antigens. *Journal of Experimental Medicine* **169** 457–467

Klein G (1975) The Epstein Barr virus and neoplasia. *New England Journal of Medicine* **293** 1353–1357

Levine AM, Meyer PR, Begandy MK *et al* (1984) Development of B-cell lymphoma in homosexual men. *Annals of Internal Medicine* **100** 7–13

Ley V, Roth C, Langlade-Demoyen P, Larsson E-L and Kourilsky P (1990) A novel approach to the induction of specific cytolytic T cells in vivo. *Research in Immunology* **141** 855–863

Ljunggren H-G, Stam NJ, Öhlén C *et al* (1990) Empty MHC class I molecules come out in the cold. *Nature* **346** 476–480

Lurquin C, Van Pel A, Mariamé B *et al* (1989) Structure of the gene coding for tum‾ transplantation antigen P91 A: a peptide encoded by the mutated exon is recognized with Ld by cytolytic T cells. *Cell* **58** 293–303

Macatonia SE, Taylor PM, Knight SC and Askovas BA (1989) Primary stimulation by dendritic cells induces antiviral proliferative and cytotoxic T cell responses in vitro. *Journal of Experimental Medicine* **169** 1255–1264

Meijer I, Jochemsen AG, De Wit CM, Bos JL, Morello D and Van Der Eb (1989) Adenovirus type 12 E1A downregulates expression of a transgene under control of a major histocompatibility complex class I promoter: evidence for transcriptional control. *Journal of Virology* **63** 4039–4042

Melief CJM (1991) Tumor eradication by adoptive transfer of cytotoxic T lymphocytes, In: Klein G and Van De Woude G (eds). *Advances in Cancer Research Academic Press,* vol 58, pp 143–175, Academic Press, Orlanda Florida

Melief CJM and Kast WM (1990) Efficacy of cytotoxic T lymphocytes against virus-induced tumours. *Cancer Cells* **2** 116–120

Melief CJM and Kast WM (1991a) Cytotoxic T lymphocyte therapy of cancer and tumour escape mechanisms. *Seminars in Cancer Biology* **2** 347–354

Melief CJM and Kast WM (1991b) T cell immunotherapy of cancer. *Research in Immunology* **142** 425–429

Melief CJM, Vasmel WLE, Offringa R *et al* (1989) Immunosurveillance of virus induced tumours. *Cold Spring Harbor Symposia on Quantitative Biology* **54** 597–603

Mellins E, Smith L, Arp B, Cotner T, Celis E and Pious D (1989) Defective processing and presentation of exogenous antigens in mutants with normal HLA class II genes. *Nature* **343** 71–74

Monaco JJ, Cho S and Attaya M (1990) Transport protein genes in the murine MHC: possible implications for antigen processing. *Science* **250** 1723–1726

Mulé JJ, Yang JC, Afrenière RL, Shu S and Rosenberg SA (1987) Identification of cellular mechanisms operational in vivo during the regression of established pulmonary metastases by the systemic administration of high dose recombinant IL-2. *Journal of Immunology* **139** 285–294

Neefjes JJ, Stollorz V, Peters PJ, Geuze HJ and Ploegh HL (1990) The biosynthetic pathway of MHC class II but not of class I molecules intersects the endocytic route. *Cell* **61** 171–183

North RJ, Awwad M and Dunn PC (1989) T cell mediated tumour regression in experimental systems, In: Melchers F (ed). *Progress in Immunology* vol VII, pp 1097–1103, Springer Verlag, Berlin

Old LJ (1989) Structural basis for tumour cell recognition by the immune system, In: Melchers F (ed). *Progress in Immunology* vol VII, pp 1053–1062, Springer Verlag, Berlin

Ostrand-Rosenberg S, Roby C, Clements VK and Cole GA (1991) Tumour-specific immunity can be enhanced by transfection of tumour cells with syngeneic MHC class II genes or allogeneic MHC class I genes. *International Journal of Cancer* (Supplement 6) 61–68

Peace DJ, Chen W, Nelson H and Cheever MA (1991) T cell recognition of transforming proteins encoded by mutated ras proto-oncogenes. *Journal of Immunology* **146** 2059–2065

Peters PJ, Neefjes JJ, Oorschot V, Ploegh HL and Geuze HJ (1991) Segregation of MHC class II molecules from MHC class I molecules in the Golgi complex for transport to lysosomal compartments. *Nature* **349** 669–676

Poiesz BJ, Ruscetti FW, Gazdar AF, Bunn PA, Minna JD and Gallo RC (1980) Detection and isolation of type C retrovirus particles from fresh and cultured lymphocytes of a patient with cutaneous T cell lymphoma. *Proceedings of the National Academy of Sciences of the USA* **77** 7415–7419

Ramsdell F and Fowlkes BJ (1990) Clonal deletion versus clonal anergy: the role of the thymus in inducing self tolerance. *Science* **248** 1342–1348

Ranges GE, Figari IS, Espevik T and Palladino MA (1987) Inhibition of cytotoxic T cell development by transforming growth factor β and reversal by tumor necrosis factor α. *Journal of Experimental Medicine* **166** 991–998

Roche PA and Cresswell P (1990) Invariant chain association with HLA DR molecules inhibits immunogenic peptide binding. *Nature* **345** 615–617

Rodriguez NR, Rowan A, Smith MEF *et al* (1990) p53 mutations in colorectal cancer. *Proceedings of the National Academy of Sciences of the USA* **87** 7555–7559

Rötzschke O, Falk F, Deres K *et al* (1990) Isolation and analysis of naturally processed viral peptides as recognized by cytotoxic T cells. *Nature* **348** 252–254

Salter RD and Cresswell P (1986) Impaired assembly and transport of HLA-A and -B antigens in a mutant T x B cell hybrid. *EMBO Journal* **5** 943–949

Schild H, Von Hoegen P and Schirrmacher V (1989) Modification of tumour cells by a low dose of Newcastle disease virus II Augmented tumour-specific T cell response as a result of CD4+ and CD8+ immune T cell cooperation. *Cancer Immunology and Immunotherapy* **28** 22–28

Schrier PI, Bernard R, Vaessen RT, Houweling A and Van Der Eb AJ (1983) Expression of class I major histocompatibility antigens switched off by highly oncogenic adenovirus 12 in transformed rat cells. *Nature* **305** 771–775

Schrier PI, Versteeg R, Peltenburg LTC, Plomp A, Van 't Veer L and Krüse-Wolters KM (1991) Sensitivity of melanoma cell lines to natural killer cells: a role for oncogene-modulated HLA class I expression? *Seminars in Cancer Biology* **2** 73–83

Schulz M, Zinkernagel RM and Hengartner H (1991) Peptide-induced antiviral protection by cytotoxic T cells. *Proceedings of the National Academy of Sciences of the USA* **88** 991–993

Schumacher TNM, Heemels M-T, Neefjes JJ, Kast WM, Melief CJM and Ploegh HL (1990) Direct binding of peptide to empty MHC class I molecules on intact cells and in vitro. *Cell* **62** 563–567

Schumacher TNM, De Bruijn MLH and Vernie LN *et al* (1991) Peptide selection by MHC class I molecules. *Nature* **350** 703–706

Shu S, Chou T and Sakai K (1989) Lymphocytes generated by in vivo priming and in vitro sensitization demonstrate therapeutic efficacy against a murine tumour that lacks apparent immunogenicity. *Journal of Immunology* **143** 740–748

Sibille C, Chomez P, Wildmann C *et al* (1990) Structure of the gene of tum⁻ transplantation antigen P198: a point mutation generates a new antigenic peptide. *Journal of Experimental Medicine* **172** 35–45

Smith MEF, Marsh SGE, Bodmer JG, Gelsthorpe K and Bodmer WF (1989) Loss of HLA-A,B,C allele products and lymphocyte function associated antigen 3 in colorectal neoplasia. *Proceedings of the National Academy of Sciences of the USA* **86** 5557–5561

Spies T and DeMars R (1991) Restored expression of major histocompatibility class I molecules by gene transfer of a putative peptide transporter. *Nature* **351** 323–325

Spies T, Bresnahan M, Bahram S *et al* (1990) A gene in the human major histocompatibility class II region controlling the class I presentation pathway. *Nature* **348** 744–747

Sprent J, Gao EK and Webb SR (1990) T cell reactivity to MHC molecules: immunity versus tolerance. *Science* **248** 1357–1363

Szikora JP, Van Pel A, Brichard V *et al* (1990) Structure of the gene of tum⁻ transplantation antigen P35B: presence of a point mutation in the antigenic allele. *EMBO Journal* **9** 1041–1050

Tanaka K, Isselbacher KJ, Khoury G and Jay G (1985) Reversal of oncogenesis by the expression of a major histocompatibility complex class I gene. *Science* **228** 26–30

Teyton L, O'Sullivan D, Dickson PW *et al* (1990) Invarious chain distinguishes between the exogenous and endogenous antigen presentation pathways. *Nature* **348** 39–44

Townsend A and Bodmer H (1989) Antigen recognition by class I restricted T lymphocytes. *Annual Review of Immunology* **7** 601–624

Townsend A, Elliott T, Cerundolo V *et al* (1990) Assembly of MHC class I molecules analyzed in vitro. *Cell* **62** 285–295

Townsend A, Öhlén C, Bastin J *et al* (1989) Association of class I major histocompatibility heavy and light chains induced by viral peptides. *Nature* **340** 443–

Townsend ARM, Rothband J, Gotch FM *et al* (1986) The epitopes of influenza nucleoprotein recognized by cytotoxic T lymphocytes can be defined with short synthetic peptides. *Cell* **44** 959–968

Trowsdale J, Hanson I, Mockridge I, Beck S, Townsend A and Kelly A (1990) Sequences encoded in the class II region of the MHC related to the ABC superfamily of transporters. *Nature* **348** 741–743

Van Bleek G and Nathenson SG (1990) Isolation of an endogenously processed immunodominant viral peptide from the class I H-2 Kb molecule. *Nature* **348** 213–216

Van Denderen J, Van Der Plas D, Meeuwsen T *et al* (1990) Immunologic characterization of the tumour-specific bcr-abl junction in Philadelphia chromosome—positive acute lymphoblastic leukemia. *Blood* **76** 136–141

Van Den Eynde B, Lethe B, Van Pel A, De Plaen E and Boon T (1991) The gene coding for a major tumour rejection antigen of tumour p815 is identical to the normal gene of syngeneic DBA/2 mice. *Journal of Experimental Medicine* **173** 1373–1384

Van Pel A, Vessière F and Boon T (1983) Protection against two spontaneous mouse leukemias conferred by immunogenic variants obtained by mutagenesis. *Journal of Experimental Medicine* **157** 1992–2001

Von Hoegen P, Weber E and Schirrmacher V (1988) Modification of tumour cells by a low dose of Newcastle disease virus: augmentation of the tumour-specific T cell response in the absence of an anti-viral response. *European Journal of Immunology* **18** 1159–1166

Wang P, Vanky F, Li S-L, Vegh ZS, Persson U and Klein E (1991) Expression of MHC class I antigen on human carcinomas and sarcomas analysed by isoelectric focusing. *International Journal of Cancer* (**Supplement 6**) 106–116

Zbar B and Rapp HJ (1974) Immunotherapy of guinea pig cancer with BCG. *Cancer Research* **34 (Supplement 4)** 1532–1540

Ziegler JL, Beckstead JA, Volberding PA *et al* (1984) Non-Hodgkin's lymphoma in 90 homosexual men. *New England Journal of Medicine* **311** 565–570

Zur Hausen H, Gissman L and Schlekofer JR (1984) Viruses in the etiology of human genital cancer. *Progress in Medical Virology* **30** 170–186

The authors are responsible for the accuracy of the references

The Role of Surface HLA-A,B,C Molecules in Tumour Immunity

P MÖLLER • G J HÄMMERLING

Institute of Pathology of the Heidelberg University and Institute of Immunology and Genetics at the German Cancer Research Centre, Im Neuenheimer Feld, D-6900 Heidelberg, Germany

Introduction
Physiological premises
    Structure of HLA molecules
    Antigen presentation by class I molecules
    Inductive and downregulating signals modulating MHC class I expression
Acquired defects causing abnormal MHC class I/β_2m expression
    Downregulation of MHC class I expression by oncogenes
    Lack of β_2m expression
    Defective assembly of class I heavy chains and β_2m
MHC class I and susceptibility of tumour cells to cytotoxic T cells and natural killer cells
In situ expression of HLA-A,B,C/β_2m molecules on tumours
Impact of mode of HLA class I expression in tumours on clinical course and prognosis
Melanoma, a tumour model for adaptive immunotherapy
Does tumour induced T lymphocyte clonal anergy prevent tumour rejection?
Summary and conclusion

INTRODUCTION

The classical work by Zinkernagel and Doherty (1974, 1979) that reactivity of cytotoxic T cells is restricted by surface molecules encoded in the class I region of the major histocompatibility complex (MHC) has stimulated the idea that these molecules are also of importance for the host defence mechanisms against autologous tumour cells. The early observation that some individual tumours lack MHC class I molecules gave rise to the immune escape theory hypothesizing that lack of class I determinants could provide a selective advantage for tumour cells because they might escape from putative tumour reactive T cell attack (Sanderson and Beverley, 1983). The existence of tumour specific antigenic determinants presented in conjunction with MHC molecules has often been supposed but was formally proven only recently in a murine tumour model (Lurquin *et al*, 1989; van den Eynde *et al*, 1991). Conversely, it was shown that a lack in class I expression on tumour cells was cor-

Cancer Surveys Volume 13: A New Look at Tumour Immunology
© 1992 Imperial Cancer Research Fund. 0-87969-370-3/92. $3.00 + .00

related with an increased susceptibility to lysis by natural killer (NK) cells (Kärre *et al*, 1986). This observation is the basis of the "missing self" concept in tumour immunology. Although there is good evidence that either mechanism is operative in laboratory systems, it seems reasonable to assume that immunoselection is not a basal mechanism in tumorigenesis because immunodeficiencies are not associated with a generally increased cancer risk (Biggar *et al*, 1989). Thus, immunodeficient mice such as nude or SCID mice or patients with inborn or acquired immunodeficiencies do not develop carcinomas at a higher rate: the only tumours with increased frequency appear to be virally induced tumours (Pelicci *et al*, 1986; Cannon *et al*, 1990; Joncas *et al*, 1990; Swinnen *et al*, 1990). This, however, does not imply that the immune system does not react against neoplasia. It is unknown which and how many human tumours are immunogenic and what percentage of these elicit an effective immune response against the tumour. It is well known that many neoplasms induce a chronic lymphohistiocytic inflammatory reaction within the tumour stroma or at the frontier of invasion. At present, we can merely state that whatever spontaneously happens in this microenvironment in terms of host versus tumour activity is in itself incapable of eliminating the neoplastic clone. This does not exclude the possibility that by manipulating this system, its effectiveness can be augmented. Since there is no a priori reason to doubt that at least some human cancers induce an immune response, it follows that MHC class I expression must be important. Therefore, we summarize here what is known about the physiology and molecular pathology of HLA class I expression on human tumour cells and its consequences on cell mediated cytotoxicity. For an overview on animal models, see Hämmerling *et al* (1987).

PHYSIOLOGICAL PREMISES

Structure of HLA Molecules

The MHC consists of an array of genes on chromosome 6p2 encoding several sets of immunoregulatory molecules. Two classes of these are polymorphic members of the immunoglobulin superfamily and serve as antigen presenting structures and restriction elements of the cellular immune response by interacting with the T cell antigen receptor (TcR) and with accessory molecules of autologous T cells.

MHC class I molecules are highly polymorphic type I integral transmembrane glycoproteins encoded by a group of closely linked loci, the best known being designated HLA-A,B,C. They are assembled with β_2-microglobulin (β_2m), which is a protein encoded on chromosome 15. The crystallographic structures of HLA-A2.1 and HLA-Aw68.1 indicate that the TcR of cytotoxic T cells interacts with the exposed helical parts of the HLA class I $\alpha1$ and $\alpha2$ domains that form the rim of a groove in which the antigenic peptide is bound (Bjorkman, 1987a,b). The size and shape of this groove seem to be sublocus and/or allotype dependent and account for the known restrictions in peptide binding (Bouillot *et al*, 1989; Chen and Parham, 1989; Falk *et al*, 1991; Winter *et al*, 1991). The $\alpha 3$ domain of the HLA class I molecule is the site of physical contact with the CD8 accessory molecule (Salter *et al*, 1989). Interaction of both TcR and CD8 with the same class I molecule is necessary for T cell activation (Conolly *et al*, 1990; Salter *et al*, 1990). The functionally relevant quarternary structure of the class I heavy chain is maintained by the association with $\beta_2 m$ (Kozlowski *et al*, 1991) and the antigenic peptide (Townsend *et al*, 1990; Schumacher *et al*, 1991; Silver *et al*, 1991). Depending on the MHC class I molecule, the class I/$\beta_2 m$ complex is labile at physiological temperatures in the absence of peptide, resulting in dissociation of $\beta_2 m$ and denaturation of the heavy chain on the cell surface (Schnabl *et al*, 1990; Benjamin *et al*, 1991; Ortiz-Navarrete and Hämmerling, 1991; Rock *et al*, 1991). For an antigen specific MHC/TcR mediated cytolysis, about 200 class I/$\beta_2 m$/peptide complexes per target cell seem to be sufficient (Christinck *et al*, 1991).

Antigen Presentation via MHC Class I Molecules

It is now well established that antigens are presented as peptide fragments. The optimum size of naturally processed peptides seems to be eight to nine aminoacid residues (Rötzschke *et al*, 1990; van Bleek and Nathenson, 1990; Falk *et al*, 1991; Schumacher *et al*, 1991). Pathways of antigen processing and presentation via class I and class II molecules (HLA-DR, HLA-DP and HLA-DQ antigens) differ fundamentally (Morrison *et al*, 1986). MHC class I molecules present predominantly endogenous (including newly synthesized viral) antigens, whereas class II molecules can present endocytosed exogenous antigen (Sweetser *et al*, 1989). Endogenous peptides, usually derived from the cytosolic compartment, are assembled within the endoplasmic reticulum with newly synthesized class I and $\beta_2 m$ (Nuchtern *et al*, 1989; Yewdell *et al*, 1989; Townsend *et al*, 1990). This complex is transported through the Golgi complex to the cell surface.

Inductive and Downregulating Signals Modulating MHC Class I Expression

MHC class I molecules are expressed constitutively in high amounts on the surface of many cell types (Daar *et al*, 1984; Natali *et al*, 1984). Several types of cells such as hepatocytes, lymph vessel endothelium and skeletal muscle, although lacking these structures under physiological conditions, express HLA-A,B,C during chronic inflammation (Barbatis *et al*, 1981; Koretz *et al*, 1987; Emslie-Smith *et al*, 1989). Other cell types such as smooth muscle cells of the gut wall constitutively lack MHC class I and are not inducible (Koretz *et al*, 1987). In the constitutively positive or inducible cell types, expression can be modulated by enhancing stimuli such as interferon (IFN)-α, -β and -γ (Heron *et al*, 1978; Wallach *et al*, 1982; Nissen *et al*, 1987; Hakem *et al*, 1989) and tumour necrosis factor—especially in synergy with IFN-γ (Collins *et al*, 1986; Avila-Carino *et al*, 1988; Eager *et al*, 1989). The same holds true for many types of tumour cells (Lampson and Fisher, 1984; Nissen *et al*, 1985; Pfizen-maier *et al*, 1987; Nisticò *et al*, 1990). In in vitro systems, IFN-α induced HLA class I expression can still be enhanced by phorbol esters (Erusalimsy *et al*, 1989). Virus infection was also shown to modulate class I expression; Epstein-Barr virus infection of normal B lymphocytes increased surface antigenic densities of HLA-A,B,C molecules threefold to sixfold (Jilg *et al*, 1991). By contrast, human immunodeficiency virus 1 (HIV-1) infection of the CD4+ T cell leukaemia line CEM-E5 caused downmodulation of class I expression during the time of virus replication (Scheppler *et al*, 1989). DNA damage in-duced by ultraviolet light C (254 nm) and the carcinogen benzo(*a*)pyrene derivate BPDE and, alternatively, administration of protein synthesis inhibitor cycloheximide (acting as DNA synthesis inhibitor) was observed to induce MHC class I protein synthesis rapidly in fibroblasts and keratinocytes; this ef-fect was shown not to be a direct consequence of an arrest of DNA synthesis but was interpreted as a still ill-defined cellular stress reaction (Lambert *et al*, 1989). The only cytokine/hormone known so far to reduce the level of class I products on the cell surface is hydrocortisone and its functionally related deri-vates. These were shown to downmodulate HLA-A,B,C molecules on periph-eral blood cells by about 15% (Hokland *et al*, 1981). Keratinocytes also display slightly decreased levels of class I mRNA and surface class I molecules upon long term treatment with dexamethasone (von Knebel-Doeberitz *et al*, 1990).

The molecular biology of MHC gene regulation will not be discussed here; for recent reviews, see Acolla *et al* (1991), Kara and Glimcher (1991) and David-Watine *et al* (1991).

ACQUIRED DEFECTS CAUSING ABNORMAL MHC CLASS I/β_2m EXPRESSION

An abnormally low number of MHC class I/β_2m molecules on the surface of neoplastic cells can be caused by numerous different mechanisms. Principally, there might be structural alterations at the genomic level localized either within HLA class I or β_2m genes or within genes regulating their transcription. Transcription may be suppressed by *trans*-acting factors governing the promo-tors. Furthermore, intracellular transport, assembly and export mechanisms may be disturbed or deficient. According to the nature of the defect, surface expression of HLA-A,B,C locus products and β_2m may be irreversibly abrogated or, in case of downregulation, normal levels may be restored by stimuli physiologically acting as inducing or enhancing signals. Defects may range from allelic loss to complete absence of functional MHC class I/β_2m complexes on the cell surface. We shall discuss examples for different defects causing abnormal HLA-A,B,C/β_2m expression in tumour cells.

Downregulation of MHC Class I Expression by Oncogenes

Bernards *et al* (1986) have shown that human neuroblastoma cell lines, known for low levels of MHC class I products (Lampson *et al*, 1983), display amplification of the N-*myc* nuclear proto-oncogene. This amplification may be causative for MHC class I downmodulation (Versteeg *et al*, 1990) or not: the constitutive overexpression of the transfected recombinant N-*myc* gene in neuroblastoma cell lines produced no consistent change in class I mRNA and surface expressed molecules (Feltner *et al*, 1989). An inverse correlation between N-*myc* and class I mRNA levels was found to be unstable depending on the stimulus by which one of them, or both, could be modulated (Gross *et al*, 1990). A similar relation was found in human melanoma between c-*myc* and class I genes (Versteeg *et al*, 1988). However, the suppressive effect of c-*myc* was more pronounced for the HLA-B locus than for the HLA-A locus (Versteeg *et al*, 1989). A regulatory phenomenon rather than a structural defect is assumed for the HLA-A11 negative Burkitt's lymphomas arising in HLA-A11 positive patients, since this lack could be overcome by interferon and tumour necrosis factor, at least in some of the tumour derived cell lines (Avila-Carino *et al*, 1988). Further support for this view comes from Marley *et al* (1989), who found a synergism of both cytokines in downregulating c-*myc* and upregulating class I/β_2m in the small cell lung carcinoma cell lines NCI-H146 and NCI-H209. Oncogene controlled suppression of class I genes may be just one of several mechanisms leading to defects in HLA-A,B,C expression. In melanoma cell lines, a stable lack of HLA-A2 locus specific mRNA has been found that was not correlated with abnormal c-*myc* mRNA levels (Wölfel *et al*, 1989; Pandolfi *et al*, 1991). Furthermore, c-*myc* does not seem to be involved in class I suppression in non-small lung carcinoma (Redondo *et al*, 1991), and Ki-*ras* mutations were not correlated with downregulation of class I molecules in colon carcinoma (Oliva *et al*, 1990). Transformation of human fibroblasts with Rous sarcoma virus led to reduced HLA-A,B,C and β_2m mRNA and protein levels (Gogusev *et al*, 1988). The same effect could be found in human cells transformed by adenovirus 12, and again this repression, which is caused by transforming proteins encoded by the viral E1A gene (Grand *et al*, 1987), could be circumvented by IFN-γ (Eager *et al*, 1989). Locus specific suppression of HLA class I expression in a panel of colon carcinoma cell lines was shown to be mediated by a loss of locus specific DNA binding transcription factors (Soong and Hui, 1991).

In conclusion, although there is strong evidence for MHC class I downregulation mediated by the adenovirus 12 derived E1A oncogene in hamster cells, the situation is less clear in other systems, and little information is available on the possible mechanisms involved.

Lack of β_2m Expression

Daudi, a Burkitt's lymphoma B cell line with deficient surface HLA-A,B,C molecules (Nilsson *et al*, 1974), lacks cytoplasmic β_2m, although mRNA for β_2m is detectable (Rosa *et al*, 1983a,b). This mRNA is not translatable because of a point mutation in the initiation codon (Rosa *et al*, 1983b). From the early studies with Daudi cells, it was concluded that β_2m is required for cell surface expression of MHC class I molecules. Indeed, transfection of the murine β_2m gene into Daudi cells restored the capability of the cell line to export class I/β_2m heterodimers (Seong *et al*, 1988). Colon carcinomas failing to bind anti-HLA-A,B,C/β_2m antibody W6/32 because they lacked β_2m did not contain β_2m mRNA as demonstrated by in situ hybridization (Momburg and Koch, 1989). Thus, an alternative defect, namely on the transcriptional level, seems to be operative. Such a defect could also be found in the human melanoma cell line FO-1. Its lack of β_2m mRNA could be traced back to a deletion of the first exon of the 5' flanking region and of a segment of the first intron of the β_2m gene (D'Urso *et al*, 1991).

Defective Assembly of Class I Heavy Chains and β_2m

Somatic mutants of lymphoblastoid B cell lines have been generated that although having their HLA-A, HLA-B and β_2m genes transcribed, have reduced levels of surface expressed class I/β_2m complexes (DeMars *et al*, 1985). Like the murine model system RMA-S (Ljunggren and Kärre, 1985; Townsend *et al*, 1989), one of these lines, LCL 721.174 (DeMars *et al*, 1984, 1985), and T2, its somatic hybrid with CEM, were shown to transcribe the HLA-A2, HLA-B5 and β_2m genes; but only some HLA-A2 molecules (about 20%) were assembled and transported to the cell surface, probably devoid of antigenic peptide. Thus, these cell lines appeared to have a defect in the supply of peptides into the endoplasmic reticulum. Furthermore, these cell lines lack MHC class II determinants because of deletions within the class II region (Salter and Cresswell, 1986; Cerundolo *et al*, 1990; Hosken and Bevan, 1990). Impaired class I/β_2m assembly and transport were shown to be due to the deletion of one or two ABC transporter genes, the products of which are probably responsible for the transport of peptides from the cytosol into the endoplasmic reticulum (Deverson *et al*, 1990; Spies *et al*, 1990; Trowsdale *et al*, 1990). In a spontaneous mouse lung carcinoma (CMT 64.5) and also in methyl-cholanthrene A induced fibrosarcoma (BC2), a defect was observed in the intracellular assembly of class I heavy chain and β_2m that could be overcome by IFN-γ (Klar and Hämmerling, 1989).

Whatever the nature of the defect causing anomalous HLA-A,B,C surface expression on tumour cells might be, the consequence is a disturbance of a potential CD8+ T cell/target cell interaction. If tumour antigens exist, they must be presented by these molecules. Principally, a point mutation in a gene encoding a self protein may lead to a new peptide that could bind to the self MHC molecules on tumour cells and thus be recognized by the immune system as foreign. Alternatively, oncofetal proteins physiologically expressed during embryogenesis before the development of T cell tolerance and re-expressed as a consequence of neoplastic transformation might be candidates for "tumour antigens". The first possibility would elicit a unique, individual anti-tumour response. The second possibility could apply more generally and would possibly be associated with the histological type of tumour.

MHC CLASS I AND SUSCEPTIBILITY OF TUMOUR CELLS TO CYTOTOXIC T CELLS AND NATURAL KILLER CELLS

Only recently, direct evidence that cell mediated cytotoxic T lymphocyte (CTL) response to a tumour specific/associated antigen might indeed happen in vivo has been reported by Boon and coworkers (Lurquin et al, 1989; Van den Eynde et al, 1991). Indirect evidence for this mechanism comes from blocking studies with anti-MHC class I antibodies. Pretreatment of tumour cells from 35 patients with different types of carcinomas and sarcomas with monoclonal antibody W6/32 abrogated CTL mediated cytolysis of allogeneic tumour cells in all experiments but cytolysis of autologous tumour cells in only some experiments (Slovin et al, 1986; Vánky et al, 1987). Induction of class I molecules in constitutively class I negative tumours was shown to stimulate autologous lymphocytes to generate autotumorotoxicity, which, in turn, could be blocked by anti-class I monoclonal antibody W6/32 (Vánky et al, 1989). More direct evidence comes from the work of Seigler's group, who raised anti-melanoma CTL that could lyse the autologous tumour and, exclusively, allogeneic melanomas that shared HLA-A2; these effects, again, could be inhibited by W6/32 (Darrow et al, 1989). It was concluded from this study and confirmed by Pandolfi et al (1991) that HLA-A2 might function as a restricting element for T cell recognition of a melanoma associated antigen. In the absence of HLA-A2, the restricting element was shown to be HLA-A1. However, in case of heterozygosity, the HLA-A2 allotype was dominant (Crowley et al, 1991). The most convincing data that tumour antigens are presented by human cancer cells are those of Itoh et al (1988) and Rosenberg and coworkers, who extracted tumour infiltrating lymphocytes (TIL) and isolated tumour reactive CD8+ T cells and generated clones that retained their capacity to lyse autologous tumour cells in vitro (see below).

Whereas it is clear that a CTL response benefits from MHC class I expression on the target cell, the reverse seems to be true for NK cells. The observation by Stern et al (1982) that embryonic carcinoma cells lacking MHC antigens are targets of NK cells has since been extended to other tumour cell types and, more precisely, was ascribed to the lack of class I molecules (Kärre et al, 1986; Storkus et al, 1987; Sturmhöfel and Hämmerling, 1990). This inverse correlation between expression of HLA class I determinants and susceptibility to NK mediated lysis was found in (mutant) cell line systems such as Epstein-Barr virus (EBV) transformed lymphoblastoid B cell lines (Storkus et al, 1987, 1989; Öhlén et al, 1989; Shimizu and DeMars, 1989) and in many other human cell lines. In the lymphoblastoid (LCL) B cell system, it could further be demonstrated that high levels of class I expression are positively correlated with lytic potential of LCL specific cytotoxic T cells and negatively correlated with NK susceptibility (Öhlén et al, 1989). In this experimental set, a striking reduction of CTL activity and an increase in NK susceptibility were already measurable at the level of a single MHC allele. Indirect evidence suggesting that class I molecules are physically involved in this mechanism was achieved by blocking experiments with anti-class I antibodies (Lobo and Spencer, 1989; Vánky *et al*, 1989; Sturmhöfel and Hämmerling, 1990), and direct evidence came from Quillet *et al* (1988), who transfected Daudi cells with the β_2m gene and not only could restore the capacity of the cell line to express class I/β_2m heterodimers but also got resistance to NK mediated lysis. After transfecting class I deficient mutant lymphoblastoid B cell lines with genes encoding different class I allotypes, Shimizu and DeMars (1989) concluded that HLA-B sublocus products might be directly involved in mediating NK resistance. This protection of target cells from NK lysis after transfection of class I genes, however, did not extend to cytotoxicity by interleukin-2 (IL-2) stimulated NK cells (Storkus *et al*, 1989). NK susceptibility could be reduced or even abrogated by pretreatment of the target cell population with IFN-γ (de Fries and Golub, 1988; Grönberg *et al*, 1989) or IFN-α (Migita *et al*, 1991). Although IFN-γ induced class I molecules in small cell lung carcinoma lines was paralleled by resistance to NK cell lysis, reduction of NK susceptibility could not be achieved by transfection with HLA-A2, HLA-B27 or HLA-B27 together with β_2m (Stam *et al*, 1989). Similarly, transfection of NK susceptible K562 and Molt-4 targets with HLA-A2 and HLA-B7 did not alter the susceptibility, although the transfectants neoexpressed class I; again, IFN-γ treatment decreased susceptibility to NK mediated cytotoxicity (Leiden *et al*, 1989). The failure of HLA-A2 to protect cells from NK lysis was further analysed by Storkus *et al* (1991). They traced down the non-protective phenotype to a histidine residue at position 74 of the α1 domain of this molecule which might sterically inhibit access to a side pocket of the peptide binding groove. By contrast, NK susceptibility was found to be independent of HLA class I expression on a comprehensive panel of astrocytoma, meningioma and lung, breast and colon carcinoma cell lines, whereas IFN-γ treatment generally increased the resistance to NK lysis (Pena *et al*, 1990). From these experiments, it was concluded that molecules which are not HLA class I antigens but IFN-γ inducible may confer NK resistance. For the time being, these data do not lead to a consistent concept on the point of whether or not Kärre's concept of "missing self" directly elicits NK mediated lysis.

IN SITU EXPRESSION OF HLA-A,B,C/β_2m MOLECULES ON TUMOURS

To determine the role of MHC class I molecules for CTL or NK mediated tumour rejection, a large number of investigators have begun in situ analysis of MHC class I expression in human tumour tissues.

The first in situ demonstrations of loss of membrane bound β_2m were reported by Fleming *et al* (1981), Turbitt *et al* (1981) and Weiss *et al* (1981) in breast carcinoma and precancerous lesions of the skin. Ever since, a number of immunohistological studies have addressed abnormal HLA expression in tumours. The data available allow some general statements, but only a few aspects can presently be regarded as settled. It was commonly assumed that class I molecules are expressed by virtually all cell types and that non-expression of these can be regarded as a loss or defect. Although this holds true for nearly all types of epithelia (except for germinal cells) and haematopoietic cells, some mesenchymal cells (eg muscle cells, adipocytes) constitutively lack HLA-A,B,C determinants (Daar *et al*, 1984; Natali *et al*, 1984; Mechtersheimer *et al*, 1990). Therefore, lack of class I antigens in seminomas (Bell *et al*, 1987) and in some mesenchymal tumours (eg leiomyoma, rhabdomyosarcoma, lipoma) has to be regarded as normal, and detection of class I antigens will consequently have to be regarded as abnormal (neoexpression). Apart from these principal problems, immunohistochemical data are qualitative, and quantitative statements are difficult to attain. Intratumoural heterogeneity is often semiquantitatively characterized as + or −; the antigenic density when found reduced with respect to intrinsic high controls (eg interstitial cells) is often indicated as weak or (+). Furthermore, the identification of the entire tumour cell population in an immunostained tissue section may be technically easy (eg in a tubular adenocarcinoma) or very difficult (eg in malignant fibrous histiocytoma). Serial section analysis with cell type specific antibodies highlighting the neoplastic population is often mandatory, and panleucocyte reagents such as CD53 are helpful in revealing the local inflammatory infiltrate (Mechtersheimer *et al*, 1990). As a consequence of these theoretical and methodological difficulties, several published results in this field have to be interpreted with caution.

Abnormal loss/hypoexpression of MHC class I antigens was found in eccrine porocarcinoma (Holden *et al*, 1984), in carcinomas of thyroid (Betterle *et al*, 1991) and larynx (Esteban *et al*, 1990), in lung carcinoma of non-small cell and small cell type (Doyle *et al*, 1985; Redondo *et al*, 1991) and other neuroendocrine tumours (Funa *et al*, 1986), in transitional cell carcinoma (Nouri *et al*, 1990; Tomita *et al*, 1990), carcinoma of the breast (Fleming *et al*, 1981; Natali *et al*, 1983a; Göttlinger *et al*, 1985; Pérez *et al*, 1986; Möller *et al*, 1989b), cervix (Connor and Stern, 1990) and ovary (Ferguson *et al*, 1985). The situation is best known for colorectal carcinoma. Since the first description of a loss of class I determinants in colon carcinoma by Csiba *et al* (1984), it has been repeatedly confirmed that about 10–15% of such cancers completely lack reactivity with the HLA-A,B,C framework antibody W6/32 (Momburg *et al*, 1986; Durrant *et al*, 1987; van der Ingh *et al*, 1987; Stein *et al*, 1988; Lopéz-Nevot *et al*, 1989). Thus, the percentages published by McDougall *et al* (1990) (28% complete loss and 68% reduced expression) seem extreme. Although defects in HLA-A,B,C expression are also sporadically detectable in benign tumours such as adenomas of the thyroid (Betterle *et al*, 1991), breast (Möller *et al*, 1989b) and colon (Smith *et al*, 1989), this abnormality is a feature of poorly differentiated carcinomas irrespective of their histotype. The same correlation may largely account for the reported associations with clinical indices such as local aggressiveness and was often used as an argument to speculate on the impact of abnormal class I expression on prognosis. Accordingly, a loss of HLA-A,B,C locus products in non-Hodgkin's lymphoma of B cell origin is highly correlated with the grade of malignancy (Möller *et al*, 1987b). The B lymphoma type almost regularly lacking class I molecules is a locally aggressive, non-disseminating lymphoma, originating in the thymus (Möller *et al*, 1986, 1987a,b, 1989a). The situation is more complex in soft tissue tumours: some neoplasms of fibrous origin and of autonomic ganglia showed an abnormal abrogation/loss of HLA-A,B,C/β_2m with respect to their cells of origin (Mechtersheimer *et al*, 1990; Sugio *et al*, 1991), whereas compared with the normal state, an induction/neoexpression of class I molecules was found in a considerable number of tumours of muscle, peripheral nerve, cartilage-forming, adipose and vascular tissues (Mechtersheimer *et al*, 1990). Mechtersheimer *et al* (1990) presented evidence that this neoexpression did, in most instances, occur in the absence of an inflammatory interstitial infiltrate and hence is most probably cytokine independent in soft tissue tumours. An abnormal induction of HLA-A,B,C molecules, mimicking neoexpression of class I in liver cells as a consequence of virus infection, was observed in hepatocellular carcinoma (Paterson *et al*, 1988). Neoexpression of HLA class I has also to be assumed for HLA-A,B,C positive seminomas (Klein *et al*, 1990).

A complete loss of reactivity with class I framework antibody W6/32, which recognizes a conformational epitope on the intact heavy chain/β_2m complex (Barnstable *et al*, 1978; Jeffries and MacPhersan, 1987; Kahn-Perles *et al*, 1987), has been shown to result from a defect in β_2m expression. This sort of defect, long known for the B cell lymphoma line Daudi (Nilsson *et al*, 1974), could be shown in situ on the protein level (our unpublished data) with monoclonal antibodies recognizing free heavy chains or β_2m and on the mRNA level (Momburg and Koch, 1989). A relative reduction of immunohistochemical reactivity (as compared with intrinsic high controls, ie interstitial reactive cells) has repeatedly been shown to be due to selective loss of HLA-A and/or HLA-B expression (Rees *et al*, 1988; Momburg *et al*, 1989; Smith *et al*, 1989; Connor and Stern, 1990; Esteban *et al*, 1990; Oliva *et al*, 1990; Andersson *et al*, 1991; Redondo *et al*, 1991). As far as specified, selective loss of HLA-A2 seems to be most frequent, followed by loss of the supertypic HLA-Bw6 antigen. Furthermore, a (focally) combined loss of two sublocus products (eg HLA-A2 together with the supertypic specificity Bw6) could be observed (Momburg *et al*, 1989; Esteban *et al*, 1990). In Burkitt's lymphoma, defective expression furthermore appears to also involve the HLA-C locus (Andersson *et al*, 1991). Loss of sublocus products result in a reduced reactivity with framework antibodies such as W6/32, which, in immunohistology, is often characterized as "hypoexpression". Considering the fact that class I hypoexpression occurs in about 35% of colorectal carcinomas (Möller *et al*, 1991a,b) and in about 50% of breast carcinomas (Möller *et al*, 1989b), it can be concluded that dysregulations within the MHC genome are commonplace at least in two epidemiologically very important cancers.

A correlation between reduction/loss of class I expression and loss/hypoexpression of class II/invariant chain (Ii) was described for B cell non-Hodgkin's lymphomas (Möller *et al*, 1987b; Momburg *et al*, 1987), breast carcinoma (Möller *et al*, 1989b) and colorectal carcinoma (Möller *et al*, 1991a), suggesting the existence of a *trans*-acting factor, normally operative regulating both gene regions together with the β_2m gene and the Ii gene (which is located on chromosome 5).

It is conceivable that elicitation of CTL mediated lysis may be either facilitated or even enabled by accessory molecules with either cosignalling properties and/or heterotypic adhesion receptor function. Therefore, recent in situ studies on the expression of surface antigens in tumours have included adhesion molecules.

Signal transducing molecules involved in efficiently eliciting an antigen driven clonal expansion of T cells may be LFA-1(CD11a/CD18)-ICAM-1(CD54) and/or LFA-3(CD56)-CD2. Lysis of IFN-γ treated keratinocytes with allogeneic class I specific CTL was recently shown to be mediated by interaction of T cell LFA-1 and keratinocyte ICAM-1 (Symington and Santos, 1991). During cognate T cell/target cell interaction, LFA-3 is most likely physically associated with the HLA proteins involved (Bierer *et al*, 1989), and antigen specific binding is substantially weakened in the absence of LFA-3 (Recny *et al*, 1990). Observations that LFA-3 is downregulated in several EBV positive Burkitt's lymphoma lines (Billaud *et al*, 1987; Gregory *et al*, 1988) and abrogated in sporadic cases of transitional cell carcinoma (Nouri *et al*, 1990) and colon carcinoma (Smith *et al*, 1989) have led to the suggestion that a loss of ICAM-1 and/or LFA-3 might contribute to the putative escape of tumours from cytotoxic T cell attack. We therefore extended the analysis of our cohort of colorectal cancer patients to the expression of ICAM-1 and LFA-3. The results obtained, however, fail to confirm this nascent hypothesis, at least with respect to colorectal carcinoma. ICAM-1 was not expressed in normal colon epithelium or colorectal carcinoma (unpublished results). By contrast, LFA-3 was regularly detectable in normal colon epithelium. In colorectal carcinoma, we found an abnormal reduction of LFA-3 in 43.6% of 149 tumours examined, whereas a complete loss of this molecule was detectable in 6.7%. There was a statistical correlation of reduction/loss of HLA-A,B,C (as determined by W6/32 binding) and a reduction/loss of LFA-3. The presence or absence of LFA-3 did not correlate with disease free survival in this group of 149 patients who underwent curative surgery (Möller *et al*, 1991b).

IMPACT OF MODE OF MHC EXPRESSION IN TUMOURS ON CLINICAL COURSE AND PROGNOSIS

Clinical studies on the MHC expressional status of malignant tumours are still scarce and controversial. A reduction of HLA-A,B,C antigens was reported to be more frequent in poorly differentiated and invasively growing transitional cell carcinomas than in well differentiated superficial ones (Ottesen *et al*, 1987; Tomita *et al*, 1990). The same correlation could be observed in squamous cell carcinoma of the larynx, although the metastatic potential of HLA-A,B,C defective tumours was not increased (Esteban *et al*, 1990). In a recent study by Concha *et al* (1991) on MHC class I expression in 94 breast carcinomas, a statistical relation between patients' survival and HLA class I negative phenotype emerged. In this cohort, about 8% completely lacked this class of molecules and about 20% showed a severely downregulated expression (which is in good agreement with our data [Möller *et al*, 1989b]). Respective survival data were calculated on a basis of 77 patients, and mean survival time was short (28 months). Conversely, it was clearly shown by Wintzer *et al* (1990) that the HLA-A,B,C expressional status had no apparent influence on disease free and overall survival in breast carcinoma. The study by Wintzer *et al* (1990) is based on 66 patients; the median follow-up time of 45 months is, although longer, still quite a short time for mammary carcinoma. Thus, the question of a prognostic potential of the modality of MHC class I expression in breast carcinoma is still debatable. A more pessimistic point of view can be derived from our own data on colorectal carcinoma. In a preliminary study, we concluded from our survival data that reduction or loss of HLA-A,B,C antigens in colorectal carcinoma is not a prognostic variable (Stein *et al*, 1988). This pilot study was based on 159 unselected patients; maximum follow-up time was 39 months and the survival data were calculated irrespective the cause of death. The mode of HLA-A,B,C expression did not influence survival within this time of observation. A subsequent prospective study on the basis of 152 curatively resected patients with a mean follow-up time of 48 months (which is sufficiently long for colorectal carcinoma) showed that presence versus absence of HLA-A,B,C/β_2m was not correlated with recurrence rate or survival (Möller *et al*, 1991a). Although these data seem reliable to us, it should be noted that the cohort as a whole showed a very favourable course: during the time of observation, a mere 28 relapsed and only 16 patients died because of their tumour. The mean age was 66 years (an age when multimorbidity is common), and causes of death unrelated to the neoplastic disease were disregarded. Nevertheless, since the classic indices indicating favourable prognosis in colorectal carcinoma (depth of invasion, lymph node status and histological differentiation) emerged as such in this study, a potential effect of the modality of HLA expression would, if existing at all for this type of tumour, indeed be slight.

So far, clinical studies have concentrated mainly on tumours with loss of HLA-A,B,C because sufficient information on tumours with loss of individual alleles has not yet been acquired. From theoretical considerations and from data obtained in murine tumour models, it is clear that on a given immunogenic tumour, in general, only one MHC class I allele presents the tumour antigen (Hämmerling *et al*, 1987). Therefore, loss of all HLA alleles is not likely to reflect immunological selective forces. Such forces are more likely to result in escape variants with loss of only one allele. What is the aim of in situ studies besides gathering basic information on the heterogeneity of tumours? The clinically relevant aim is certainly to establish a direct correlation between loss of HLA and malignancy of a tumour in order to draw conclusions on a continuing anti-tumour immune response and to delineate variables of prognostic value with the hope of using this kind of information for therapeutic interventions. It is obvious that a very large number of human tumours will have to be screened for loss of individual HLA alleles and respective clinical studies will have to be done, which will require considerable effort. Even if such studies demonstrate immunoselection in one or other case, the question remains whether this kind of information is clinically useful or whether it would be more promising to concentrate directly on the demonstration or induction of a host anti-tumour response. Indeed, in the course of infectious mononucleosis, the T cell system is capable of eliminating macroscopical masses of EBV transformed lymphoblastoid cells that, in case of immunodeficiency, can give rise to the so-called lymphoproliferative syndrome, which is a highly aggressive disease closely mimicking high grade malignant non-Hodgkin's lymphoma (Pelicci et al, 1986; Cannon et al, 1990; Joncas et al, 1990; Swinnen et al, 1990). This situation doubtlessly justifies further therapeutic efforts to sensitize and stimulate T cells in order to control minimum residual disease after conventional tumour surgery.

MELANOMA, A TUMOUR MODEL FOR ADAPTIVE IMMUNOTHERAPY

Not every human tumour type is suitable for clinical research in immunotherapy. The ideal tumour should have its highest incidence in young adulthood (which keeps to a minimum comorbidity); it should be highly metastatic, life expectancy should be limited and conventional radio/chemotherapy should be either ineffective or, at least, not curative. In such a situation, new therapeutic approaches are ethically justified, patients' consent will be easy to obtain and the grade of effectiveness of the immunotherapeutic regimen will disclose itself within a reasonable period of time. In this respect, malignant melanoma is optimum.

Melanocytes and naevomelanocytes in benign hyperplasia and dermal naevocellular naevi are devoid of class I/β_2m (Ruiter et al, 1982; Bröcker et al, 1985) but have a propensity to neoexpress this molecular complex in junctional naevi (Bröcker et al, 1985) and melanoma (Ruiter et al, 1982). Since class I/β_2m negativity was more often noted in metastatic tumour than in tumour primaries, a secondary loss of this neoexpression was assumed (Ruiter et al, 1984), which, in turn, was postulated to be associated with tumour progression. As reported by van Duinen et al (1988), lack of HLA-A,B,C might have contributed to the unfavourable clinical course of a cohort of 39 melanoma patients whose metastases were investigated in this respect. Natali et al (1983b) and Taramelli et al (1986), however, did not find such a correlation comparing primary and metastatic lesions. Class I expression can be induced or enhanced by interferon in melanoma cell lines (Houghton et al, 1984; Maio et al, 1989) and short term cultures of tumour cell isolates (Taramelli et al, 1986). As we have mentioned (see above), CTL recognition of autologous and allogeneic melanoma cells was non-randomly restricted to the HLA-A2 locus and, in the absence of HLA-A2, to HLA-A1 (which, however, is dominated by HLA-A2 in heterozygosity) (Darrow *et al*, 1989; Crowley *et al*, 1991). Isolation of TIL from metastatic melanoma revealed the presence of tumour specific CTL that were predominantly CD8+ and CD16–; cytotoxicity could be blocked by either CD3 monoclonal antibody or by anti-HLA-A,B,C antibody. These tumour specific CTL could be propagated with IL-2 alone while retaining their specificity (Itoh *et al*, 1988). These observations were confirmed by Topalian *et al* (1989) and Knuth *et al* (1989). Rosenberg's group (Topalian *et al*, 1989) isolated by cell separation highly effective CTL out of the crude TIL preparation. The clones obtained were CD8+/CD57–. Knuth *et al* (1989) identified by subcloning HLA-A2 as the restriction element for three different melanoma associated antigens (Wölfel *et al*, 1989). This group of workers reported that in their hands, effective lysis was still dependent on IFN-γ pretreatment of target cells. The touchstone in this system, the melanoma specific/associated antigen or antigenic peptide, has not yet been identified as such, although it was suggested by different laboratories that tumour specific antigens exist on melanoma cells. On the basis of these observations, the Rosenberg group decided to treat melanoma patients with autologous tumour specific CTL isolated from TIL. The administration was carried out together with systemic IL-2 treatment (Rosenberg *et al*, 1988). A recent report on 28 months clinical trial (Aebersold *et al*, 1991) states that 23 of 55 melanoma patients responded to TIL therapy in terms of tumour regression, whereas the remainder were regarded as non-responders. This response rate was regarded as better than that observed upon systemic IL-2 alone. Lysis of tumour cells by TIL (which was not due to LAK cell activity) was significantly higher for responding patients than for non-responding patients. In other words, there are interindividual differences in immunoreactivity of melanoma patients probably correlated with differences in CTL reactivities.

DOES TUMOUR INDUCED T LYMPHOCYTE CLONAL ANERGY PREVENT TUMOUR REJECTION?

Self tolerance is a basic homoeostatic principle of the immune system. It is mediated through mechanisms controlling the T and B cells. In early ontogeny, clonal deletion during the negative selection process in the thymus reduces the number of potentially autoreactive T cells. Furthermore, clonal anergy due to intrathymic and peripheral self tolerance induction prevents the normal immune system from acting against self determinants not presented in the thymus (Ramsdell and Fowlkes, 1990; Schwartz, 1990; Hämmerling *et al*, 1991). Restrictions in autoreactivity seem to be far more elaborate on the T cell than on the B cell level, and this might be due to the highly developed B cell dependency on T cell help (Goodnow *et al*, 1990; Kronenberg, 1991; Nossal, 1991). It has been shown in vitro that longlasting anergy of a peripheral T cell can be the consequence of an antigen-MHC complex recognition in the absence of costimulatory signals delivered by the antigen presenting cell (Schwartz, 1990).

In double-transgenic mice with exclusive expression of a target antigen in the periphery outside the thymus, a surprising variety of peripheral tolerance mechanisms was observed, dependent on the tissue expressing the target antigen (Hämmerling *et al*, 1991; Schönrich *et al*, 1991). When expression of a foreign MHC class I antigen (H-2K^b) was directed exclusively into the liver with an albumin promoter, the mice were tolerant in vivo. The potentially self reactive T cells were present, but tolerance was manifested by an irreversible downregulation of the K^b specific TcR and CD8. In another transgenic mouse with expression of the MHC model antigen in extrathymic cells of neuroectodermal origin, a reversible downregulation of TcR and CD8 was found, whereas in mice with exclusive expression in extrathymic keratinocytes, anergy was seen without downmodulation of the TcR. In other studies, peripheral deletion of T cells has been reported. Thus, in the periphery, distinct stages of tolerance can be induced depending on the anatomical site of antigen expression. In the transgenic model systems we mention, tolerance is induced in immature T cells shortly after exit from the thymus. However, there is also evidence that mature T cells are likewise susceptible for peripheral tolerance induction (Rocha and von Boehmer, 1991). A recent finding fitting this concept is that specific antigen bound to the TcR of a HLA-A2+ cytotoxic T cell line in the absence of antigen presenting cells downmodulates CD8 (Robbins and McMichael, 1991). An alternative mechanism for tolerance induction was proposed by Walden and Eisen (1990), who showed that cognate peptide alone induces self destruction of cloned CD8+ cytolytic T lymphocytes.

In addition, in view of the in vitro data illustrating the need for additional molecules on the target cell conferring costimulatory signals in order to elicit a cytotoxic T cell response, it can be speculated that cells (and tumours derived therefrom) lacking these structures may induce anergy in vivo. The fact that peripheral tolerance can be induced with relative ease not only is important for organ specific autoimmunity but also raises the intriguing question of whether or not a growing tumour induces peripheral tolerance and thereby prevents an effective T cell response. It will be of interest to address this possibility not only in animal systems but, in particular, with respect to those human tumours against which no obvious cytotoxic T cell activity is generated. In animal systems, many examples exist that the peripheral T cell anergy observed in vivo can be overcome in vitro, for example by addition of IL-2 (Schwartz, 1990; Otten and Germain, 1991). This raises the hope that appropriate manipulations can reverse clonal anergy in tumour patients. It becomes obvious that research in the field of autoimmunity and tumour immunology focuses on the two sides of the same coin: whereas research in autoimmunity attempts to prevent the breaking of self tolerance and the induction of an autoimmune response, tumour immunology concentrates on the generation of an immune response against the tumour, possibly by breaking tumour specific, tumour induced anergy.

SUMMARY AND CONCLUSION

It is well established that MHC class I molecules present peptides from endogenous proteins, such as virus or tumour antigens, to CD8+ T lymphocytes. This implies that expression of MHC class I molecules on tumours is also mandatory for an effective T cell response against neoplasias. Indeed, numerous murine models exist (such as IC9, 3LL, P815) in which the existence of MHC presented tumour antigens and a protective CTL response have been well documented (reviewed in Hämmerling et al, 1987). However, the key question of whether cytolytic T cell attack has a role in human cancer remains unsolved. Similarly, the role of NK cells is unclear; these seem to lyse cells with low levels of MHC class I expression more efficiently. So far, human tumour specific antigens that can be presented by HLA molecules have not been identified on the molecular level. For a subpopulation of patients with malignant melanoma, the existence of tumour antigen can be deduced from the existence of tumour specific cytotoxic T cells isolated from TIL. However, for other epidemiologically more important tumours such as carcinomas of the colon, breast and lung, even indirect evidence is still missing. It is thus unknown how many tumours express tumour specific antigen at all and whether these putative antigens are of unique specificity or are shared by certain groups of (histologically related) neoplasias. Most reports agree that malignant cells in general have a more or less pronounced propensity to express class I molecules abnormally and often in the sense of hypoexpression or (sublocus selective) loss. Mechanisms inducing aberrant expression are numerous. Immunohistochemical studies revealed that an abnormal content in surface class I/β_2m may be associated with other aspects of dedifferentiation of the tumour and hence may eventually correlate with biological signs of an increased grade of malignancy. Consequences of defective MHC class I expression for the survival of a malignant clone may theoretically consist of an escape from cytotoxic T cell attack or in an increased susceptibility for NK mediated lysis.

In view of the fact that a particular antigen in a cell will be presented only by one or few HLA alleles on the cell, one would not expect that immunoselection would lead to a loss of all HLA alleles. It can be deduced from the few existing clinical studies on the prognostic impact of aberrant MHC class I expression that immunoselection by one way or the other is not a relevant mechanism in terms of tumour biology. All published studies, however, are far from being complete because the battery of allele specific monoclonal antibodies required for a complete analysis of all class I alleles is still missing. New techniques such as the generation of allelic HLA antibodies in HLA transgenic mice (Hämmerling et al, 1990; Tahara et al, 1990) could greatly facilitate the production of such a set of typing antibodies. Even with such an antibody panel available, the critical question has to be asked whether the results to be expected are worth the immense effort. Probably, many hundreds of tumours of a particular histotype would have to be screened for loss of individual HLA alleles, and careful clinical studies including tumour monitoring by (repeated) tumour biopsy and survival analysis would be mandatory before definite conclusions can be drawn whether immunoselection really takes place and alters the clinical course of a given neoplastic disease. From the present knowledge, it seems likely that even such data will be difficult to interpret because they will be obscured by the fact that many human neoplasias seem to switch on or off many genes randomly, including HLA, resulting in intratumoural heterogeneity without the involvement of immunoselective forces.

Although such studies are likely to provide interesting and basic insights into the heterogeneity of tumour populations in vivo, it seems more appropriate to concentrate on cellular host versus tumour responses in various human cancers, to test for possible tolerance mechanisms, to induce an effective anti-tumour response and to find indices that indicate which tumours might be immunogenic and therefore are suitable candidates for an immune intervention. Such studies will also require the analysis of HLA antigens, the search for preferential restriction molecules and possibly for ways to enhance their expression.

References

Acolla RS, Auffray C, Singer DS and Gaurdiola J (1991) The molecular biology of MHC genes. *Immunology Today* **12** 97–99

Aebersold P, Hyatt C, Johnson S *et al* (1991) Lysis of autologous melanoma cells by tumor-infiltrating lymphocytes: association with clinical response. *Journal of the National Cancer Institute* **83** 932–937

Andersson ML, Stam NJ, Klein G, Ploegh HL and Masucci MG (1991) Aberrant expression of HLA class I antigens in Burkitt lymphoma cells. *International Journal of Cancer* **47** 544–550

Avila-Carino J, Torsteindottir S, Bejarano MT, Klein G, Klein E and Masucci MG (1988) Combined treatment with interferon (IFN)-γ and tumor necrosis factor (TNF)-α up-regulates the expression of HLA class I determinants in Burkitt lymphoma lines. *Cellular Immunology* **117** 303–311

Barbatis C, Woods J, Morton JA, Fleming KA and McGee JO'D (1981) Immunohistochemical analysis of HLA (A,B,C) antigens in liver disease using a monoclonal antibody. *Gut* **22** 985–991

Barnstable CJ, Bodmer WF, Brown G *et al* (1978) Production of monoclonal antibodies to group A erythrocytes, HLA and other human cell surface antigens—new tools for genetic analysis. *Cell* **14** 9–20

Bell DA, Flotte TJ and Bhan AK (1987) Immunohistochemical characterization of seminoma and its inflammatory cell infiltrate. *Human Pathology* **18** 511–520

Benjamin RJ, Madrigal JA and Parham P (1991) Peptide binding to empty HLA-B27 molecules of viable cells. *Nature* **35** 174–177

Bernards R, Dessain SK and Weinberg RA (1986) N-*myc* amplification causes down-modulation of MHC class I antigen expression in neuroblastoma. *Cell* **47** 667–674

Betterle C, Presotto F, Carnetto A *et al* (1991) Expression of class I and II human leukocyte antigens by thyrocytes and lymphocytic infiltration on human thyroid tumors: an immunofluorescence study. *Cancer* **67** 977–983

Bierer BE, Golan DE, Brown CS, Herrmann SH and Burakoff SJ (1989) A monoclonal antibody to LFA-3, the CD2 ligand, specifically immobilizes major histocompatibility complex proteins. *European Journal of Immunology* **19** 661–665

Biggar RJ, Burnett W, Mikl J and Nasca P (1989) Cancer among New York men at risk of acquired immunodeficiency syndrome. *International Journal of Cancer* **43** 979–985

Billaud M, Calender A, Seigneurin J-A and Lenoir GM (1987) LFA-1, LFA-3, and ICAM-1 expression in Burkitt's lymphoma. *Lancet* **ii** 1327–1328

Bjorkman P, Saper M, Samraoui B, Bennett W, Strominger J and Wiley D (1987a) Structure of the human class I histocompatibility antigen HLA-A2. *Nature* **329** 506–512

Bjorkman P, Saper M, Samraoui B, Bennett W, Strominger J and Wiley D (1987b) The foreign antigen-binding site and T cell recognition regions of class I histocompatibility antigens. *Nature* **329** 512–518

Bouillot M, Choppin J, Cornille F *et al* (1989) Physical association between MHC class I molecules and immunogenic peptides. *Nature* **339** 473–475

Bröcker E-B, Suter L, Brüggen J, Ruiter DJ, Macher E and Sorg C (1985) Phenotypic dynamics of tumor progression in human malignant melanoma. *International Journal of Cancer* **36** 29–35

Cannon MJ, Pisa P, Fox RI and Cooper NR (1990) Epstein-Barr virus induces aggressive lymphoproliferative disorders of human B cell origin in SCID/hu chimeric mice. *Journal of Clinical Investigation* **85** 1333–1337

Cerundolo V, Alexander J, Anderson K *et al* (1990) presentation of viral antigen controlled by a gene in the major histocompatibility complex. *Nature* **345** 449–452

Chen BP and Parham P (1989) Direct binding of influenza peptides to class I HLA molecules. *Nature* **337** 743–745

Christinck ER, Luscher MA, Barber BH and Williams DB (1991) Peptide binding to class I MHC on living cells and quantitation of complexes for CTL lysis. *Nature* **352** 67–70

Concha A, Cabrera T, Ruiz-Cabello F and Garrido F (1991) Can the HLA phenotype be used as a prognostic factor in breast carcinoma? *International Journal of Cancer* **6** [**Supplement**] 146–154

Conolly JM, Hansen TH, Ingold AL and Potter TA (1990) Recognition by CD8 on cytotoxic T lymphocytes is ablated by several substitutions in the class I α3 domain: CD8 and the T-cell receptor recognize the same class I molecule. *Proceedings of the National Academy of Sciences of the USA* **87** 2137–2141

Connor ME and Stern PL (1990) Loss of MHC class-I expression in cervical carcinomas. *International Journal of Cancer* **46** 1029–1034

Collins T, Lapierre LA, Fiers W, Strominger JL and Pober JS (1986) Recombinant human tumor necrosis factor increases mRNA levels and surface expression of HLA-A,B antigens in vascular endothelial cells and dermal fibroblasts *in vitro*. *Proceedings of the National Academy of Sciences of the USA* **83** 446–450

Crowley NJ, Darrow TL, Quinn-Allen MA and Seigler HF (1991) MHC-restricted recognition of autologous melanoma by tumor-specific cytotoxic T cells: evidence for restriction by a dominant HLA-A allele. *Journal of Immunology* **146** 1692–1699

Csiba A, Whitwell HL and Moore M (1984) Distribution of histocompatibility and leucocyte differentiation antigens in human colon and in benign and malignant colonic neoplasms. *British Journal of Cancer* **50** 699–709

Daar AS, Fuggle SV, Fabre JW, Ting A and Morris PJ (1984) The detailed distribution of HLA-A,B,C antigens in normal human organs. *Transplantation* **38** 287–292

Darrow TL, Slingluff CL and Seigler HF (1989) The role of HLA class I antigens in recognition of melanoma cells by tumor-specific cytotoxic T lymphocytes: evidence for shared tumor antigens. *Journal of Immunology* **142** 3329–3335

David-Watine B, Israel A and Kourilsky P (1991) The regulation and expression of MHC class I genes. *Immunology Today* **11** 286–292

de Fries RU and Golub SH (1988) Characteristics and mechanisms of IFN-γ-induced protection of human tumor cells from lysis by lymphokine-activated killer cells. *Journal of Immunology* **140** 3686–3693

DeMars R, Chang CC, Shaw S, Reitnauer PJ and Sondel PM (1984) Homozygous deletions that simultaneously eliminate expression of class I and class II antigens of EBV-transformed B-lymphoblastoid cells. *Human Immunology* **11** 77–97

DeMars R, Rudersdorf R, Chang CC *et al* (1985) Mutations that impair a posttranscriptional step in expression of HLA-A and -B antigens. *Proceedings of the National Academy of Sciences of the USA* **82** 8183–8187

Deverson EV, Gow IR, Coadwell WJ *et al* (1990) MHC class II region encoding proteins related to the multidrug resistance family of transmembrane transporters. *Nature* **348** 738–741

Doyle A, Martin WJ, Funa K *et al* (1985) Markedly decreased expression of class I histocompatibility antigens, protein, and mRNA in human small cell lung cancer. *Journal of Experimental Medicine* **161** 1135–1151

Durrant LG, Ballantyne KC, Armitage NC *et al* (1987) Quantitation of MHC antigen expression on colorectal tumours and its association with tumour progression. *British Journal of Cancer* **56** 425–432

D'Urso CM, Wang Z, Cao Y, Takate R, Zeff RA and Ferrone S (1991) Lack of HLA class I antigen expression by cultured melanoma cells FO-1 due to a defect in β_2m gene expression. *Journal of Clinical Investigation* **87** 284–292

Eager KB, Pfitzenmaier K and Ricciardi RP (1989) Modulation of major histocompatibility complex (MHC) class I genes in adenovirus 12 transformed cells: interferon-γ increases class I expression by a mechanism that circumvents E1A induced-repression and tumor necrosis factor enhances the effect of interferon-γ. *Oncogene* **4** 39–44

Emslie-Smith AM, Arahata K and Engel AG (1989) Major histocompatibility complex class I antigen expression, immunolocalization of interferon subtypes, and T cell-mediated cytotoxicity in myopathies. *Human Immunology* **20** 224–231

Erusalimsy JD, Kefford RF, Gilmore DJ and Milstein C (1989) Phorbol esters potentiate the induction of class I HLA expression by interferon α. *Proceedings of the National Academy of Sciences of the USA* **86** 1973–1976

Esteban F, Concha A, Delgado M, Pérez-Ayala M, Ruiz-Cabello F and Garrido F (1990) Lack of MHC class I antigens and tumour aggressiveness of the squamous cell carcinoma of the larynx. *British Journal of Cancer* **62** 1047–1051

Falk K, Rötzschke O, Stevanovic S, Jung G and Rammensee H-G (1991) Allele-specific motifs revealed by sequencing of self-peptides eluted from MHC molecules. *Nature* **351** 290–296

Feltner DE, Cooper M, Weber J, Israel MA and Thiele CJ (1989) Expression of class I histocompatibility antigens in neuroectodermal tumors in independent of the expression of a transfected neuroblastoma *myc* gene. *Journal of Immunology* **143** 4292–4299

Ferguson A, Moore M and Fox H (1985) Expression of MHC products and leukocyte differentiation antigens in gynaecological neoplasms: an immunohistological analysis of the tumor cells and infiltrating leucocytes. *British Journal of Cancer* **52** 551–563

Fleming KA, McMichael A, Morton JA, Woods J and McGee JO'D (1981) Distribution of HLA class I antigens in normal human tissue and in mammary cancer. *Journal of Clinical Patholology* **34** 779–784

Funa K, Gazdar AF, Minna JD and Linnola RI (1986) Paucity of β_2-microglobulin expression on small cell lung cancer, bronchial carcinoids, and certain other neuroendocrine tumors. *Laboratory Investigation* **55** 186–193

Gogusev J, Teutsch B, Morin MT *et al* (1988) Inhibition of HLA class I antigen and mRNA expression induced by Rous sarcoma virus in transformed human fibroblasts. *Proceedings of the National Academy of Sciences of the USA* **85** 203–207

Goodnow CC, Adelstein S and Basten A (1990) The need for central and peripheral tolerance in the B cell repteroire. *Science* **248** 1373–1379

Göttlinger HG, Rieber P, Gokel JM, Lohe KJ and Riethmüller G (1985) Infiltrating mononuclear cells in human breast carcinoma: predominance of T4+ monocytic cells in the tumor stroma. *International Journal of Cancer* **35** 199–205

Grand RJA, Rowe M, Byrd PJ and Gallimore PH (1987) The level of expression of class-I MHC antigens in adenovirus-transformed human cell lines. *International Journal of Cancer* **40** 213–219

Gregory CD, Murray RJ, Edwards CF and Rickinson AB (1988) Downregulation of cell adhesion molecules LFA-3 and ICAM-1 in Epstein-Barr virus-positive Burkitt's lymphoma underlies tumor cell escape from virus-specific T cell surveillance. *Journal of Experimental Medicine* **167** 1811–1824

Grönberg A, Ferm M, Tsai L and Kiessling R (1989) Interferon is able to reduce tumor cell susceptibility to human lymphokine-activated killer (LAK) cells. *Cellular Immunology* **118** 10–21

Gross N, Beck D and Favre S (1990) *In vitro* modulation and relationship between N-*myc* and HLA class I RNA steady-state levels in human neuroblastoma cells. *Cancer Research* **50** 7532–7536

Hakem R, le Bouteiller P, Barad M *et al* (1989) IFN-mediated differential regulation of the expression of HLA-B7 and HLA-A3 class I genes. *Journal of Immunology* **142** 297–305

Hämmerling GJ, Klar D, Plüm W, Momburg F and Moldenhauer G (1987) The influence of major histocompatibility complex class I antigens on tumor growth and metastasis. *Biochimica Biophysica Acta* **907** 245–259

Hämmerling GJ, Chamberlaine JW, Dill O *et al* (1990) Self-tolerance to HLA focuses the response of immunized H1A-transgenic mice on production of antibody to precise polymorphic HLA alloantigens. *Proceedings of the National Academy of Sciences of the USA* **87** 235–239

Hämmerling GJ, Schönrich G, Momburg F *et al* (1991) Non-deletional mechanisms of peripheral and central tolerance: studies with transgenic mice with tissue specific expression of a foreign MHC class I antigen. *Immunological Reviews* **122** 47–68

Heron I, Hokland M and Berg K (1978) Enhanced expression of β_2-microglobulin and HLA antigens on human lymphoid cells by interferon. *Proceedings of the National Academy of Sciences of the USA* **75** 6215–6219

Holden CA, Shaw M, McKee PH, Sanderson AR and MacDonald DM (1984) Loss of membrane β_2 microglobulin in eccrine porocarcinoma: its association with the histopathologic and clinical criteria of malignancy. *Archives of Dermatology* **120** 732–735

Hokland M, Larson B, Heron I and Plessner T (1981) Corticosteroids decrease the expression of β_2-microglobulin and histocompatibility antigens on human peripheral blood lymphocytes in vitro. *Clinical and Experimental Immunology* **44** 239–246

Hosken NA and Bevan MJ (1990) Defective presentation of endogenous antigen by a cell line expressing class I molecules. *Science* **248** 367–37

Houghton AN, Thomson TM, Gross D, Oettgen HF and Old LJ (1984) Surface antigens of melanoma and melanocytes: specificity of induction of Ia antigens by human γ-interferon. *Jounal of Experimental Medicine* **160** 255–269

Itoh K, Platsucas CD and Balch CM (1988) Autologous tumor-specific cytotoxic T lymphocytes in the infiltrate of human metastatic melanomas: activation by interleukin-2 and autologous tumor cells and involvement of the T cell receptor. *Journal of Experimental Medicine* **168** 1419–1441

Jeffries WA and MacPherson GG (1987) Expression of the W6/32 HLA epitope by cells of rat, mouse, human and other species: critical dependence on the interaction of specific MHC heavy chains with human or bovine β_2-microglobulin. *European Journal of Immunology* **17** 1257–1263

Jilg W, Voltz R, Markert-Hahn C, Mairhofer H, Münz I and Wolf H (1991) Expression of class I major histocompatibility complex antigens in Epstein-Barr virus-carrying lymphoblastoid cell lines and Burkitt lymphoma cells. *Cancer Reseach* **51** 27–32

Joncas JH, Russo P, Brochu P *et al* (1990) Epstein-Barr virus polymorphic B-cell lymphoma associated with leukemia and with congenital immunodeficiencies. *Journal of Clinical Oncology* **8** 378–384

Kahn-Perles B, Bowyer C, Arnold B, Sanderson AR, Ferrier P and Lemonnier FA (1987) Acquisition of HLA class I W6/32 defined antigenic determinant by heavy chains from different species following association with bovine β_2-microglobulin. *Journal of Immunology*

138 2190–2196

Kara CJ and Glimcher LH (1991) Regulation of MHC class II gene transcription. *Current Opinion in Immunology* **3** 16–21

Kärre K, Ljunggren HG, Piontek G and Kiessling R (1986) Selective rejection of H-2-deficient lymphoma variants suggests alternative immune defence strategy. *Nature* **319** 675–678

Klar D and Hämmerling GJ (1989) Induction of assembly of MHC class I heavy chains with $\beta_2$microglobulin by interferon-γ. *EMBO Journal* **8** 475–481

Klein B, Klein T, Konichenzky M *et al* (1990) The expression of HLA class I antigens in germ cell testicular cancer. *American Journal of Clinical Pathology* **93** 202–207

Knuth A, Wölfel T, Klehmann E, Boon T and Meyer zum Büschenfelde K-H (1989) Cytolytic T-cell clones against an autologous human melanoma: specificity study and definition of three antigens by immunoselection. *Proceedings of the National Academy of Sciences of the USA* **86** 2804–2808

Koretz K, Momburg F, Otto HF and Möller P (1987) Sequential induction of MHC antigens on autochthonous cells of the ileum affected by Crohn's disease. *American Journal of Pathology* **129** 493–502

Kozlowski S, Takeshita T, Boehnke W-H *et al* (1991) Excess β_2 microglobulin promoting functional peptide association with purified slouble class I MHC molecules. *Nature* **349** 74–77

Kronenberg M (1991) Self-tolerance and autoimmunity. *Cell* **65** 537–542

Lambert ME, Ronai ZA, Weinsten IB and Garrels JI (1989) Enhancement of major histocompatibility class I protein synthesis by DNA damage in cultured human fibroblasts and keratinocytes. *Molecular and Cellular Biology* **9** 847–850

Lampson LA and Fisher CA (1984) Weak HLA and β_2-microglobulin expression of neural cell lines can be modulated by interferon. *Proceedings of the National Academy of Sciences of the USA* **81** 6476–6480

Lampson LA, Fisher CA and Whelan JP (1983) Striking paucity of HLA-A,B,C and β_2-microglobulin on human neuroblastoma cell lines. *Journal of Immunology* **130** 2471–2478

Leiden JM, Karpinsky BA, Gottschalk L and Kornbluth J (1989) Susceptibility to natural killer-mediated cytolysis is independent of the level of target cell class I HLA expression. *Journal of Immunology* **142** 2140–2147

Ljunggren H-G and Kärre K (1985) Host resistance directed selectively against H-2-deficient lymphoma variants: analysis of the mechanism. *Journal of Experimental Medicine* **162** 1745–1759

Lobo PI and Spencer CE (1989) Use of anti-HLA antibodies to mask major histocompatibility complex gene products on tumor cells can enhance susceptibility of these cells to lysis by natural killer cells. *Journal of Clinical Investigation* **83** 278–287

López-Nevot MA, Esteban F, Ferrón A *et al* (1989) HLA class I gene expression on human primary tumours and autologous metastases: demonstration of selective loss of HLA antigens on colorectal, gastric, and laryngeal carcinomas. *British Journal of Cancer* **59** 221–226

Lurquin C, van Pel A, Mariamé B *et al* (1989) Structure of the gene of tum⁻ transplantation antigen P91A: the mutated exon encodes a peptide recognized with Ld by cytolytic T cells. *Cell* **58** 293–301

Maio M, Gulwani B, Langer JA *et al* (1989) Modulation by interferons of HLA antigen, high-molecular-weight melanoma-associated antigen, and intercellular adhesion molecule 1 expression by cultured melanoma cells with different metastatic potential. *Cancer Research* **49** 2980–2987

Marley GM, Doyle LA, Ordóñez JV, Sisk A, Hussain A and Chiu Yen R-W (1989) Potentiation of interferon induction of class I major histocompatibility complex antigen expression by human tumor necrosis factor in small cell lung cancer cell lines. *Cancer Research* **49** 6232–6236

McDougall CJ, Ngoi SS, Goldman IS *et al* (1990) Reduced expression of HLA class I and II antigens in colon cancer. *Cancer Research* **50** 8023–8027

Mechtersheimer G, Staudter M, Majdic O, Dörken B, Moldenhauer G and Möller P (1990) Expression of HLA-A,B,C, β$_2$-microglobulin (β$_2$m), HLA-DR, -DP, -DQ and of HLA-D-associated invariant chain (Ii) in soft tissue tumors. *International Journal of Cancer* **46** 813–823

Migita K, Eguchi K, Akiguchi I *et al* (1991) Synergistic effects of phorbol ester and interferon-α: target cell class I HLA antigen expression and restistance to natural killer and lymphokine-activated killer cell-mediated cytolysis. *Cellular Immunology* **134** 325–335

Möller P, Lämmler B, Herrmann B, Otto HF, Moldenhauer G and Momburg F (1986) The mediastinal clear cell lymphoma of B-cell type has variable defects in MHC antigen expression. *Immunology* **59** 411–417

Möller P, Moldenhauer G, Momburg F *et al* (1987a) Mediastinal lymphoma of clear cell type is a tumor corresponding to terminal steps of B cell differentiation. *Blood* **69** 1087–1095

Möller P, Herrmann B, Moldenhauer G and Momburg F (1987b) Defective expression of MHC class I antigens is frequent in B-cell lymphomas of high grade malignancy. *International Journal of Cancer* **40** 32–39

Möller P, Hofmann WJ, Mielke B and Otto HF (1989a) Das primär mediastinale, hellzellige B-Zell-Lymphom ist ein epithelassoziiertes Thymuslymphom. *Der Pathologe* **10** 234–239

Möller P, Mattfeldt T, Gross C *et al* (1989b) Expression of HLA-A, B, C, -DR, -DP, -DQ and of HLA-D-associated invariant chain (Ii) in non-neoplastic mammary epithelium, fibroadenoma, adenoma, and carcinoma of the breast. *American Journal of Pathology* **135** 73–83

Möller P, Momburg F, Koretz K *et al* (1991a) Influence of major histocompatibility complex class I and II antigens on survival in colorectal carcinoma. *Cancer Research* **51** 729–736

Möller P, Koretz K, Schlag P and Momburg F (1991b) Frequency and abnormal expression of HLA-A,B,C and HLA-DR molecules, invariant chain, and LFA-3 (CD58) in colorectal carcinoma and its impact on tumor recurrence. *International Journal of Cancer* **6** [Supplement] 155–162

Momburg F and Koch S (1989) Selective loss of β$_2$-microglobulin mRNA in human colon carcinoma. *Journal of Experimental Medicine* **169** 309–314

Momburg F, Degener T, Bacchus E, Moldenhauer G, Hämmerling GJ and Möller P (1986) Loss of HLA-A,B,C and *de novo* expression of HLA-D in colorectal carcinoma. *International Journal of Cancer* **38** 459–464

Momburg F, Herrmann B, Moldenhauer G and Möller P (1987) B-cell lymphomas of high-grade malignancy frequently lack HLA-DR, -DP, and DQ antigens and the associated invariant chain. *International Journal of Cancer* **40** 598–603

Momburg F, Ziegler A, Harpprecht J, Möller P, Moldenhauer G and Hämmerling GJ (1989) Selective loss of HLA-A or HLA-B antigen expression in colon carcinoma. *Journal of Immunology* **142** 352–358

Morrison LA, Lukacher AE, Braciale VL, Fan DP and Braciale TJ (1986) Differences in antigen presentation to MHC class I and Class II-restricted influenza virus-specific cytolytic T lymphocyte clones. *Journal of Experimental Medicine* **163** 903–921

Natali PG, Giacomini P, Bigotti A *et al* (1983a) Heterogeneity in the expression of HLA and tumor-associated antigens by surgically removed and cultured breast carcinoma cells. *Cancer Research* **43** 660–668

Natali PG, Cavaliere R, Bigotti A *et al* (1983b) Antigenic heterogeneity of surgically removed primary and autologous metastatic human melanoma lesions. *Journal of Immunology* **130** 1462–1466

Natali PG, Bigotti A, Nicotra MR, Viora M, Manfredi D and Ferrone S (1984) Distribution of human class I (HLA-A,B,C) histocompatibility antigens in normal and malignant tissues of nonlymphoid origin. *Cancer Research* **44** 4679–4687

Nilsson K, Evrin PE and Welsh KI (1974) Production of β2-microglobulin in normal and malignant human cell lines and peripheral lymphocytes. *Transplantion Reviews* **21** 53–84

Nissen MH, Larsen JK, Plesner T, Olesen BK and Ernst P (1985) α-Interferon induces enhanced expression of HLA-A,B,C antigens and β-2-microglobulin *in vivo* and *in vitro* in various subsets of human lymphoid cells. *Clinical and Experimental Immunology* **69** 632–

638

Nisticò P, Tecce R, Giacomini P *et al* (1990) Effect of recombinant human leukocyte, fibroblast, and immune interferons on expression of class I and II major histocompatibility complex and invariant chain in early passage human melanoma cells. *Cancer Research* **50** 7422–7429

Nossal GJV (1991) B-cell selection and tolerance. *Current Opinion in Immunology* **3** 193–198

Nouri AMF, Smith D, Crosby D and Oliver RTD (1990) Selective and non-selective loss of immunoregulatory molecules (HLA-A,B,C antigens and LFA-3) in transitional cell carcinoma. *British Journal of Cancer* **62** 603–606

Nuchtern JG, Bonifacio JS, Biddison WE *et al* (1989) Brefeldin A implicates egress from endoplasmic reticulum in class I restricted antigen presentation. *Nature* **339** 223–226

Öhlén C, Bejarano M-T, Grönberg A *et al* (1989) Studies of sublines selected for loss of HLA expression from an EBV-transformed lymphoblastoid cell line: changes in sensitivity to cytotoxic T cells activated by allostimulation and natural killer cells activated by IFN or IL-2. *Journal of Immunology* **142** 3336–3341

Oliva MR, Cabrera T, Esquivias J *et al* (1990) K-*ras* mutations (codon 12) are not involved in down-regulation of MHC class-I genes in colon carcinomas. *International Journal of Cancer* **46** 426–431

Ortiz-Navarette V and Hämmerling GJ (1991) Surface appearance and instability of empty H-2 class I molecules under physiological conditions. *Proceedings of the National Academy of Sciences of the USA* **88** 3594–3597

Otten GR and Germain RN (1991) Split anergy in a CD8+ T cell: receptor-dependent cytolysis in the absence of interleukin-2 production. *Science* **251** 1228–1231

Ottesen SS, Kieler J and Christensen B (1987) Changes in HLA A,B,C expression during spontaneous transformation of human urothelial cells in vitro. *European Journal of Clinical Oncology* **23** 991–995

Pandolfi F, Boyle LA, Trentin L, Kurnick JT, Isselbacher KJ and Gattoni-Celli S (1991) Expression of HLA-A2 antigen in human melanoma cell lines and its role in T-cell recognition. *Cancer Research* **51** 3164–3170

Paterson AC, Sciot R, Kew MC, Callea F, Dusheiko GM and Desmet VJ (1988) HLA expression in human hepatocellular carcinoma. *British Journal of Cancer* **57** 369–373

Pelicci P-G, Knowles II DM, Arlin ZA *et al* (1986) Multiple monoclonal B cell expansions and c-*myc* oncogene rearrangements in acquired immune deficiency syndrome-related lymphoproliferative disorders: implications for lymphomagenesis. *Journal of Experimental Medicine* **164** 2049–2076

Pena J, Anlonso C, Solana R, Serrano R, Carracedo J and Ramirez R (1990) Natural killer susceptibility is independent of HLA class I antigen expression on cell lines obtained from human solid tumours. *European Journal of Immunology* **20** 2445–2449

Pérez M, Cabrera T, Lopéz-Nevot MA *et al* (1986) Heterogeneity of the expression of class I and II HLA antigens in human breast carcinoma. *Journal of Immunogenetics* **13** 247–253

Pfizenmaier K, Scheurich P, Schlüter C and Krönke M (1987) Tumor necrosis factor enhances HLA-A,B,C and HLA-DR gene expression in human tumor cells. *Journal of Immunology* **138** 975–980

Quillet A, Presse F, Marchiol-Fournigault C *et al* (1988) Increased resistance to non-MHC-restricted cytotoxicity related to HLA A B expression: direct demonstration using β_2-microglobulin-transfected Daudi cells. *Journal of Immunology* **141** 17–20

Ramsdell F and Fowlkes BJ (1990) Clonal deletion versus clonal anergy: the role of the thymus in inducing self tolerance. *Science* **248** 1342–1348

Recny MA, Neidhardt EA, Sayre PH, Ciardelli TL and Reinherz EL (1990) Structural and functional charcterization of the CD2 immunoadhesion domain. *Journal of Biological Chemistry* **265** 8542–8549

Redondo M, Ruiz-Cabello, Concha A *et al* (1991) Altered HLA class I expression in non-small cell lung cancer is independent of c-*myc* activation. *Cancer Research* **51** 2463–2468

Rees RC, Buckle AM, Gelsthorpe K *et al* (1988) Loss of polymorphic A and B locus HLA antigens in colon carcinoma. *British Journal of Cancer* **57** 374–377

Robbins PA and McMichael AJ (1991) Immune recognition of HLA molecules downmodulates CD8 expression on cytotoxic T lymphocytes. *Journal of Experimental Medicine* **173** 221–230

Rocha B and von Boemer H (1991) Peripheral selection of the T cell repertoire. *Science* **251** 1225–1228

Rock KL, Gamble S, Rothstein L, Gramm C and Benacerraf B (1991) Dissociation of β2-microglobulin leads to the accumulation of a substantial pool of inactive class I MHC heavy chains on the cell surface. *Cell* **65** 611–620

Rosa F, Fellous M, Dron M, Tovey M and Revel M (1983a) Presence of an abnormal β2-microglobulin mRNA in Daudi cells: induction by interferon. *Immunogenetics* **17** 125–131

Rosa R, Berissi H, Weissenbach J, Maroteaux L, Fellous M and Revel M (1983b) The β$_2$-microglobulin mRNA in human Daudi cells has a mutated initiation codon but is still inducible by interferon. *EMBO Journal* **2** 239–243

Rosenberg SA, Packard BS, Aebersold PM *et al* (1988) Use of tumor-infiltrating lymphocytes and interleukin-2 in the immunotherapy of patients with metastatic melanoma: a preliminary report. *New England Journal of Medicine* **319** 1676–1680

Rötzschke O, Falk K, Deres K *et al* (1990) Isolation and analysis of naturally processed viral peptides as recognized by cytotoxic cells. *Nature* **348** 252–254

Ruiter DJ, Bhan AK, Harrist TJ, Sober AJ and Mihm MC Jr (1982) Major histocompatibility antigens and mononuclear inflammatory infiltrate in benign nevomelanocytic proliferations and malignant melanoma. *Journal of Immunology* **129** 2808–2815

Ruiter DJ, Bergmann W, Welvaart K *et al* (1984) Immunohistochemical analysis of malignant melanomas and nevocellular nevi with monoclonal antibodies to distinct monomorphic determinants of HLA antigens. *Cancer Research* **44** 3930–3935

Salter RD and Cresswell P (1986) Impaired assembly and transport of HLA-A and -B antigens in a mutant TxB cell hybrid. *EMBO Journal* **5** 943–949

Salter RD, Norment AM, Chen BP *et al* (1989) Polymorphism in the α3 domain of HLA-A molecules affects binding to CD8. *Nature* **338** 345–347

Salter RD, Benjamin RJ, Wesley PK *et al* (1990) The binding site for the T-cell co-receptor CD8 in the α3 domain of HLA-A2. *Nature* **345** 41–46

Sanderson AR and Beverley PCL (1983) Interferon, β-2-microglobulin and immunoselection in the pathway to malignancy. *Immunology Today* **4** 211–213

Scheppler JA, Nicholson JKA, Swan DC, Ahmed-Ansari A and McDougal JS (1989) Down-modulation of MHC-I in a CD4+ T cell line, CEM-E5, after HIV-1 infection. *Journal of Immunology* **143** 2858–2866

Schnabl E, Stockinger H, Majdic O *et al* (1990) Activated human T lymphocytes express MHC class I heavy chains not associated with β2-microglobulin. *Journal of Experimental Medicine* **171** 1431–1442

Schönrich G, Kalinke U, Momburg F *et al* (1991) Down-regulation of T cell receptors on self-reactive T cells as a novel mechanism for extrathymic tolerance induction. *Cell* **65** 293–304

Schumacher TNM, deBruijn MLH, Vernie LN *et al* (1991) Peptide selection by MHC class I molecules. *Nature* **350** 703–706

Schwartz RH (1990) A cell culture model for T lymphocyte clonal anergy. *Science* **248** 1349–1356

Seong RH, Clayberger CA, Krensky AM and Parnes JR (1988) Rescue of Daudi cell HLA expression by transfection of the mouse β2-microglobulin gene. *Journal of Experimental Medicine* **167** 288–299

Shimizu Y and DeMars R (1989) Demonstration by class I gene transfer that reduced susceptibility of human cells to natural killer cell-mediated lysis is inversely correlated with HLA class I antigen expression. *European Journal of Immunology* **19** 447–451

Silver ML, Parker KC and Wiley DC (1991) Reconstitution by MHC-restricted peptides of

HLA-A2 heavy chain with β2 microglobulin, *in vitro. Nature* **350** 619–622

Slovin SF, Lackman RD, Ferrone S, Kiely PE and Mastrangelo MJ (1986) Cellular immune response to human sarcomas: cytotoxic T cell clones reactive with autologous sarcomas I: development, phenotype, and specificity. *Journal of Immunology* **137** 3042–3048

Smith MEF, Marsh SGE, Bodmer JG, Gelsthorpe K and Bodmer WF (1989) Loss of HLA-A,B,C allele products and lymphocyte function-associated antigen 3 in colorectal neoplasia. *Proceedings of the National Academy of Sciences of the USA* **86** 5557–5561

Soong TW and Hui KM (1991) Identification of locus-specific DNA-binding factors for the regulation of HLA class-I genes in human colorectal cancer. *International Journal of Cancer* **6 [Supplement]** 131–137

Spies T, Bresnahan M, Bahram S *et al* (1990) A gene in the major histocompatibility complex class II region controlling the class I antigen presentation pathway. *Nature* **348** 744–747

Stam NJ, Kast MW, Voordouw AC *et al* (1989) Lack of correlation between levels of MHC class I antigen and susceptibility to lysis of small cellular lung carcinoma (SCLC) by natural killer cells. *Journal of Immunology* **142** 4113–4117

Stein B, Momburg F, Schwarz V, Schlag P, Moldenhauer G and Möller P (1988) Reduction or loss of HLA-A,B,C antigens in colorectal carcinoma appears not to influence survival. *British Journal of Cancer* **57** 364–368

Stern P, Gidlund M, Örn A and Wigzell H (1982) Natural killer cells mediate lysis of embryonal carcinoma cells lacking MHC. *Nature* **285** 341–342

Storkus WJ, Howell DN, Salter RD, Dawson JR and Cresswell P (1987) NK susceptibility varies inversely with target cell class I HLA antigen expression. *Journal of Immunology* **138** 1657–1659

Storkus WJ, Alexander J, Payne JA, Dawson JR and Cresswell P (1989) Reversal of natural killing susceptibility in target cells expressing transfected class I HLA genes. *Proceedings of the National Academy of Sciences of the USA* **86** 2361–2364

Storkus WJ, Salter RD, Alexander J *et al* (1991) Class I-induced resistance to natural killing: identification of nonpermissive residues in HLA-A2. *Proceedings of the National Academy of Sciences of the USA* **88** 5989–5992

Sturmhöfel K and Hämmerling GJ (1990) Reconstitution of H-2 class I expression by gene transfection decreases susceptibility to natural killer cells of an EL4 class I loss variant. *European Journal of Immunology* **20** 171–177

Sugio K, Nakagawara A and Sasazuki T (1991) Association of expression between N-*myc* gene and major histocompatibility complex class I gene in surgically resected human neuroblastoma. *Cancer* **67** 1384–1388

Sweetser MT, Morrison LA, Braciale VL and Braciale TJ (1989) Recognition of pre-processed endogenous antigen by class I but not class II MHC-restricted T cells. *Nature* **342** 180–182

Swinnen LJ, Costanzo-Nordin MR, Fisher SG *et al* (1990) Increased incidence of lymphoproliferative disorder after immunosuppression with the monoclonal antibody OKT3 in cardiac-transplant recipients. *New England Journal of Medicine* **323** 1723–1728

Symington FW and Santos EB (1991) Lysis of human keratinocytes by allogeneic HLA class I-specific cytotoxic T cells: keratinocyte ICAM-1 (CD54) and T cell LFA-1 (CD11a/CD18) mediate enhanced lysis of IFN-γ-treated keratinocytes. *Journal of Immunology* **146** 2169–2175

Tahara T, Young SY, Khan R, Abish S, Hämmerling GJ and Hämmerling U (1990) HLA antibody responses in HLA-class I transgenic mice. *Immunogenetics* **32** 351–360

Taramelli D, Fossati G, Mazzocchi A, Delia D, Ferrone S and Rarmiani G (1986) Classes I and II HLA and melanoma-associated antigen expression and modulation on melanoma cells isolated from primary and metastatic lesions. *Cancer Research* **46** 433–449

Topalian SL, Solomon D and Rosenberg SA (1989) Tumor-specific cytolysis by lymphocytes infiltrating human melanomas. *Journal of Immunology* **142** 3714–3725

Tomita Y, Matsumoto Y, Nishiyama T and Fujiwara M (1990) Reduction of major histocompatibility complex class-I antigens on invasive and high-grade transitional cell carcinoma.

Journal of Pathology **162** 157–164

Townsend A, Öhlén C, Bastin J, Ljunggren HG and Kärre K (1989) A mutant cell in which association of class I heavy and light chains is induced by viral peptides. *Cold Spring Habor Symposia on Quantitative Biology* **54** 299–308

Townsend A, Elliot T, Cerundolo V, Foster L, Barber B and Tse A (1990) Assembly of MHC class I molecules analyzed in vitro. *Cell* **62** 285–295

Trowsdale J, Hanson I, Mockridge I, Beck S, Townsend A and Kelly A (1990) Sequence encoded in the class II region of the MHC related to the "ABC" superfamily of transporters. *Nature* **348** 741–744

Turbitt ML and Mackie RM (1981) Loss of β_2 microglobulin from the cell surface of cutaneous malignant and premalignant lesions. *British Journal of Dermatology* **104** 507–513

Van Bleek G and Nathenson SG (1990) Isolation of an endogenously processed immunodominant viral peptide from the class I H-K^b molecule. *Nature* **348** 213–216

van den Eynde B, Lethé B, van Pel A, de Plaen E and Boon T (1991) The gene coding for a major tumor rejection antigen of tumor P815 is identical to the normal gene of synthetic DBA/2 mice. *Journal of Experimental Medicine* **173** 1373–1384

van den Ingh HF, Ruiter DJ, Griffioen G, van Muijen GNP and Ferrone S (1987) HLA antigens in colorectal tumors—low expression of HLA class I antigens in mucinous colorectal carcinomas. *British Journal of Cancer* **55** 125–130

van Duinen SG, Ruiter DJ, Broecker EB et al (1988) Level of HLA antigens in locoregional metastases and clinical course of the disease in patients with melanoma. *Cancer Research* **48** 1019–1025

Vánky F, Roberts T, Klein E and Willems J (1987) Auto-tumor immunity in patients with solid tumors: participation of CD3 complex and MHC class I antigens in the lytic interaction. *Immunology Letters* **16** 21–26

Vánky F, Stuber G, Rotstein S and Klein E (1989) Auto-tumor recognition following in vitro induction of MHC antigen expression on solid tumors: stimulation of lymphocytes and generation of cytotoxicity against the original MHC-antigen-negative tumor cells. *Cancer Immunology and Immunotherapy* **28** 17–21

Versteeg R, Noordermeer IA, Krüse-Wolters M, Ruiter DJ and Schrier PI (1988) c-*myc* downregulates class I HLA expression in human melanomas. *EMBO Journal* **7** 1023–1029

Versteeg R, Krüse-Wolters KM, Plomp AC et al (1989) Suppression of class I human histocompatibility leukocyte antigen by c-*myc* is locus specific. *Journal of Experimental Medicine* **170** 621–635

Versteeg R, van der Minne C, Plomp A, Sijts A, van Leeuven A and Schrier P (1990) N-*myc* expression switched off and class I human leukocyte antigen expression switched on after somatic cell fusion of neuroblastoma cells. *Molecular and Cellular Biology* **10** 5416–5423

von Knebel-Doeberitz M, Koch S, Drzonek H and zur Hausen H (1990) Glucocorticoid hormones reduce the expression of major histocompatibility class I antigens on human epithelial cells. *European Journal of Immunology* **20** 35–40

Walden PR and Eisen HN (1990) Cognate peptides induce self-destruction of CD8$^+$ cytolytic T lymphocytes. *Proceedings of the National Academy of Sciences of the USA* **87** 9015–9019

Wallach D, Fellous M and Revel M (1982) Preferential effect of γ interferon on the synthesis of HLA antigens and their mRNAs in human cells. *Nature* **299** 833–836

Weiss MA, Michael JG, Pesce AJ and DiPersio L (1981) Heterogeneity of β2-microglobulin in human breast carcinoma. *Laboratory Investigation* **45** 46–57

Winter CC, Carreno BM, Turner RV, Koenig S and Biddison WE (1991) The 45 pocket of HLA-A2.1 plays a role in presentation of influenza virus matrix peptide and alloantigens. *Journal of Immunology* **146** 3508–3512

Wintzer H-O, Benzing M and von Kleist S (1990) Lacking prognostic significance of β2-microglobulin, MHC class I and class II antigen expression in breast carcinomas. *British Journal of Cancer* **62** 289–295

Wölfel T, Klehmann, E, Müller C, Schütt KH, Meyer zum Büschenfelde K-H and Knuth A

(1989) Lysis of human melanoma cells by autologous cytolytic T cell clones: identification of human histocompatibility leukocyte antigen A2 as an restriction element for three different antigens. *Journal of Experimental Medicine* **170** 797–810

Yewdell JW and Bennik JR (1989) Brefeldin A specifically inhibits presentation of protein antigens to cytotoxic T lymphocytes. *Science* **244** 1072–1075

Zinkernagel RM and Doherty PC (1974) Restriction of in vitro T cell-mediated cytotoxicity in lymphocytic choriomeningitis within a syngeneic or semiallogeneic system. *Nature* **248** 701–702

Zinkernagel RM and Doherty PC (1979) MHC-restricted cytotoxic T cells: studies on the biological role of polymorphic major transplantation antigens determining T cell restriction —specificity, function and responsiveness. *Advances in Immunology* **27** 51–177

The authors are responsible for the accuracy of the references.

Immunity and Metastasis: In situ Activation of Protective T Cells by Virus Modified Cancer Vaccines

VOLKER SCHIRRMACHER

Institut für Immunologie und Genetik, Deutsches Krebsforschungszentrum, Im Neuenheimer Feld 280, 6900 Heidelberg 1, Germany

INTRODUCTION

Treatment of metastases poses great problems to clinical oncologists. By the time many cancers are diagnosed, metastasis has already occurred, and the presence of multiple metastases makes complete eradication by surgery, radiation or cytostatic drugs impossible. Immunotherapy appears to be a logical adjunct for the treatment of minimal residual disease after destruction of the major tumour bulk by other types of therapy, because the tumour mass that must be destroyed by host defences is smallest at that point. The possible involvement of the immune system in the control of tumour development and metastasis formation in humans is still a matter of some debate. According to the fifth cancer patient survival report (Axtell *et al*, 1976), at least 9% of breast cancer patients (about 3700 per year in the USA) live with dormant metastases for more than 10 years. Similar observations of long term patient survival have been made for some other common cancers (Hankey and Steinhorn, 1982) and suggest a long term host resistance to micrometastasis (Zajicek, 1985, 1987). The natural environment of cancer cells is not an optimized cell culture system but rather one of a responding host manifesting at least some degree of immunocompetence. The development of a primary tumour may have primed the immune system, but without appropriate secondary stimulation of primed or memory cells (eg via two signal stimulation), there may be no maturation into active immune effector cells. Metastases could therefore develop concomitantly with primed but inactive immune effector cells. It is also possible that those tumour cells that have managed to survive passage through the circulation have been able to escape or avoid immune surveillance mechanisms. The molecular basis of such immune escape mechanisms is receiving increasing attention (Goodenow *et al*, 1985) and may open new approaches to immune modulation.

Numerous investigators have studied the possibilities that innate host immune mechanisms offer for control of cancer metastasis. For immunological treatment strategies to be successful, at least three major points have to be considered: the heterogeneous nature of malignant neoplasms (Aukerman and Fidler, 1987; Nicolson, 1987), the intrinsic antigenicity/immunogenicity of metastatic tumour cells (Fidler *et al*, 1979; Klein, 1980) and the ability of the autologous host to recognize and destroy susceptible tumour cells (Stötter and Lotze, (1990). In recent years, therapeutic strategies have been developed that attempt to boost the function of the immune system in patients with cancer. The three basic strategies that are currently being employed are: (a) in vivo treatment with tumour vaccines, immunotoxins and/or biological response modifiers (BRM) (Foon, 1989); (b) ex vivo treatment of patient plasma in an attempt to remove suppressor factors and/or activate endogenous anti-tumour factors (Stevenson *et al*, 1984); and (c) ex vivo treatment of patient leukocytes in an attempt to expand their numbers (or to augment their anti-tumour function) followed by reinfusion into the patient (Rosenberg *et al*, 1988; Bolhuis, 1989; Osband *et al*, 1990).

The exploitation of the immune system with gene technology has led to the identification, isolation and mass production of cloned molecules such as cytokines, including haematopoietic growth factors with potent immuno-modulating capabilities. Some of these factors have allowed the in vitro cloning, expansion and activation of T lymphocytes, which are the most important cells involved in the regulation of the immune response. The T cells discriminate self from non-self and determine whether an antigen is to be ignored or an immune response is to be initiated and thus play a key part in tumour cell recognition and rejection. The use of monoclonal antibodies has defined a range of cell surface molecules—antigen specific T cell receptors (TCR), major histocompatibility complex (MHC) molecules and cell adhesion molecules (CAM), which are of major importance in T lymphocyte function. The TCR complex is the entity that most clearly defines T cells and controls their function; MHC and CAM have important roles in antigen presentation, cell-cell interactions, signal transduction and lymphocyte homing (Springer, 1990).

In spite of this progress in cellular immunology and molecular biology, our understanding of the function of T cells in vivo is still rather limited. More than other components of the immune system, T cells are affected by and exert their effects on cells with which they are in intimate contact. This is obvious when considering the interactions of CD4 helper T cells with antigen presenting cells or CD8 cytotoxic T cells with virus infected or tumour target cells. Such cell-cell interactions are likely to involve lymphokines, which can be focused to perform their function in short ranges and short time intervals. The analysis of such in vivo functions requires adoptive cell transfer studies among others. Such studies, which would also be pertinent to our understanding of cancer rejection mechanisms, are, however, hampered by the availability of in vitro cloned T cells and by the frustrating experience that such in vitro propagated T cells perform relatively badly in vivo, most likely because of downregulation of their homing receptors (Dailey *et al*, 1982; Mitchison, 1989). Also important in this context is the role of the extracellular matrix (ECM), which constitutes the extracellular milieu in vivo and which can markedly affect the response of cells, for instance, to cytokines. Recent evidence, summarized by Nathan and Sporn (1991), documents at least seven types of interactions between cytokines, ECM and cell adhesion phenomena.

Several reviews on different aspects of cancer immunology and immunotherapy have been published recently (Foon, 1989; Bystryn, 1990; Parmiani, 1990; Rosenberg, 1990). My comments and discussion focus on the role of the host specific T cell immunity system as a key mechanism in cancer rejection (Kedar and Klein, in press; Melief, in press) and its possible exploitation for strategies in the treatment of metastases. I shall discuss and compare procedures of in situ activation with in vitro activation and expansion and shall consider the feasibility, effectiveness and side effects of active specific immunotherapy (ASI) procedures with tumour vaccines.

UNDERSTANDING CANCER REJECTION MECHANISMS: GUIDELINES FOR IMMUNOTHERAPEUTIC STRATEGIES

Clinical Observations

Clinical trials aimed at intervening in malignant diseases with either active or passive/adoptive immunotherapies have had variable success. Success with cancer immunotherapy seems to depend on (a) tumour properties (eg histological origin, immunogenicity and metastatic capacity); (b) tumour location, burden and disease stage; (c) heterogeneity of the tumour cell population; and (d) ability of the host immune system to mount a cell mediated anti-tumour response. I focus on the first and last points and discuss the possible role of tumour immunogenicity and host T cell responses. In tests of the clinical efficacy of interleukin-2 (IL-2) treatment with or without application of lymphokine activated killer (LAK) cells, significant clinical responses have been observed, mostly in patients with melanoma or renal cell carcinoma (Rosenberg, 1990). However, considerable toxicity is involved with IL-2 therapy (Siegel and Pori, 1991). Even in these two diseases, only about a quarter or fewer of the patients responded to the treatment. Similar response rates were obtained in melanoma patients with less toxic immunological strategies, such as active immunization with cancer vaccines (Cassel *et al*,

1983; Euhus *et al,* 1989; Berd *et al,* 1990; Mitchell *et al,* 1990) or treatment with interferon-α (IFN-α) with or without chemotherapy (Kedar and Klein, in press). It has not been possible so far either to identify and preselect potential responder patients or to explain why a particular immunotherapy was successful in one patient, whereas the same procedure did not work in another patient. Because of this uncertainty, it is important to improve our understanding of basic mechanisms of cancer rejection and to orient immunological procedures through monitoring assays that correlate with protective immunity and clinical prognosis.

The following hypothesis could be proposed: patients who respond to immunotherapy are those whose tumours are immunogenic and who have the capacity to produce an endogenous, low level anti-tumour response when sufficiently stimulated. Potentially immunogenic human tumours include melanoma and renal cell carcinoma, in addition to virus associated cancers (Burkitt's lymphoma and cervical carcinoma). Non-virally induced human tumours can be expected to be either non-immunogenic (like some spontaneous murine tumours [Hewitt *et al,* 1976]) or weakly immunogenic (like the murine tumours induced by low dose chemical stimuli or ultraviolet light). Patients who fail to respond may carry non-immunogenic tumours or lack relevant T cell clones. Failure to respond to immunotherapy may also be due to active suppression via suppressor cells or soluble inhibitory factors. Prior tumour debulking may reduce the levels of suppressor cells or factors, but additional measures may be needed. Measures to eliminate suppression can include inhibitors of the cyclo-oxygenase pathway (indomethacin, ibuprofen, aspirin), the histamine H2 receptor blocker cimetidine, low dose chemotherapy (cyclophosphamide, adriamycin, cisplatin) or filtration by plasmapheresis (Kedar and Klein, in press).

Absence of immunogenicity does not necessarily mean absence of tumour associated antigens. It could be due to inappropriate localization of the tumour, to absence of expression of helper determinants that may be needed for effective T-T cell interaction or to poor expression of CAMs or MHC antigens. The role of MHC antigens for presentation of antigenic peptides and for recognition of tumour associated transplantation antigens (TATA) and the putative roles of MHC molecules in malignant cell progression and metastases are discussed by T Boon *et al,* C Melief and W Kast, and P Möller and G Hämmerling in this issue.

Experimental Studies

The importance of tumour immunogenicity and T cell mediated specific immune responses in cancer rejection mechanisms is substantiated by the results of studies in animal models. This can be illustrated with our own observations and results obtained in the murine ESb tumour model (Schirrmacher, 1989). ESb is a spontaneous highly metastatic variant of the L5178Y/E lymphoma of the DBA/2 mouse. The site of tumour cell inoculation and its microenviron-

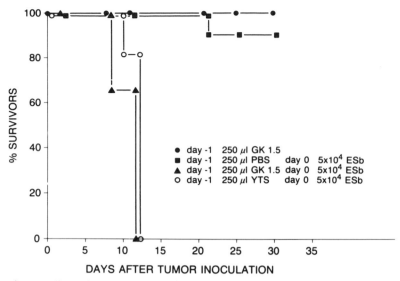

Fig. 1. Effect of in vivo depletion of either CD4 or CD8 T lymphocytes on the survival of DBA/2 mice inoculated into the ear pinna with syngeneic ESb lymphoma cells. Depleting monoclonal antibodies against CD4 (GK 1.5) or CD8 (YTS) (250 μg immunoglobulin) or phosphate buffered saline (PBS) were injected intraperitoneally into groups of mice 24 hr before the tumour cells. Non-T-cell depleted mice survived because of induction of systemic anti-tumour immunity (Schild *et al*, 1987)

ment play an important role in tumour/host interactions, such as invasion, angiogenesis and immune responses (Schirrmacher *et al*, 1982). Although the tumour cells are highly invasive in vitro (Erkell and Schirrmacher, 1988) and highly metastatic from most sites in vivo, some sites such as the ear pinna are privileged for tumour rejection. Syngeneic host immune T cells are able to recognize a distinct TATA that can induce protective immunity and tumour specific cytolytic T lymphocytes (CTL) after appropriate restimulation. In defining the parameters for induction of effective protective anti-tumour immunity in syngeneic mice, we could demonstrate a strict dependency of tumour rejection (a) on the presence of regulatory CD4 T cells and effector CD8 T cells and (b) on the site of tumour inoculation. Syngeneic mice injected with 5×10^4 live ESb cells into the ear pinna survived during the entire observation period without outgrowth of tumour cells, whereas mice depleted of either CD4 or CD8 T cells by pretreatment with the respective depleting monoclonal antibodies (MAbs) developed tumours and metastases and died within 2 weeks (Fig. 1). In vitro, an analogous requirement for immune CD4 T cells for induction of CD8 tumour specific cytotoxic T cells was found (Schild *et al*, 1988). These results thus demonstrate a role for regulatory CD4 T cells and T-T cell cooperation in the in vivo induction of protective anti-tumour immunity and tumour rejection and point to possible therapeutic interventions in the afferent phase of anti-tumour immune responses. On the basis of these and other findings, we postulate that the TATA detected in immunization/pro-

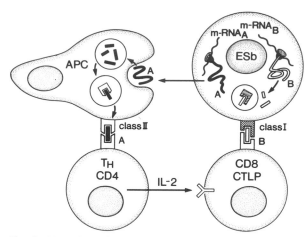

Fig. 2. Hypothetical model for recognition of ESb specific TATA via two cognate interactions. CD8 CTL recognize an MHC class I restricted epitope B and CD4 helper T cells recognize an MHC class II restricted epitope A. A is presented via antigen presenting cells (APC) and B as an endogenous peptide by the tumour cells. Arrows indicate the non-cognate interactions, ie endocytosis of shed tumour proteins by APC and interaction of cytokine with cytokine receptor

tection experiments may consist of two epitopes, A and B, that associate with class II or class I MHC molecules, respectively (Fig. 2). If so, there are several possibilities, namely (a) A=B (eg one mutated peptide); (b) A≠B (two different epitopes from the same protein) or (c) A≠B (two different epitopes derived from two different proteins). Epitope A may be recognized as an exogenous protein (as material from dead tumour cells or as shed or secreted material via antigen presenting cells), whereas epitope B may be recognized as an endogenous peptide.

Results from cytokine mediated immunotherapy experiments in animal models also point towards immune T cell responses as having a key role for protection: (a) Marked anti-tumour effects were obtained in mice with advanced weakly immunogenic tumours by treatment with either IL-2 +/– LAK cells or tumour infiltrating lymphocytes (TIL), with or without adjunct chemotherapy, or with cytokine combinations (IL-2, IFN-α, tumour necrosis factor-α [TNF-α]). In contrast, such treatment regiment proved to be ineffective against non-immunogenic tumours (Mulé *et al*, 1987; Kedar *et al*, 1990). (b) Depletion in vivo of either CD4 or CD8 T cells but not of NK cells (asialo GM 1+) before IL-2 treatment reduced the therapeutic effects in tumour bearing mice (Cameron *et al*, 1988). (c) Mice cured of transplanted weakly immunogenic tumours by treatment with IL-2 were shown to possess long term specific immunity. (d) Spleen cells taken from such mice 3–6 months after they had been cured with IL-2 based treatments could confer specific immunity to naive recipients, with most of the protective activity residing in the CD8 T cell subset (Kedar *et al*, 1989, 1990). (e) The frequency of anti-tumour CTL precursors among spleen cells of such cured mice was five to ten times greater than among spleen cells from control mice (Kedar E, personal communication).

The question of how protective T cells function can be studied by adoptive cell transfer: (a) transfer of specifically sensitized helper or cytotoxic T cell populations or T cell clones together with IL-2 was shown to cause rejection of transplanted immunogenic tumours (Cheever *et al*, 1986; Kast *et al*, 1989; Melief, in press); (b) comparative studies of autologous LAK cells and more specific TIL revealed that the latter had a better protective capacity in animal models and better tumour targeting properties in patients (Griffith *et al*, 1989); (c) the production of lymphokines, such as IFN-γ and TNF by adoptively transferred non-cytotoxic CD4 (Kitagawa *et al*, 1991) or CD8 (Barth *et al*, 1991) immune T cells can also play an important part in tumour or allograft rejection; and (d) in vitro expanded IL-2 dependent T cells have impaired in vivo homing properties resulting from downmodulation of homing receptors (Dailey *et al*, 1982).

Because of these impaired functions of in vitro propagated T cells, we tried to activate syngeneic tumour specific T cells under more physiological conditions in situ. The first successful in situ activation of tumour specific CTL was achieved in vascularized polyurethane matrices which had been preimplanted subcutaneously into ESb tumour immune animals. The application of irradiated ESb cells as tumour vaccine into such vascularized sponges led to the activation of mature CD8 CTL that could (a) directly and specifically lyse the ESb tumour cells, (b) recruit circulating host leukocytes to the site of antigen contact and (c) transfer complete anti-tumour protective capacity. Figure 3 illustrates results obtained in such an adoptive transfer system with in situ activated sponge cells (ASC) or with in vitro activated LAK cells, two populations of cytotoxic cells that had similar cytotoxic anti-tumour activity in vitro. Recipient animals also carried vascularized implanted sponge grafts into which 10^5 live ESb tumour cells were injected (day 0). The ASC were directly pressed out from sponges of the donor mice 3 days after in situ vaccination. When ASC immune cells were injected on day 0 directly into the sponges, they completely protected the animals against the outgrowth of the tumour cells. Complete protection was also achieved with CD4 T cell depleted ASC cells. In contrast, no protection was seen with CD8 T cell depleted ASC or with non-specific LAK cells (Fig. 3a). Figure 3b shows similar results obtained with tail vein injection of the ASC effector cells. This demonstrates that the in situ activated cells maintained not only their protective immune capacity but also their homing properties to detect the tumour cells in the sponges. The protective effects were seen without exogenous cytokines. This indicates that the experimental conditions simulated physiological conditions in situ.

We have also been able to generate tumour protective T cells in situ in the peritoneal cavity (Schirrmacher *et al*, 1991a). It was possible to generate syngeneic tumour specific CTL in situ within no more than 9 days by priming in the ear pinna and restimulating in the peritoneal cavity. These were the optimum sites for T cell induction (afferent arm, priming) and restimulation (ef-

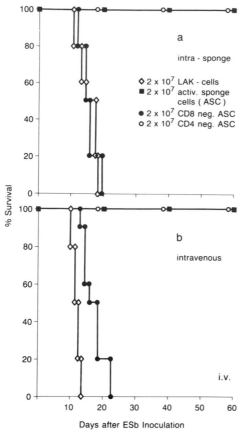

Fig. 3. Diagrammatic representation of the two adhesion pathways that can mediate CTL-target cell conjugation and thereby facilitate immunologically specific recognition via the T cell receptor/HLA-peptide complex. Adhesion can occur via interaction of LFA 1 on the CTL surface with ICAM 1 on the target, and via interaction of CD2 on the CTL with LFA 3 in the target; these interactions are independent of immunologically specific recognition but may be enhanced by it

ferent arm, effector cell activation), respectively. The peritoneal CD8 effector T cells (PEC) recognized the ESb TATA in association with the K^d class I antigen and were able to transfer protective immunity without exogenous IL-2 into normal syngeneic mice.

Tables 1 and 2 summarize the main findings of protective T cell immunity and cancer rejection mechanisms as analysed in the metastatic ESb tumour system. It seems appropriate to differentiate between induction (priming) requirements (Table 1) and activation (secondary stimulation) requirements (Table 2) of protective immune cells and to draw attention to differences in vivo and in vitro. As an example, monoclonal antibodies against CD2 have been reported to activate T cells in vitro via an alternative pathway. In contrast, we recently observed that non-depleting anti-CD2 monoclonal antibodies, when injected in vivo before antigen, could lead to long lasting T cell unresponsiveness (Gückel *et al*, 1991). Furthermore, we have not been able

---

TABLE 1. Induction requirements for protective immunity in a metastasizing animal tumour model (ESb)

---

a) Upon transplantation into syngeneic immunocompetent mice, it depends on the site of injection whether there will be progressive tumour growth and metastasis (eg subcutaneous, intraperitoneal) or predominant induction of anti-tumour immunity and no tumour growth (eg pinna)

b) Induction of protective immunity in the pinna can be abrogated by depletion of T cells and requires cooperative interactions between CD4 and CD8 T cells, tumour cells and possibly potent antigen presenting cells

c) Induction of protective immunity in the pinna can also be abrogated by pretreatment with a non-depleting monoclonal antibody against mouse CD2, suggesting that antigen non-specific CD2-LFA-3 like interactions are important in situ in T cell immune responses and tumour rejection

---

to prime tumour specific T cells in vitro, even when combining the antigen with APC and a variety of cytokines, whereas priming in vivo seemed to occur quite regularly, even when the tumour cells were injected at sites where they grew and metastasized. Finally, tumour specific CTL can be activated by secondary stimulation both in vitro and in vivo, but there seem to be differences in their in vivo migratory and tumour targeting properties.

DESIGN OF CANCER VACCINES FOR ACTIVE IMMUNIZATION

Animal Tumour Model Studies

While working in metastasizing animal tumour models over many years, we have realized that in order to influence the balance between immunity and

---

TABLE 2. Activation requirements and adoptive transfer of protective immunity in a metastasizing animal tumour model (ESb)

---

a) Protective immunity of immunized mice is based on cell mediated and not humoral immunity and can be adoptively transferred with CD8 immune T cells into normal or preirradiated syngeneic mice

b) Optimum stimulation of protective T cells requires at least two steps, namely priming and activation. Microenvironmental requirements for these two steps differ: whereas priming has been possible so far only in vivo, activation can be achieved both in vitro (mixed lymphocyte-tumour cell cultures) and in vivo (vascularized sponge, peritoneal cavity). In situ activated T cells have good tumour targeting properties and do not require exogenous cytokines for protective function.

c) Activated CD8 T cells recognize a class I associated TATA and exert direct and tumour specific cytotoxic activity as well as delayed type hypersensitivity like reactivity in vivo

d) Animals bearing progressively growing tumours have primed T cells. These, however, cannot be activated as easily as T cells from tumour immune mice to become CTL by antigen alone and require additional costimulatory factors. These findings are relevant for the design of appropriate cancer vaccines

---

metastasis, there has to be early intervention, and it has to be selective in activating the tumour specific clones. If tumour rejection cannot be achieved, there is still the possibility of induction of tumour dormancy, in which there seems to be balance between control by the immune system and tumour cell growth. Tumour dormancy was often observed at particular sites such as the footpad or ear pinna or upon transfer of tumour cells into preimmunized hosts. Sometimes this balance was overcome by the outgrowth of immuno-resistant tumour cell variants. In the ESb tumour model, this has been seen reproducibly after subcutaneous tumour cell inoculation or after intrasplenic inoculation of tumour cells into preimmunized hosts. Such immune escape variants could not be recognized and lysed by tumour specific CTL but still expressed the K^d restricting MHC molecules. These TATA$^-$ immune escape variants appeared to be gene regulatory variants rather than mutants or gene loss variants (Altevogt *et al*, 1986). Such variants were never observed in situations where effective anti-tumour responses or no anti-tumour responses occurred. For instance, no immune escape variants were seen upon injection of tumour cells (a) into nu/nu mice (no T cell responses) or (b) into the pinna of syngeneic or allogeneic MHC congenic mice (strong T cell responses). Anti-tumour immune cells from the latter could transfer protective immunity into syngeneic mice without allowing the generation of immune escape variants (Schirrmacher *et al*, 1991b).

These findings encouraged us to try tumour vaccination studies to allow for more effective anti-tumour T cell responses to circumvent immune escape problems. We favoured the use of non-oncogenic viruses, in particular of membrane budding myxo-viruses such as influenza A or Newcastle disease virus (NDV), to infect tumour cells in order to augment their immunogenicity. The rationale for this approach has been discussed elsewhere (Schirrmacher *et al*, 1986). We followed three different concepts for application of viruses in tumour therapy, namely (a) oncolysis by lytic viruses (Sinkovics, 1986), (b) tumour xenogenization by non-lytic viruses aimed at T helper cell activation (Kobayashi, 1986) and (c) second signal immune stimulation, ie use of viruses adsorbed to the tumour cell surface for local induction of costimulatory signals to immune T cells interacting with a tumour antigen (Schirrmacher *et al*, 1986). Most experiments were performed with the NDV strain Ulster, which is a non-lytic avirulent strain well suited to concepts (b) and (c). This negative stranded RNA virus possesses an external envelope with spike glycoproteins of two types: HN, a glycoprotein with haemagglutinating and neuraminidase activity, which binds to ubiquitous sialic acid containing gangliosides on cell surfaces, and F, a glycoprotein with membrane fusing ability. Figure 4 illustrates and summarizes the main parameters for cell surface modification of tumour cells by NDV Ulster. In comparison with influenza virus, NDV is more restricted in its host range and is much less hazardous for humans (Ahlert and Schirrmacher, 1990). Because of its low neurotropism, the use of NDV as an anti-neoplastic agent was proposed in 1965 by Cassel (Cassel and Garret, 1965), who since then has vaccinated more than 5000 melanoma patients with

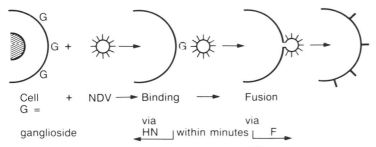

Cell   +   NDV ⟶ Binding   ⟶   Fusion

G =

                       via   via

ganglioside   ⟵ HN ⟶ within minutes ⟵ F ⟶

Fig. 4. Tumour cell infection by NDV. Binding of ^{125}I-labelled NDV to tumour cells is rapid (a few minutes) and specific (inhibition by antibody or cold virus). After 4 hr, infected cells express de novo synthesized viral antigens and produce non-infectious viral particles. For tumour vaccine modification, only 32 haemagglutinating units /10^7 cells are used, which correspond to approximately 3 ng viral protein

NDV melanoma oncolysates. This local active specific immunotherapy (ASI) protocol was well tolerated, and significant improvements in 5 year survival rates were reported (Cassel *et al*, 1983) and reproduced in a second unpublished study (Cassel WA, personal communication). The authors also observed enhanced inflammatory cell responses in cerebral metastases during concurrent therapy with viral oncolysates (Cassel *et al*, 1986). With its potency to induce IFN-α and IFN-β, TNF-α, adrenocorticotropic hormone, TIMP (tissue inhibitor of metalloproteinases) and heat shock proteins (Schirrmacher *et al*, 1986), NDV attached to tumour cell surfaces could be considered to be a potent biological response modifier in such a tumour vaccine.

Major contributions to the understanding of the principles of ASI were made in the L10 guinea pig hepatocarcinoma (Hanna *et al*, 1982) and in the ESb mouse lymphoma (Heicappell *et al*, 1986; Schirrmacher *et al*, 1986, 1989). The similarities between the optimum protocols developed in these two metastasizing tumours and the therapeutic results are obvious from the comparison shown in Fig. 5. In the L10 tumour, a series of studies demonstrated that BCG, admixed with tumour cells, could induce a degree of systemic tumour immunity that would eliminate a small, disseminated tumour burden when the vaccine was carefully controlled for such variables as the number of viable but non-tumorigenic tumour cells (10^7 optimal), the ratio of viable BCG organisms to tumour cells (1:1) and the vaccination regimen (three vaccines, 1 week apart). Whereas in the L10 tumour, postoperative immunotherapy with irradiated autologous tumour cells admixed with BCG protected against lymph node and lung metastases, in the ESb tumour, postoperative treatment with irradiated NDV infected autologous tumour cells protected against haematogenous metastases. Important variables for optimum therapeutic effects were the time of operation of the primary tumour, the residual disseminated tumour burden and the dose of virus added to a standard dose of 10^7 irradiated tumour cells (Heicappell *et al*, 1986). The site of vaccination also appeared to be important: in the L10 guinea pig model, three vaccinations injected intradermally protected against lymphatic spread, whereas in the ESb

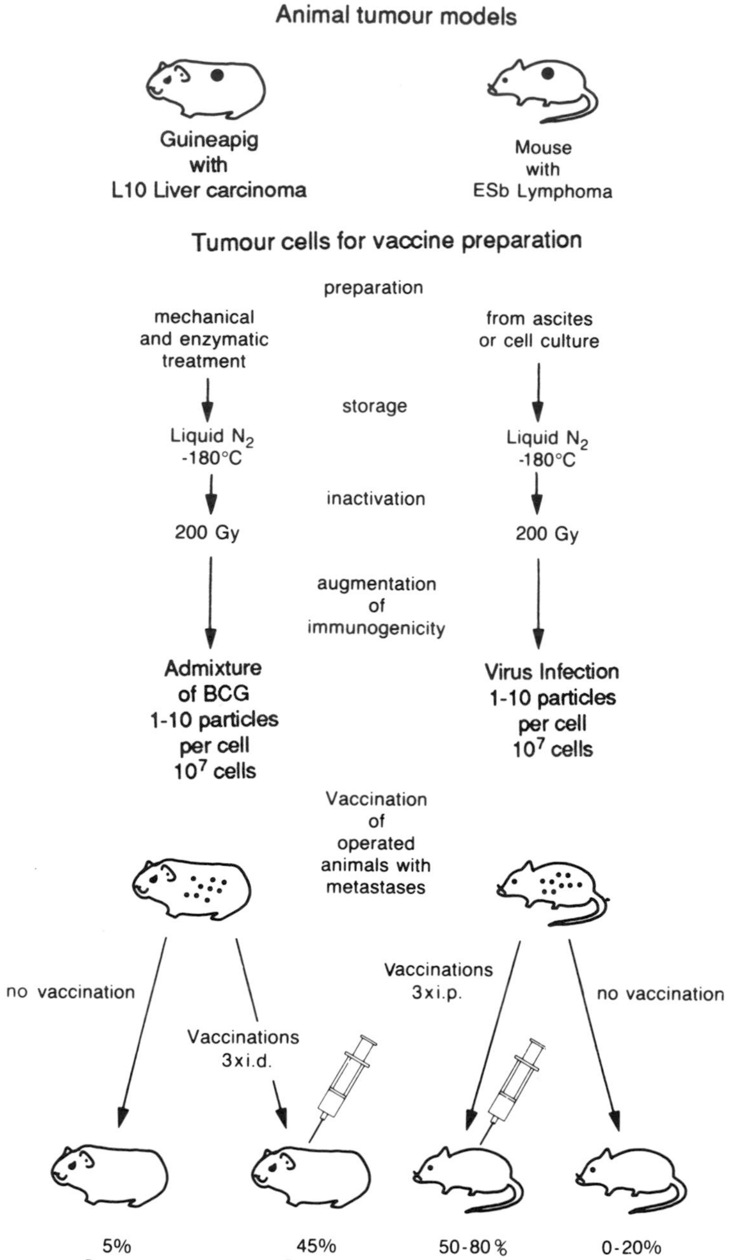

Fig. 5. Comparison of active specific immunotherapy (ASI) protocols developed in two different animal tumour models for postoperative treatment of micrometastatic disease

mouse model, intraperitoneal application of the vaccine had the strongest protective effect against visceral metastases (Fig. 6). In both models, postoperative vaccination with inactivated viable tumour cells without viral or bacterial adjuvants had no therapeutic effect. Figure 6 shows the survival curves of dif-

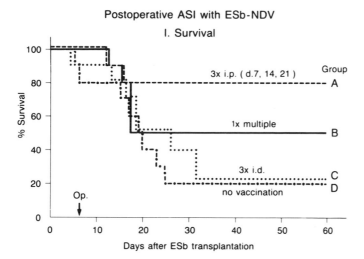

Postoperative ASI with ESb-NDV

I. Survival

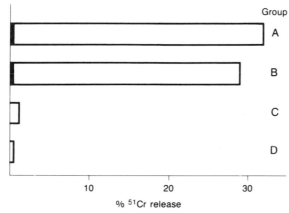

II. PEC-Cytotoxicity against ESB (□) and Eb (■)

Fig. 6. Results from a postoperative immunotherapy study with NDV modified tumour cell vaccine. Intradermally growing ESb tumours were removed (Op.) when 5-7 mm in diameter. The mice were either vaccinated according to different protocols (A-C) or remained untreated (D). I, survival curves. II, in situ generated tumour specific cytotoxicity from peritoneal exudate cells (PEC) 3 days after the first vaccination

ferent groups of animals that had been transplanted intradermally with ESb tumour cells and operated on 1 week later. Without further treatment, most animals died from metastases (group D), whereas about 50% of the mice survived when treated once postoperatively with the vaccine distributed at multiple sites (group B). Three intraperitoneal injections at weekly intervals led to 80% survival (group A), whereas the same regimen applied intradermally had no therapeutic benefits (group C). The different levels of protective immunity generated in these groups of mice seemed to correlate with the in situ activation of tumour specific CTL as tested from peritoneal exudate cells (PEC) taken 3 days after the first vaccination (Fig. 6, lower part). The cytotoxic activity of PEC was specific for the ESb tumour and mediated by CD8 T cells recognizing a K^d associated TATA (Schirrmacher et al, 1991a). The findings corroborate the above reported adoptive transfer studies in which in situ activated effector T cells could transfer protective immunity against ESb metastases.

The efficiency of the anti-metastatic effect of vaccination was dependent on the size of the metastases, their vascularization and the total tumour burden. In both tumour models, it was shown that vaccination leads to a local inflammatory reaction, which extends to the draining lymph nodes and eventually leads to a systemic immunity and inflammatory reactions at sites of metastases. The interconnections between local vaccine reaction and systemic immunity were evaluated in the guinea pig model by means of removal of the local reaction sites of the skin or of the draining lymph nodes at different times and testing the effects on postoperative survival. The stronger the local reaction the better the extend of systemic immunity induced. The combination of autologous tumour cells and BCG in the vaccine had a synergistic effect both on the intensity of the local reaction and on the protective immunity. In these studies, it was also documented that the viability of the inactivated tumour cells was of decisive importance and that the cells had to be frozen under controlled conditions; otherwise, their immunogenicity was greatly decreased. In the ESb tumour system, we found that simple freezing/thawing of the tumour cells completely destroyed their immunogenicity with regard to stimulating tumour specific CTL in mixed lymphocyte-tumour cell (MLTC) cultures. This defect could not be restored by the addition of cytokines such as IL-1, IL-2, IFN-γ or IL-4. The stronger immunogenicity of intact tumour cells compared with membrane preparations could be due to accessory adhesive and/or signalling molecules (Springer, 1990).

It is not easy to compare the mechanism of function of the two non-specific vaccine components NDV and BCG because no specific T cell responses were analysed in vitro in the L10/BCG system. When we compared the two vaccines in the L10 model, they were found to have similar efficacy. A combination of the two types of vaccines did not lead to better protective immune effects. BCG induces long lasting ulcers in animals and patients, whereas NDV does not. Another advantage of NDV may be its more precise localization at the tumour cell surface where immune cell/tumour cell interactions take place. We analysed in the ESb model the effect of NDV modification of tumour cells with respect to effects on the tumour specific T helper and CTL responses. We could confirm the findings of Kobayashi (1986), who reported for other viruses that viral xenogenization of tumour cells can increase immunogenicity dramatically. Animals immunized with ESb-NDV in the pinna developed strong systemic immunity and rejected in a quantitative TD_{50} assay a 250-fold higher dose of live ESb tumour cells upon challenge in the back than animals immunized against non-modified ESb tumour cells (Schirrmacher et al, 1986). When we analysed in detail the immune response

TABLE 3. Costimulatory activity of NDV bound to tumour cells on priming in vivo and restimulation in vitro of tumour specific CTL and effects of anti-interferon α, β antibodies and IL-2 on the CTL response

Exp.	Group	In vivo[a]	MLTC in vitro[b]	CTL activity[c] ESb	CTL activity[c] Eb	Reciprocal CTLP frequency ESb	Reciprocal CTLP frequency Eb
1	A	ESb	ESb	19.6	3	16 000	>100 000
	B	ESb+anti-IFN-α	ESb	0	0	65 000	>100 000
	C	ESb-NDV	ESb-NDV	54.1	2	6500	>100 000
	D	ESb+anti-IFN-α	ESb-NDV	11.0		27 000	>100 000
2	A	ESb	ESb	3	0	nd	
	B	ESb	ESb+IL-2	75	12		
	C	ESb	IL-2	12	11		
	D	ESb	ESb-NDV	81	9		

nd = not done

[a]*Experiment 1.* Mice were immunized on day 0 with 5×10^4 ESb cells intra-pinna. Animals of groups B and D received on day -2 and +4 anti-IFN specific antiserum. *Experiment 2.* CTL activation from spleen cells of tumour bearing mice. Mice were inoculated with 5×10^4 ESb cells intradermally in the flank and the growing tumour was removed on day 8

[b]On day 9 immune spleen cells were restimulated in bulk cultures or in limiting dilutions in micro-MLTC cultures or in limiting dilutions in micro-MLTC cultures together with IL-2 and mitomycin C inactivated stimulator cells for 4 days (MLTC) or 7 days (micro-MLTC LDA cultures for frequencies)

[c]CTL activity was determined in a 4 hr ^{51}Cr release assay at an effector:target cell ratio of 30:1 (*experiment 1*) or 50:1 (*experiment 2*) and is expressed as % specific release. Eb is a related lymphoma line expressing a different TATA

of animals inoculated in the pinna with either live ESb or live ESb-NDV cells, we found three levels where NDV exerted an amplifying effect on the immune response: (a) an increased CD4+ T cell mediated helper response (Schild *et al*, 1989), (b) an increased frequency of tumour specific cytotoxic T lymphocyte precursors (von Hoegen *et al*, 1988), and (c) an increased stimulatory capacity of NDV modified ESb cells for activating tumour specific cytotoxic T lymphocyte precursers (CTLP) to mature CTL in vitro (von Hoegen *et al*, 1990).

Table 3 summarizes some of findings on the potentiation of tumour specific CTL responses. Experiment 1 shows the increased cytolytic capacity generated in secondary MLTC cultures with immune spleen cells primed and restimulated by ESb-NDV (group C) compared with immune cells primed and restimulated by ESb (group A). The immune CTLP frequency at the beginning of the cultures was 1 in 6500 for ESb-NDV immune cells, compared with 1 in 16 000 of the ESb immune cells. All CTL clones analysed were still tumour specific, and under these immunization conditions, there were no CTL clones with specificity for the virus or for Eb cells, which express a different TATA (von Hoegen *et al*, 1988). The priming effect of in vivo immunization was strongly affected by application of an anti-serum to IFN-α/β that could neutralize endogenous as well as locally induced interferon. There was a strong reduction in CTLP frequency and in CTL activity, suggesting that interferons play an important part in the generation of tumour specific CTL activity as well as for the augmentation effect of NDV modification. The reduction in the generation of CTL by anti-IFN-α/β could be overcome with excess interferon, especially when using ESb-NDV as stimulator cells (von Hoegen et al, 1990). In experiment 2, we investigated the postoperative activation of tumour specific CTLP from mice with metastases. Spleen cells from such mice behaved like spleens from suboptimally immunized mice. Stimulation in MLTC cultures with the specific antigen was not sufficient to generate CTL activity. The activation of tumour specific CTLP required stimulation with the specific antigen plus additional costimulator. Such costimulator function was observed with exogenous IFN-α,β (von Hoegen et al, 1990) or IL-2 (group B). Interleukin-2 alone only increased non-specific cytolytic activity. As can be seen from a comparison of group D with A, a good costimulatory activity was also exerted by infection of the stimulator cells with NDV, which led to a selective increase of the tumour specific response.

Clinical Studies

The primary aim of active immunotherapy is to potentiate selectively the patient's immune reaction against the tumour and to establish long lasting immune memory. Reagents used in cancer patients for active immunizations include intact irradiated autologous tumour cells (Hoover et al, 1985; Rao et al, 1988; Schulof et al, 1988; Berd et al, 1990; McCune et al, 1990), allogeneic fresh or cultured tumour cells of the same histological type or allogeneic tumour cell homogenates (Morton, 1986; Mitchell et al, 1990), tumour oncolysates (Cassel et al, 1983) and soluble tumour antigens (Hollinshead et al, 1987; Bystryn, 1990). Various groups reported positive results with active immunization as a postsurgical adjuvant treatment (Cassel et al, 1983; Hollinshead et al, 1987) or in patients with progressive advanced disease (Tallberg et al, 1985; Morton, 1986; Berd et al, 1990; Mitchell et al, 1990).

A variety of methods and procedures to modify cancer vaccines have been developed to increase their immunogenicity: chemical and enzymatic modification (Rao et al, 1988); xenogenization with viruses (Kobayashi, 1986; Schirrmacher et al, 1986); modification by mutagens (Boon et al, 1989); transfection of genes coding for MHC class I antigens (Gopas et al, 1989); upregulation of the expression of MHC antigens, integrins and tumour associated antigens by in vitro exposure to IFN-γ and TNF-α (Vanky et al, 1990); use of the vaccine together with low doses of IL-1 (McCune and Marquis, 1990), IL-2 (Naito et al, 1988) or IFN-γ (Giovarelli et al, 1986); and using molecularly engineered tumour cells carrying genes for lymphokines (Fearon et al, 1990; Russel, 1990). Potentiation of immune stimulation can also be expected with unmodified or modified tumour cells combined with various natural and synthetic immunoadjuvants (Lise and Audibert, 1989). In many of these studies with improved modified cancer vaccines, a beneficial effect was reported in many patients, and the treatment was well tolerated.

On the basis of the ASI concept developed in the ESb tumour model, we have established a corresponding vaccination protocol for cancer patients. The vaccine consists of freshly isolated autologous intact tumour cells inactivated by irradiation and modified by coincubation with a small predetermined amount of NDV (Ulster). In various types of cancer patients, new protocols for postoperative ASI treatment were worked out in either "adjuvant" or "advanced disease" situations. We felt encouraged to do so by our findings that several autologous T cell clones against a human melanoma recognized not only one but several individually distinct antigenic specificities expressed on separate tumour derived proteins. The tumour was thus characterized as expressing multiple distinct antigenic specificities, which could activate different CD4 and CD8 anti-tumour T cell clones (Notter and Schirrmacher, 1990). For preparation of tumour cell vaccines, optimum procedures were first developed for the isolation and inactivation of live tumour cells from freshly operated specimens of primary tumours or metastases. This was done for malignant melanoma, hypernephroma, breast carcinoma, ovarian carcinoma and colon cancer. For preparation of a vaccine, irradiated cells stored in liquid nitrogen were thawed and coincubated at 37°C for 1 hour with live or inactivated NDV. The virus modified cells were characterized with immunological, biochemical and electron microscopical methods. Sterile and other quality controls were included (Lehner *et al*, 1990). Results from phase I studies have been reported (Schirrmacher, *et al*, 1989; Bohle *et al*, 1990; Liebrich *et al*, 1991; Pomer *et al*, in press).

The first evaluation of clinical response to adjuvant ASI treatment with autologous tumour cell vaccines modified by NDV infection (ATV-NDV) was done in colorectal cancer patients following resection of liver metastases (Schlag P, Manasterski M, Gerneth T *et al*, unpublished). In this high risk group of patients, adjuvant chemotherapy has only limited success and 70–80% relapse within 5 years from the outgrowth of micrometastasis not detectable at the time of liver resection. The objective of the study was to investigate whether ASI influences (a) the immune response to autologous tumour cells and (b) the recurrence free and overall survival of vaccinated patients compared with non-vaccinated matched controls. We also wanted to see whether delayed-type hypersensitivity (DTH) reactivity correlated with clinical outcome. After a follow-up of at least 12 months, tumour recurrence developed in 7 of 23 patients in comparison to 13 from 23 patients treated with surgery only. The recurrence free interval for patients with relapse was strongly correlated with the increase in DTH reactivity against autologous tumour cells. It was not correlated with DTH reactivity against standard antigens of the Merieux test or other tested controls. Figure 7A illustrates this correlation between DTH reactivity and recurrence free interval as found in our colorectal carcinoma study. A similar correlation was recently found in a melanoma study by Berd *et al* (1990) (Fig. 7B). Furthermore, in renal cell car-

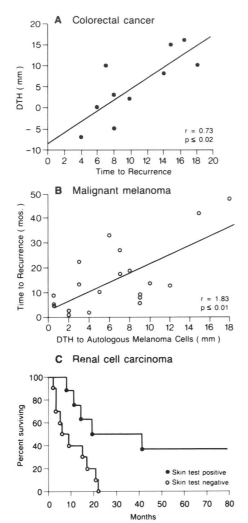

Correlation of survival with skin testing
by autologous tumor cells

Fig. 7. Three studies showing a correlation between delayed type hypersensitivity (DTH) skin test response to autologous tumour cells and clinical response, in terms of time to recurrence (A,B) or survival (C). A, colorectal cancer (after Schlag P, Manasterski M, Gerneth T *et al*, unpublished). B, malignant melanoma (after Berd *et al*, 1990). C, renal cell carcinoma (after McCune *et al*, 1990)

cinoma (Fig. 7C) patients, McCune reported improvement in 5 year survival of ASI treated DTH positive patients compared with ASI treated DTH negative patients (McCune *et al*, 1990).

There was thus a clear advantage in our studies for patients who underwent postoperative vaccination with ATV-NDV. Evidence of recurrent disease in the first 12 months after liver resection could be reduced by 27%. Subgroup analysis showed a further trend for improved survival in immunological responder patients with an augmented DTH to autologous tumour cells.

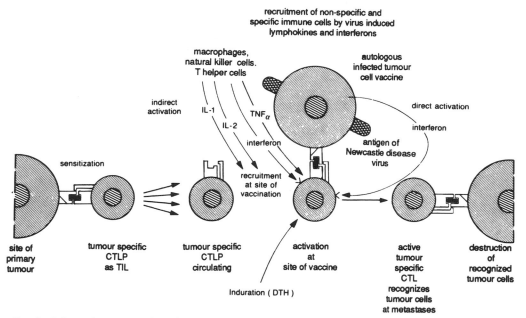

recruitment of non-specific and
specific immune cells by virus induced
lymphokines and interferons

macrophages,
natural killer cells.
T helper cells

autologous
infected tumour
cell vaccine

indirect
activation   IL-1   direct activation
              IL-2   TNFα
                              interferon
              interferon

sensitization   antigen of
                                            Newcastle disease
                                                  virus

recruitment
at site of
vaccination

site of   tumour specific   tumour specific   activation   active   destruction
primary   CTLP   CTLP   at   tumour   of
tumour   as TIL   circulating   site of vaccine   specific   recognized
                                                                  CTL   tumour cells
                                                                  recognizes
                                                                  tumour cells
                                                                  at metastases

Induration (DTH)

Fig. 8. Schematic presentation of the concept and mechanism of action of virus modified autologous tumour vaccine. For further details, see text

Figure 8 illustrates how we anticipate the mechanism of function of the ASI treatment. To the left is shown the site of the primary tumour, where priming of virgin T cells may take place. This process may involve complex cell-cell interactions and three or four cell type clusters (Mitchison and O'Malley, 1987), as illustrated in Fig. 2. The middle part shows the activation of primed or memory T cells in the skin at the site of ATV-NDV vaccine application. Since memory cells show distinct pathways of lymphocyte recirculation (MacKay *et al*, 1990) and express skin homing receptors (Picker *et al*, 1990), they probably can be easily recruited during an inflammatory DTH reaction to the site of antigen application. NDV induced IFN-α and IFN-β may be important initial mediators of lymphocyte migration in the absence of immune memory T cells, whereas in the presence of immune T cells, IFN-γ seems to account for most of the DTH related lymphocyte recruitment (Issekutz *et al*, 1988). NDV induced, locally produced cytokines also may function as costimulatory signal 2 in conjunction with the antigen receptor mediated signal 1 according to the two-signal pathway of T cell activation proposed by Schwartz (1990). In support of this assumption, we demonstrated that the NDV mediated potentiation of tumour specific DTH activity could be inhibited by anti-interferon antibodies (Table 3; von Hoegen *et al*, 1990). NDV may also increase via its haemagglutinin-neuraminidase glycoprotein adhesive host/tumour cell interactions and thereby increase their binding affinity and/or avidity. Finally, activated antigen specific effector cells may recirculate and, upon recognition of antigen at the site of metastases, shown to the right, may

TABLE 4. Rationale for using NDV infected autologous tumour cells (ATV-NDV) as vaccine for postoperative ASI treatment

Variable	ATV-NDV	Limitations
Specificity	high: includes individually distinct MHC associated tumour antigens; closest match to the patient's own cancer	non-antigenic tumours; proportion of stroma cells and infiltrating host cells
Immunogenicity	high: intact cells, in particular virus infected cells superior to subcellular material for T cell responses	immunoresistant tumour cell variants
Valency	as a polyvalent reagent such a vaccine better suited than monovalent reagents to treat heterogeneous cellular disease such as cancer	standardization
Tolerability/ side effects	both components well tolerated; side effects very few	tumour enhancement, induction of suppression
Effectiveness	local immune reactions: apparent synergistic interaction of ATV and NDV in skin reactivity to the vaccine	non-responding patients
	systemic reactions: increased DTH reactivity to challenge with autologous tumour cells, reactions at sites of residual disease, reduced recurrence rate	possibly tumour mass
Practicability	can be prepared within 6–12 hr from fresh specimens; feasible for a central laboratory with trained staff. Mail service possible within 24 hr	amount of materials; general availability

induce there anti-tumour immune responses. Secretion of IFN-γ seems to be important also at this step, since the effectiveness of TIL when adoptively transferred to mice bearing micrometastasis correlated better with their ability secrete interferon specifically than with their cytotoxicity in vitro (Barth *et al*, 1991).

Table 4 summarizes the rationale for using ATV-NDV in cancer patients. Variables of importance for any kind of cancer vaccine, such as specificity, immunogenicity, valency, tolerability, effectiveness and practicability, are considered. We have already mentioned that in our hands viable tumour cells are superior to cell membranes with respect to activating tumour specific CTLP. This is corroborated with a defined immunoglobulin idiotype, which served as tumour antigen. Immunization with idiotype positive viable tumour cells induced protective immunity, whereas immunization with equivalent amounts of idiotype presented in soluble form gave no protection but rather caused tumour enhancement (Ghosh *et al*, 1990). Although arguments in favour of the use of ATV-NDV are summarized, we also draw attention to possible limitations of their use. Limitations may exist with regard to (a) responsiveness of the patient, (b) amount of available material, (c) residual tumour mass and/or recurrent tumour mass and (d) antigenic heterogeneity and immunoresistance. We are fully aware that this type of treatment must be combined with other modalities, but this is true also for other immunotherapeutic approaches. As a local form of treatment, ASI is better tolerated by cancer patients than systemic high dose cytokine treatment or adoptive LAK or TIL therapy. Intensive research in this promising area of clinical tumour immunology is warranted to increase our strategies for treatment of metastatic disease.

SUMMARY AND CONCLUSIONS

Data from animal models and clinical observations from immunotherapy trials suggest that tumour reactive host T cells can have an important role in the control of metastasis and tumour rejection. If tumour cells express tumour associated antigens recognizable by T cells, their antigenicity/immunogenicity is usually weak, and accessory molecules are required to stabilize the T cell/tumour cell interaction and to deliver the antigen/T cell receptor (TCR) mediated signal (signal 1) together with costimulatory signals (signal 2). The sum of these intracellular signals received by the corresponding T cells with the fitting TCR may determine the intensity of the anti-tumour response. A deficiency of anti-tumour T cell responsiveness in cancer patients could thus be due to a lack of signal 1 and/or signal 2 or to inappropriate timing between the two signals. A further point to consider is the distinction between primary and secondary T cell responses: between priming of virgin T cells and activation of primed memory T cells. Our experience with a metastasizing animal tumour suggests that the microenvironmental requirements for these two steps differ. This means that the site of a primary (or secondary) tumour may be good for one type of response (eg priming) but not for the other (eg memory response). One purpose of active immunotherapy could therefore consist of exposing the cancer patient's immune system to its own tumour cells in the context of a new microenvironment that may be well suited for activating memory type responses.

On the basis of these considerations, we discuss the possibilities of immunological intervention and propose the use of a two-component cancer vaccine for active immunization and two signal stimulation of endogenous memory T cells in tumour bearing animals or cancer patients. As a specific component, we favour the use of intact, viable, radiation inactivated autologous tumour cells, which should represent the closest match to the patient's own cancer. If this is not possible, cells from allogeneic corresponding tumours or tumour cell lines could be used. On a longer time scale of treatment, one may consider an induction therapy with autologous vaccine followed by maintenance therapy (when autologous material has run out) with allogeneic material. As a second non-specific component, we favour and have good experience with a virus, NDV, which can easily attach to the cells of the vaccine and facilitate the delivery of costimulatory signals to tumour reactive T cells following postoperative vaccination of tumour bearing hosts. We summarize the rationale of this approach as well as the results from animal model and clinical studies. Finally, we discuss the advantages and disadvantages or limitations of active immunization with virus modified autologous tumour cells.

The rational application of active specific immunotherapy to human cancer will depend to a large extent on a better definition of tumour associated antigens in human neoplasms and on methods for augmenting immune responses against these antigens. Patients with earlier disease are more likely to respond to any immunotherapeutic manoeuvres, since the cancer patient's general immune competence is greatest when the disease is localized and will often be impaired due to metastases. Future directions of study should aim at improvements of immune monitoring of cancer patients (a) to discriminate as early as possible between potential responder and non-responder patients so that only the former are included in immunotherapy trials, (b) to correlate immunological variables (such as skin reactivity to autologous cancer cell and fluorescence activated cell sorter analysis of peripheral blood lymphocyte subpopulations) with clinical prognosis and (c) to enable individualized therapies and follow-up studies that can be oriented along immunological response parameters. Immunotherapy studies should be done by those centres that have the knowledge and means to monitor the patient's immune response concomitantly with the immunotherapeutic trials.

Acknowledgements

These studies were supported by the Dr Mildred Scheel Foundation, the German Cancer Research Centre and the Tumour Centre Heidelberg/Mannheim. I thank a number of collaborators, both experimental and clinical, for their help and contributions, in particular Dr T Ahlert, Dr P Schlag, Dr W Liebrich, Dr G Bastert, Dr M Manasterski, Dr B Lehner, Dr V Möbus, Dr S Pomer as clinical partners and Dr P von Hoegen, Dr R Heicappell, Dr H J Schild, Dr U Zangemeister, Dr B Kyewski, Dr P Altevogt, Dr B Gückel and Dr Ch. Ertel from our Division.

References

Ahlert T and Schirrmacher V (1990) Isolation of a human melanoma adapted Newcastle Disease Virus mutant with highly selective replication patterns. *Cancer Research* **50** 5962–5968

Altevogt P, von Hoegen P and Schirrmacher V (1986) Immuno-resistant metastatic tumor variants can re-express their tumor antigen after treatment with DNA methylation-inhibiting agents. *International Journal of Cancer* **38** 707–711

Aukerman SL and Fidler IJ (1987) The heterogeneous nature of metastatic neoplasms: relevance to biotherapy, In: Oldham RK (ed). *Principles of Cancer Biotherapy*. In: Oldham RK (ed). *Principles of Cancer Biotherapy*, pp 21-47, Raven Press Ltd, New York

Axtell LM, Ardyce J, Asire MS and Meyers MH (1976) Cancer patient survival report No 5, pp 795–992, *Department of Health Education and Welfare Publication (National Institutes of Health)*, Bethesda, Maryland

Barth RJ, Mulé JJ, Spiess PJ and Rosenberg SA (1991) Interferon γ and tumor necrosis factor have a role in tumor regressions mediated by murine CD8$^+$ tumor-infiltrating lymphocytes. *Journal of Experimental Medicine* **173** 647–658

Berd D, Maguire HC, McCue P and Mastrangelo MJ (1990) Treatment of metastatic melanoma with an autologous tumor-cell vaccine: clinical and immunologic results in 64 patients. *Journal of Clinical Oncology* **8** 1858–1867

Bohle W, Schlag P, Liebrich W *et al* (1990) Postoperative active specific immunization in colorectal cancer patients with virus modified autologous tumor cell vaccine. *Cancer* **66** 1517–1523

Bolhuis RLH (1989) T cell responses to cancer, In: Feldmann M, Lamb J and Owen MJ (eds). *T Cells*, pp 347–364, John Wiley and Sons, Chichester

Boon T, van Pel A and de Plaen E (1989) Tum$^-$ transplantation antigens, point mutations, and antigenic peptides: a model for tumor-specific transplantation antigens? *Cancer Cells* **1** 25–28

Bystryn JC (1990) Tumor vaccines. *Cancer Metasasis Reviews* **9** 81–91

Cameron RB, McIntosh IK and Rosenberg SA (1988) Synergistic antitumor effects of combination immunotherapy with recombinant interleukin-2 and a recombinant hybrid α-interferon in the treatment of established murine hepatic metastases. *Cancer Reasearch* **48** 5810–5817

Cassel WA and Garret RE (1965) Newcastle Disease Virus as an antineoplastic agent. *Cancer* **18** 863

Cassel WA, Murray DR and Phillips HS (1983) A phase II study on the postsurgical management of stage II malignant melanoma with a Newcastle Disease Virus Oncolysate. *Cancer* **52** 856–860

Cassel WA, Weidenheim KM, Campbell WG and Murray DR (1986) Malignant melanoma: inflammatory mononuclear cell infiltrates in cerebral metastases during concurrent therapy with viral oncolysate. *Cancer* **57** 1302–1312

Cheever MA, Thompson DB, Klarnet IP and Greenberg P (1986) Antigen-driven long-term cultured T cells proliferate in vivo, distribute widely, mediate specific tumor therapy and persist long-term as functional memory T cells. *Journal of Experimental Medicine* **163** 1100–1112

Dailey MO, Fathmann G, Butcher EC, Pillemer E and Weissmann I (1982) Abnormal migration of T lymphocyte clones. *Journal of Immunology* **128** 2134–2136

Erkell L and Schirrmacher V (1988) A quantitative in vitro assay for tumor cell invasion through extracellular matrix or into protein gels. *Cancer Research* **48** 6933–6937

Euhus DM, Gupta RK and Morton DL (1989) Induction of antibodies to a tumor-associated antigen by immunization with a whole melanoma cell vaccine. *Cancer Immunology and Immunotherapy* **29** 247–254

Fidler IJ, Gersten DM and Kripke ML (1979) Influence of immune status on the metastasis of three murine fibrosarcomas of different immunogenicities. *Cancer Research* **39** 3816–3821

Fearon ER, Pardoll DM, Itaya T *et al* (1990) Interleukin-2 production by tumor cells bypasses T helper function in the generation of an anti-tumor response. *Cell* **60** 397

Foon KA (1989) Biological response modifiers: the new immunotherapy. *Cancer Research* **49** 1621–1639

Ghosh SK, White LM, Gosh R and Baukert RB (1990) Vaccination with membrane-associated idiotype provides greater and more prolonged protection of animals from tumor challenge than the soluble form of idiotype. *Journal of Immunology* **145** 365

Giovarelli M, Cofano F, Vecchi A *et al* (1986) Interferon activated tumor inhibition in vivo: small amounts of interferon-gamma inhibit tumor growth by eliciting host systemic immunoreactivity. *International Journal of Cancer* **37** 141–148

Goodenow RS, Vogel JM and Linsk RL (1985) Histocompatibility antigens on murine tumor cells. *Science* **230** 777–783

Gopas J, Rager-Zisman B, Bar-Eli M, Hämmerling GJ and Segal S (1989) The relationship between MHC antigen expression and metastasis. *Advances in Cancer Research* **53** 89–115

Griffith KD, Read EJ, Carrasquillo JA *et al* (1989) In vivo distribution of adoptively transferred indium-111-labeled tumor infiltrating lymphocytes and peripheral blood lymphocytes in patients with metastatic melanoma. *Journal of the National Cancer Institute* **81** 1709–1717

Gückel B, Berek C, Altevogt P, Schirrmacher V and Kyewski BA (1991) Anti-CD2 antibodies induce T cell unresponsiveness in vivo. *Journal of Experimental Medicine* **174** 957–967

Hankey BF and Steinhorn SC (1982) Long-term patient survival for some more frequently occurring cancers. *Cancer* **60** 1904–1912

Hanna MG, Pollack VA, Peters LC and Hoover HC (1982) Active specific immunotherapy of established micrometastases with BCG plus tumor cell vaccines. *Cancer* **49** 659–664

Heicappel R, Schirrmacher V, von Hoegen P, Ahlert T and Appelhans B (1986) Prevention of metastatic spread by postoperative immunotherapy with virally modified autologous tumor cells. *International Journal of Cancer* **37** 569–577

Hewitt HB, Blake ER and Walder S (1976) A critique of the evidence for active host defence against cancer, based on personal studies of 27 murine tumors of spontaneous origin. *British Journal of Cancer* **33** 241–259

Hollinshead A, Stewart THM, Takita H, Dalbow M and Concannon J (1987) Adjuvant specific active lung cancer immunotherapy trials. *Cancer* **60** 1249–1262

Hoover HC, Surdyke M, Dangel RB, Peters LC and Hanna MG (1985) Prospectively randomized trial of adjuvant active-specific immunotherapy for human colorectal cancer. *Cancer* **55** 1236–1243

Issekutz TB, Stoltz UM and Meide P (1988) Lymphocyte recruitment in delayed-type hypersensitivity: the role of IFN-γ. *Journal of Immunology* **140** 2989–2993

Kast WM, Offringa R, Peters PJ *et al* (1989) Eradication of adenovirus E1-induced tumors by E1A-specific cytotoxic T lymphocytes. *Cell* **59** 603–614

Kedar E and Klein E Cancer immunotherapy: are the results discouraging? can they be improved ? *Advances in Cancer Research* (in press)

Kedar E, Ben-Aziz R, Epstein E and Leshem B (1989) Chemo-immunotherapy of murine tumors using interleukin-2 (IL-2) and cyclophosphamide. *Cancer Immunology and Immunotherapy* **29** 74–78

Kitagawa S, Sato S, Azuma T, Schimizu I, Hamaoka T and Fujiwara H (1991) Heterogeneity of CD4 T cells involved in anti-allo-class I H-2 responses functional discrimination between the major proliferating cells and helper cells assisting cytotoxic T cell responses. *Journal of Immunology* **146** 2513

Klein G (1980) Immune and non-immune control of neoplastic development: contrasting effects of host and tumor evolution. *Cancer* **45** 2486–2499

Kobayashi H (1986) The biological modification of tumor cells as a means of inducing their regression: an overview. *Journal of Biological Response Modifiers* **5** 1–11

Lehner B, Schlag P, Liebrich W and Schirrmacher V (1990) Postoperative active specific immunization in curatively resected colorectal cancer patients with virus-modified autologous tumor cell vaccine. *Cancer Immunology and Immunotherapy* **32** 173–178

Liebrich W, Schlag P, Manasterski M *et al* (1991) In vitro and clinical characterization of a Newcastle Disease Virus-modified autologous tumor cell vaccine for treatment of colorectal cancer patients. *European Journal of Cancer* **27** 703–710

Lise LD and Audibert F (1989) Immunoadjuvants and analogs of immunomodulatory bacterial structures. *Current Opinion in Immunology* **2** 269–274

MacKay CR, Marston W and Dudler L (1990) Naive and memory T cells show distinct pathways of lymphocyte recirculation. *Journal of Experimental Medicine* **171** 801–817

McCune CS and Marquis DM (1990) Interleukin 1 as an adjuvant for active specific immunotherapy in a murine tumor model. *Cancer Research* **50** 1212–1215

McCune CS, O'Donnell RW, Marquis DM and Sahasrabudhe PM (1990) Renal cell carcinoma treated by vaccines for active specific immunotherapy: a correlation of survival with skin testing by autologous tumor cells. *Cancer Immunology and Immunotherapy* **32** 62–66

Melief CJM Tumor eradication by adoptive transfer of cytotoxic T lymphocytes. *Advances in Cancer Research* (in press)

Mitchell MS, Hare W, Kempf RA *et al* (1990) Active specific immunotherapy for melanoma. *Journal of Clinical Oncology* **8** 856–869

Mitchison A and O'Malley C (1987) Three-cell-type clusters of T cells with antigen-presenting cells best explain the epitope linkage and noncognate requirements of the in vivo cytolytic response. *European Journal of Immunology* **17** 1579–1583

Mitchison NA (1989) Introduction, In: Feldmann M, Lamb J and Owen MJ (eds). *T Cells*, pp 1–7, John Wiley and Sons, New York

Morton DL (1986) Active immunotherapy against cancer: present status. *Seminars in Oncology* **13** 180–185

Mulé JJ, Yang JC, Afreniere RL, Shu S and Rosenberg SA (1987) Identification of cellular mechanisms operational in vivo during the regression of established pulmonary metastases by the systemic administration of high-dose recombinant IL-2. *Journal of Immunology* **139** 285–294

Naito K, Pellis NR and Kahan BD (1988) Effect of continuous administration of interleukin 2 on active specific chemoimmunotherapy with extracted tumor-specific transplantation antigen and cyclophosphamide. *Cancer Research* **48** 101–108

Nathan C and Sporn M (1991) Cytokines in context. *Journal of Cellular Biology* **113** 981–986

Nicolson GL (1987) Tumor cell instability, diversification, and progression to the metastatic phenotype: from oncogene to oncofetal expression. *Cancer Research* **47** 1473–1487

Notter M and Schirrmacher V (1990) Tumor specific T cell clones recognize different protein determinants of autologous human malignant melanoma cells. *International Journal of Cancer* **45** 834–841

Osband ME, Lavin PT *et al* (1990) Effect of autolymphocyte therapy on survival and quality of life in patients with metastatic renal cell carcinoma. *Lancet* **335** 994–998

Parmiani G (1990) An explanation of the variable clinical response to interleukin-2 and LAK cells. *Immunology Today* **11** 113–115

Picker LJ, Terstappon LWMM, Rott LS, Streeter PR, Stein H and Butcher E (1990) Differential expression of homing-associated adhesion molecules by T cell subsets in man. *Journal of Immunology* **145** 3247–3255

Pomer S, Thiele R, Daniel V *et al* Sequential treatment of patients with advanced renal cell carcinoma with autologous tumor vaccine and subcutaneous administration of recombinant interleukin-2 and interferon-K-2b. *World Journal of Urology* (in press)

Rao VS, Wiseman C, Mazumder A *et al* (1988) Effect of cholesteryl-hemisuccinate (CHS) on cell-mediated immunity in melanoma patients treated with active specific intralymphatic immunotherapy. *Proceedings of the American Association of Cancer Research* **29** 409

Rosenberg SA (1990) Adaptive immunotherapy for cancer. *Scientific American* **262** 62–69

Rosenberg SA, Schwarz SL and Spiess PJ (1988) Combination immunotherapy for cancer: synergistic antitumor interactions of interleukin-2, alfa interferon and tumor-infiltrating lymphocytes. *Journal of the National Cancer Institute* **80** 1393–1397

Russel SJ (1990) Lymphokine gene therapy for cancer. *Immunology Today* **11** 196–200

Schild H-J, Kyewski B, von Hoegen P and Schirrmacher V (1987) CD4+ helper T cells are required for resistance to a highly metastatic murine tumor. *European Journal of Immunology* **17** 1863–1866

Schild H-J, von Hoegen P and Schirrmacher V (1989) Modification of tumor cells by a low dose of Newcastle Disease Virus II Augmented tumor specific T cell response as a result of CD4+ and CD8+ immune T cell cooperation. *Cancer Immunology and Immunotherapy* **28** 22–28

Schirrmacher V (1989) Immunobiology and immunotherapy of cancer metastases: ten year studies in an animal model resulting in the design of an immunotherapy procedure now under clinical testing. *Interdisciplinary Science Reviews* **14** 291–303

Schirrmacher V, Fogel M, Russmann E, Bosslet K, Altevogt P and Beck L (1982) Antigenic variation in cancer metastasis: immune escape versus immune control. *Cancer Metastasis Reviews* **1** 241–272

Schirrmacher V, Ahlert T, Heicappell R, Appelhans B and von Hoegen P (1986) Successful application of non-oncogenic viruses for antimetastatic cancer immunotherapy. *Cancer Reviews* **5** 19–49

Schirrmacher V, von Hoegen P, Schlag P et al (1989) Active specific immunotherapy with autologous tumor cell vaccines modified by Newcastle Disease Virus: experimental and clinical studies, In: Schirrmacher V, Schwartz-Albiez R (eds). *Cancer Metastasis*, pp 157–170, Spinger Verlag, Berlin-Heidelberg-New York

Schirrmacher V, Leidig S and Griesbach A (1991a) In situ activation of syngeneic tumor specific cytotoxic T-lymphocytes: importance of site of antigen stimulation. *Cancer Immunology and Immunotherapy* **33** 299–306

Schirrmacher V, von Hoegen P, Griesbach A and Zangemeister-Wittke U (1991b) Specific eradication of micrometastases by transfer of tumor immune T-cells from MHC congenic mice. *Cancer Immunology and Immunotherapy* **32** 373–381

Schulof RS, Mai D, Nelson MA et al (1988) Active specific immunotherapy with an autologous tumor cell vaccine in patients with resected non-small cell lung cancer. *Molecular Biotherapy* **1** 30–36

Schwartz RH (1990) A cell culture model for T lymphocyte clonal anergy. *Science* **248** 1349–1356

Siegel JP and Pari RK (1991) Interleukin-2 toxicity. *Journal of Clinical Oncology* **9** 694–704

Sinkovics J (1986) Oncolytic viruses and viral oncolysates. *Annales Immunologicae Hungaricae* **26** 271–290

Springer TA (1990) The sensation and regulation of interactions with the extracellular environment: the cell biology of lymphocyte adhesion receptors. *Annual Reviews of Cellular Biology* **6** 359–402

Stevenson HC, Foon KA, Kanapa DJ, Favilla T, Beman I and Oldham RK (1984) The potential value of cytapheresis for adoptive immunotherapy of cancer patients. *Plasma Therapy and Transfusion Technology* **5** 237–250

Stötter H and Lotze MT (1990) Cytolytic effector cells against human tumors: distinguishing phenotype and function. *Cancer Cells* **2** 44–55

Tallberg T, Tykkä H, Mahlberg K et al (1985) Active specific immunotherapy with supportive measures in the treatment of palliatively nephrectomized, renal adenocarcinoma patients: a thirteen-year follow-up study. *European Urology* **11** 233–243

Vanky F, Wang P, Pattaroy M and Klein E (1990) Adhesion molecule ICAM-1 and major histocompatibility complex class-1 antigen on human tumor-cells is required for their interaction with autologous lymphocytes in vitro. *Cancer Immunology and Immunotherapy* **31** 19–27

von Hoegen P, Weber E and Schirrmacher V (1988) Modification of tumor cells by a low dose of Newcastle Disease Virus; augmentation of the tumor-specific T cell responses in the absence of an anti-viral response. *European Journal of Immunology* **18** 1159–1166

von Hoegen P, Zawatzky R and Schirrmacher V (1990) Modification of tumor cells by a low dose of Newcastle Disease Virus III Potentiation of tumor specific cytolytic T cell activity via induction of interferon, alfa, beta. *Cellular Immunology* **126** 80–90

Zajicek G (1985) The estimation of host-resistance in cancer. *Medical Hypothesis* **18** 79–89

Zajicek G (1987) Long survival with micrometastasis: at least 9 % of breast cancer patients carry metastases for more than 10 years. *Cancer Journal* **1** 414–415

The author is responsible for the accuracy of the references.

MHC Loss in Colorectal Tumours: Evidence for Immunoselection?

LOUKAS KAKLAMANIS[1] • ANN HILL[2]

[1]*Nuffield Department of Pathology and* [2]*Cancer Immunology Laboratory, ICRF Institute of Molecular Medicine, John Radcliffe Hospital, Oxford*

Introduction
HLA class I antigens
   HLA class I expression in human tumours
   HLA class I expression in colorectal cancer
Aetiology of MHC loss
   Loss of MHC class I expression could be of selective advantage to the tumour
   Loss of MHC class I expression could be secondary to another factor
   that is of selective advantage to the tumour
   Significance of allelic rather than total MHC loss
   Can the genetic mechanisms of MHC class I loss provide clues
   to its aetiology?
Summary and conclusions

INTRODUCTION

The discovery of the nature of major histocompatibility complex (MHC) restricted recognition of antigen by T cells led to the concept that T cells recognize tumour cells as "altered self" and that a major function of the immune system is to recognize and destroy potentially malignant mutant cells. This concept of "immune surveillance" seems to be even more probable in the light of recent awareness that cytotoxic T cells recognize antigen derived from internal proteins rather than cell surface proteins (Townsend *et al*, 1989a). However, convincing evidence that this process occurs in vivo to any significant extent has been hard to obtain. It is obvious from animal models that cytotoxic T lymphocytes (CTL) can recognize syngeneic tumour cells and can control and reject transplanted syngeneic tumours (Maryanski and Boon, 1982; Hammerling *et al*, 1987; De Plaen *et al*, 1988; Lurquin *et al*, 1989; Van den Eynde *et al*, 1991). Cytotoxic T lymphocytes recognizing autologous tumour cells have been found in humans as well (Herin *et al*, 1987; Knuth *et al*, 1989), and in a few malignancies, dense lymphocytic infiltration and the occasionally observed spontaneous remission suggest that immune mediated tumour destruction can occur. Furthermore, the frequent finding of low or absent HLA class I expression on tumour cells has been interpreted as providing se-

Cancer Surveys Volume 13: *A New Look at Tumour Immunology*
© 1992 Imperial Cancer Research Fund. 0-87969-370-3/92. $3.00 + .00

lective advantage to the tumour in avoiding immune mediated destruction (Hammerling *et al*, 1987; Smith *et al*, 1989). However, the very frequency of HLA class I loss implies that immune activation against autologous tumours is an extremely common event and suggests that without a functioning immune system, many more tumours would occur. This rests uneasily with the absence of reports of an increased incidence of non-virally induced tumours in long term immunosuppressed humans and animals. In this chapter, we review HLA class I loss in tumours and ask whether it is possible to draw conclusions from it about the role of immune surveillance in the natural history of tumours.

HLA CLASS I ANTIGENS

HLA class I antigens are transmembrane polymorphic glycoproteins composed of two polypeptide chains. The heavy chain that spans the membrane bilayer is encoded at the highly polymorphic A, B and C loci in the HLA region of the short arm of chromosome 6. Its extracellular portion is divided into three domains, α_1, α_2 and α_3, each about 90 aminoacids long. The light chain is β_2-microglobulin (β_2m), encoded by a gene on chromosome 15. β_2-Microglobulin and heavy chain must associate to allow cell surface expression (Arce Gomez *et al*, 1978; Krangel *et al*, 1979, 1982; Lancet *et al*, 1979; Ploegh *et al*, 1981; Bodmer, 1987).

Antigen, in the from of short peptides derived by processing of intracellular proteins, binds to a groove formed by the α_1 and α_2 domains of the heavy chain (Bjorkman *et al*, 1987a,b). This interaction of antigenic peptides with the binding site of class I molecules is usually required for correct folding of the heavy chain, interaction with β_2m and transport of the peptide-HLA complex to the cell surface (Townsend *et al*, 1989b). Specialized peptide transporters deliver peptide to the endoplasmic reticulum (Trowsdale *et al*, 1990; Spies and DeMars, 1991); other specialized molecules including proteases (Glynne *et al*, 1991; Kelly *et al*, 1991) and chaperone molecules (Degen and Williams, 1991) are postulated to be necessary for the correct assembly and surface expression of class I molecules. It is this peptide/heavy chain/β_2m complex that interacts with the T cell receptor of CD8+ T cells, presenting the T cells with a continuous survey of intracellular proteins. Peptide fragments thus presented that are not recognized as self can elicit T cell activation with subsequent destruction of the cell.

HLA Class I Expression in Human Tumours

A growing number of monoclonal antibodies to HLA-A, B and C antigens recognizing both polymorphic and shared determinants have allowed the study of HLA expression in different tissues and tumours by immunohistochemistry of frozen sections or cell lines (Brodsky *et al*, 1979b). Early studies on tumour cell lines often revealed defective class I expression. One of the first lines to be studied was Daudi, derived from a Burkitt's lymphoma. Complete lack of expression of class I was due to the absence of β_2m, and although HLA-A,B,C products were synthesized, they were not functionally expressed on the cell surface (Rosa et al, 1983). The same defect has also been observed in the colorectal adenocarcinoma cell line LoVo (Brodsky et al, 1979a; Travers et al, 1986). Studies on tumours in frozen section also showed aberrant HLA expression. Defective expression of class I molecules has been described in breast carcinomas (Fleming et al, 1981; Whitwell et al, 1984), in cutaneous malignant lesions (Turbitt and Mackie, 1981), in ovarian carcinomas (Kabawat et al, 1983) and in B cell lymphomas of high grade malignancy (Möller et al, 1987). By contrast, renal cell carcinomas (with the exception of the granular cell type) showed preservation of HLA class I, and it has been postulated that this allows the higher rate of spontaneous regression seen in cases of renal cell carcinoma (Tomita et al, 1990b). Reduction of class I antigens was significantly correlated with a decreased degree of tumour cell differentiation and the presence of invasion in transitional cell carcinomas (Tomita et al, 1990a).

HLA Class I Expression in Colorectal Cancer

Loss of HLA class I expression in colorectal carcinoma was first reported by Csiba and Moore (1984). Further reports (Momburg et al, 1986) suggested an inverse correlation between the loss of these antigens and the degree of differentiation. Other studies supported an association of this loss with the mucinous type of colorectal carcinoma, by itself an unfavourable prognostic feature (Van den Ingh et al, 1987). Recent data, however, suggest that the presence or absence of HLA class I molecules does not seem to modify tumour behaviour or to influence survival (Stein et al, 1988).

The development of monoclonal antibodies for specific HLA-A,B,C allelic products and polymorphic determinants has allowed a more detailed evaluation of the expression and tissue distribution of the different alleles. Several recent studies (Rees et al, 1988; Momburg et al, 1989; Natali et al, 1989; Smith et al, 1989) have found that in addition to the approximately 10% of colorectal carcinomas that lack expression of any HLA class I antigens, many more tumours display loss of expression of some class I alleles with the retention of others. Complete tumour HLA-A2 loss was observed more frequently than complete loss of HLA-A1 or HLA-A3 (Smith et al, 1989). These findings imply that selective loss might be more important in escape from tumour immunity. There is, however, no detailed information about the underlying defects causing these findings.

Our study of HLA expression in 60 colorectal adenocarcinomas was undertaken to provide a more comprehensive survey of allelic loss in colorectal tumours and if possible to probe the underlying mechanisms. The study is part of a larger project aimed to identify tumour specific cytotoxic T cells in colorectal cancer. Immunocytochemistry was performed on frozen sections of

TABLE 1. Summary of HLA losses seen in 60 colorectal tumours: failure to express any HLA Class I (W6/32-ve)

Underlying mechanism			
Free heavy chain[a]	β_2m[b]	Generalized loss[c]	Focal loss[d]
Absent	Absent	3/7	1/3
Present	Absent	1/7	1/3
Absent	Present	1/7	1/3
A present; B and C absent	Absent	2/7	–

[a]Free heavy chains detected with the monoclonal antibodies HCA2 (recognizing most HLA-A locus encoded heavy chains) and HC10 (recognizing HLA-B and C locus heavy chains)
[b]β_2m was detected with monoclonal antibody BBM-1, which recognized β_2m both free and associated with heavy chain
[c]Loss over entire section = 7/60
[d]Focal loss = 3/60

TABLE 2. Loss of some allelic HLA products with retention of others

Antibody	Specificity	Loss over entire section[a]	Focal loss[a]
MA2.1	A2/B17[b]	2/27	0/27
BB7.2	A2/Aw69[c]	1/27	0/27
142.2	A1/Aw36	3/23	3/23
3G11	All A alleles except those with Bw4 motif[d]	1/47	3/47
BB7.1	B7[c]	1/8	3/8
116.5.28	Bw4	5/32	1/32
126.39	Bw6	7/43	3/43

[a]W6/32 - ve tumours excluded from this analysis
[b]McMichael et al, 1980
[c]Brodsky et al, 1979b
[d]de Waal, 1988

Fig. 1. Photomicrographs of frozen tissue sections from two illustrative cases of colorectal adenocarcinoma. Staining was with monoclonal antibodies and the APAAP technique, counterstained with haematoxylin and not eosin. Positively staining cells are red. (*Case 1*; a) (x200) Stained with W6/32 (recognizing β_2m associated class I molecules); normal epithelium on left of section and stroma +ve, malignant epithelium (–ve) on right. (b) (x400) BBM1 (recognizing β_2m either free or associated with heavy chain), tumour –ve, stroma +ve. (c) (x400) HCA2 (recognizing A locus free heavy chain), +ve. (d) (x400) HC10 (recognizing B and C locus free heavy chain), tumour –ve, stroma +ve; this case represents an example of presumed transcriptional regulation simultaneously involving B/C locus heavy chain and β_2m, while sparing at least one A locus heavy chain. (*Case 2*; a) (x100) W6/32, tumour and stroma +ve. (b) (x200) 3G11 (recognizing all assembled A locus products except those bearing the Bw4 epitope), –ve. (c) (x200) Bw4, –ve. (d) (x200) HCA2 (A locus heavy chain), +ve; this case shows no mature A locus product despite the presence of mature B or C locus product, but free A locus heavy chain is detected, suggesting an assembly defect selectively sparing B and/or C locus product(s)

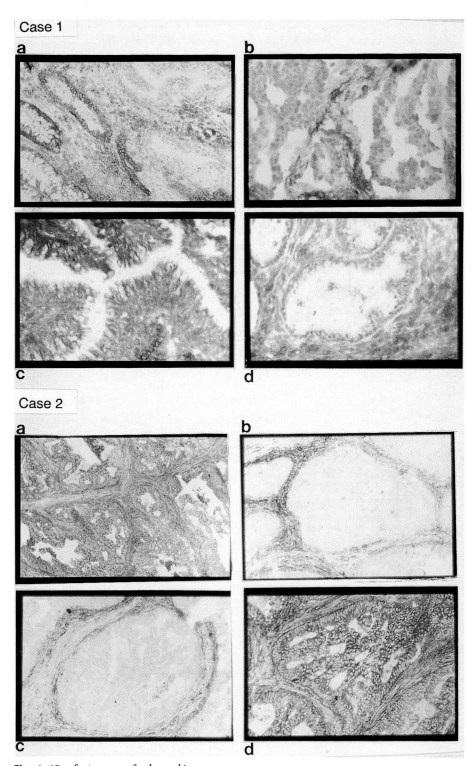

Fig. 1. (*See facing page for legend.*)

metaplastic polyps (5 cases), adenomas (15 cases) and adenocarcinomas (60 cases), and the neoplastic tissue was compared with adjacent normal stroma and nearby normal mucosa. A panel of 11 monoclonal antibodies was used in conjunction with the alkaline phosphatase/anti-alkaline phosphatase staining method (APAAP) (Cordell et al, 1984).

In no case was any difference seen between the allelic products identified in the stroma (representing connective tissue, vascular and lymphoid elements) and the non-malignant colonic epithelial tissue. None of the adenomas studied showed either focal or complete loss of all of the HLA class I molecules. However, two showed focal loss of allelic products in approximately 10% of the section. In one case, loss of an allele recognized by an anti-Bw6 antibody was seen, and a second case showed simultaneous loss of staining by 142.2 (recognizing HLA-A1) and anti-Bw6.

The findings in the 60 adenocarcinomas studied are summarized in Tables 1 and 2. Complete loss of class I expression, as detected by the antibody W6/32, which recognizes β_2m associated class I (Brodsky et al, 1979b), was seen in seven cases (11%), and focal loss was seen in a further three (5%). Staining with antibodies HCA2 and HC10, which recognize free class I heavy chains of predominantly A or B and C loci, respectively (Stam and Ploegh, 1986; Stam et al, 1990) and with BBM1 (recognizing β_2m) (Brodsky et al, 1979a) allowed some assessment of the underlying mechanisms. As shown in Table 1 and Fig. 1, case 1, loss of class I could be attributed to loss of expression of β_2m, heavy chain or both. Of the remaining 50 cases, a further 25 showed selective loss of one or more allelic products. Complete (as opposed to focal) loss of HLA-A1 was seen in 3 of the 20 individuals whose stroma was positive for this determinant, loss of A2 in 1 of 27, B7 in 1 of 8, Bw4 in 7 of 32 and Bw6 in 7 of 43. A further 14 cases showed focal allelic losses (3 A1, 3 B7, 6 Bw4 and 3 Bw6). As the antibody panel used did not cover all class I alleles, it is likely that the true frequency of selective loss is even higher. The details of selective loss are summarized in Table 2. We have thus failed to confirm the earlier suggestion that certain alleles are lost more frequently than others. In addition, we did not find any correlation between the stage or grade of the tumour and selective allelic losses. Our study differs from earlier studies, however, both in the immunohistological technique and in the source of patients.

AETIOLOGY OF MHC LOSS

The frequency of loss of MHC expression in colorectal cancers implies that this phenomenon must have biological significance. Essentially, two types of explanations are possible. Either the loss of MHC is of direct selective advantage to the tumour or the loss of MHC is an indirect consequence of another factor that is of selective advantage to the tumour. The remainder of this review focuses on these two classes of explanations and discusses ways by which they might be distinguished.

Loss of MHC Class I Expression Could Be of Selective Advantage to the Tumour

The simplest and most appealing explanation for MHC class I loss is that tumour cells without MHC class I molecules have a selective advantage over those with MHC class I molecules. The only established function of MHC class I molecules is to interact with the T cell receptors of CD8+ CTL, and CTL are known to be able to cause tumour regression (Engers *et al*, 1984; De Plaen *et al*, 1988). It is assumed that mutations causing loss of MHC are advantageous in the face of selective pressure due to an active CTL response (see reviews by Boon *et al*, Knuth *et al* and Möller and Hämmerling in this issue).

It is apparent that CTL can be identified that recognize autologous tumours; this has been well documented in mouse models, as has tumour escape from destruction by CTL by loss of the MHC class I allele that restricted the anti-tumour response (Hammerling *et al*, 1987). A handful of cases have been reported in which such CTL have been derived from human patients (see recent review by Knuth *et al* in this issue). Most reports have been from patients with melanoma, although there are isolated reports of responses to other tumours, including fibrosarcoma (Slavin *et al*, 1986). The predominance of reports of CTL to melanoma may simply be due to technical factors, in that a major block to identifying anti-tumour CTL has been the difficulty in establishing tumour cell lines, and this has proved easier for melanoma than for most human epithelial tumours. On the other hand, there is good clinical evidence for an immune response to melanoma, in that melanomas have a particularly high level of infiltrating lymphocytes and not uncommonly undergo spontaneous regression. Colorectal tumours are not known to undergo spontaneous regression and furthermore do not appear in increased frequency in patients undergoing prolonged immunosuppression, such as long term transplant recipients. Melanomas also constitutively express MHC class II and hence are capable of stimulating a helper T cell response, which may be necessary for the generation of CTL in vivo: in one animal model, the lack of immune response to a syngeneic colorectal tumour line was rectified by transfecting the cell line with interleukin-2, suggesting that lack of help may sometimes be limiting in vivo (Fearon *et al*, 1990). Thus, although the case for tumour immunity to melanoma seems to be relatively strong, the response to colorectal tumours remains more uncertain. In this light, the frequency of MHC downregulation we and others have found in colorectal cancers, especially allelic losses, is important if it can be taken to imply that colorectal tumours frequently provoke an immune response.

The frequency of focal loss is particularly intriguing. According to the hypothesis, focal loss should represent immunoselection in action, ie at the time of surgical resection, a recent immune attack has provided clones with loss of particular MHC alleles with a selective advantage over those retaining expression of these alleles. We have, however, never noticed an increased lymphocytic infiltration with tumour necrosis in the adjacent areas that are still positive for the lost allele. Of course, it is possible that other mutations—for instance, in adhesion molecules or in nominal antigen, or the secretion of immunosuppressive factors such as transforming growth factor-β (TGF-β) (Torre Amione et al, 1990)—could have occurred in these areas, rendering them non-immunogenic. Nevertheless, the absence of lymphocytic infiltration is puzzling. If selective pressure applied by a CTL response is the cause of the observed loss of MHC, its very frequency implies that colorectal tumours are the site of a continuous and intense immunological battle.

Evidence for non-immunological roles for MHC class I molecules is scant. However, transfection of MHC genes into MHC negative tumour lines has been reported either to enhance (Sunday et al, 1989) or to suppress (Gattoni Celli et al, 1988) their clonability in vitro. Although these reports are extremely limited, there remains an outside chance that some unexplored functions of MHC in modulating growth may provide selective advantage to certain tumours to downregulate MHC expression.

Loss of MHC Class I Expression Could Be Secondary to Another Factor That Is of Selective Advantage to the Tumour

It is possible to imagine two ways in which loss of MHC could be incidental to something else which is of actual selective advantage to the tumour. Firstly, the MHC or β$_2$m gene, or another gene such as one encoding an MHC specific transcription factor, could lie in close proximity to a tumour suppressor gene. There is no evidence currently to support this, and the variety of mechanisms underlying MHC loss seen in our series makes it an unlikely explanation. Secondly, MHC loss could be secondary to altered transcriptional regulation, which would have other advantages to the tumour.

The process of malignant transformation involves loss of function of tumour suppressor genes (in colon cancer including *DCC*, *APC* and wild type *p53*) and activation of oncogenes by mutation or other mechanisms (mutant *p53* and *ras* act as oncogenes in colorectal cancer) (Fearon and Vogelstein, 1990). In addition, altered methylation of DNA is seen early in the process of malignant transformation of colonic epithelium (Goelz et al, 1985; Silverman et al, 1989). These changes result in a profound rearrangement of the cell's transcriptional regulation. As many transcription factors have a wide variety of target genes, it is possible that loss of detectable MHC expression is an incidental consequence of altered transcriptional programming whose selective advantage to the cell is unregulated growth.

Regulation of MHC class I gene expression is complex (comprehensively reviewed in Singer and Maguire, 1990). MHC class I molecules are constitutively expressed on most somatic cells of the adult but are absent on the fertilized egg and during early embryogenesis; placental trophoblast cells do not express classical class I molecules, but they do express the non-classical class I molecule, HLA-G. Throughout fetal life, MHC levels gradually increase, reaching adult levels near birth. In the adult, MHC class I levels differ widely between different tissues. Class I expression is highly inducible, notably by the interferons (IFNs) and tumour necrosis factor-α (TNF-α), with IFN-γ and TNF-α having a synergistic effect. Thus, MHC class I gene regulation allows developmental, tissue specific and cytokine responsive regulation. The mechanisms are beginning to be elucidated and are predictably complex.

As described above, cell surface MHC class I expression is dependent not only on the presence of newly synthesized heavy chain and β$_2$m but also on peptide transporters and probably specialized proteases and chaperone molecules. Each of these genes is subject to separate transcriptional regulation, although there are many common features such as interferon responsiveness. The peptide transporter RING 4 is constitutively expressed in lymphoid cells, but northern blots failed to detect messenger RNA (mRNA) in colorectal cancer cell lines in the absence of IFN-γ (Trowsdale *et al*, 1990). Defective expression of any of these genes can be presumed to affect cell surface class I expression (see below for examples).

The regulation of expression of class I MHC genes appears to occur at several levels. Evidence for *cis*-acting regulation comes from studies on tumour cell lines (see below) (Singer and Maguire, 1990). This supragenic regulation may be mediated by chromatin configuration or by the DNA methylation state of the gene. The possibility that these mechanisms operate not only in tumour lines but also during developmental non-expression of class I is raised by studies with the trophoblast tumour line JAR (Boucraut *et al*, in press). This has the class I phenotype of the normal human trophoblast, ie it expresses HLA-G but no classical class I MHC; hence, it is reasonable to assume that the mechanism of downregulation of classical class I in JAR reflects the mechanism operative in the normal trophoblast. Transfected class I genes are expressed normally in JAR. The lack of expression of classical class I genes in JAR is thought to be due to hypermethylation (Boucraut *et al*, in press).

Much more is known about *trans*-acting regulation of class I gene expression. Several regulatory sequences have been identified in the 5′ flanking region of class I genes (reviewed in Singer and Maguire, 1990). The promoter (RNase polymerase II binding site), which contains CAAT and TATA boxes, lies 26–57 bases upstream of the initiation of translation site. Two enhancer sites have been identified, enhancer A (169–181 bp upstream) and enhancer B (76–82 bp upstream). Enhancer A is overlapped by an interferon response element. In addition, a negative regulatory element responsive to *trans*-acting factors has been identified 675–769 bp upstream of the swine class I gene, PD1. A number of different factors have been identified as binding to the enhancer A region. These include KBF1, KBF2, H2TF1, NFκB, GRP3, AP1 (product of the oncogenes *fos* and *jun*), AP2 and GREB/ATF (reviewed in Singer and Maguire, 1990). KBF1 activity is absent in embryonic carcinoma (EC) cell lines that do not express class I but is induced on differentiation with concomitant class I expression. In contrast, KBF2 activity is present in EC cells. Some of these factors have been implicated in the response to TNF-α and interferon. An additional interferon response element downstream from the transcription initiation site has been identified for HLA (Schmidt *et al*, 1990). The β_2m gene enhancer region also binds KBF1 and KBF2 and contains an interferon responsive element, suggesting a common regulatory pathway. However, the fact that human trophoblasts can express HLA-G (which is β_2m associated) without expressing classical class I genes shows that β_2m and the heavy chain genes can be differentially regulated. The oncogene c-*myc*, which encodes a leucine zipper type transcription factor, has been reported to downregulate HLA-B locus expression (Versteeg *et al*, 1989). Many genes are additionally regulated at the level of mRNA stability. This has been little studied for class I, but there are suggestions that posttranscriptional regulation may occur (Chen *et al*, 1986).

MHC class I heavy chain transcription is thus achieved by a complex interaction of transcription factors, some of which are involved in the regulation of many genes other than MHC. Other than predicted interferon responsiveness, very little is known about the regulation of most of the other genes necessary for class I expression. Colorectal cancer cells are less well differentiated than the epithelial cells from which they were derived. As described above, MHC is poorly expressed in the developing embryo, a stage at which many genes that act as oncogenes in transformed cells are constitutively expressed at high levels (Slamon and Cline, 1984). It seems plausible that lack of MHC expression in tumours could be a consequence of an altered transcriptional regulatory programme which more resembles that of embryogenesis than fully differentiated adult tissue.

Significance of Allelic Rather Than Total MHC Loss

The loss of individual allelic products in contrast to total loss of MHC seems to provide support for the theory that MHC downregulation is due to immunoselective pressure. As most individuals are heterozygous for MHC class I heavy chain alleles, a single mutational event—either point mutation or deletion—in either the coding or the regulatory sequence could lead to loss of expression. The chance of a single mutation occurring, allowing an advantageous phenotype in the face of an active immune response, is obviously much greater than the likelihood of mutations occurring simultaneously in both copies of non-polymorphic genes such as β_2m or transcription factors (Smith *et al*, 1988). Thus, loss of individual allelic products would be predicted to be the most common mechanism by which a tumour could evade an immune response in a heterozygous individual, and the mechanism of such loss would be predicted to involve the heavy chain genes directly.

Furthermore, transcriptional regulatory changes of the sort described in the previous section could be assumed to apply equally to all class I alleles, leading to generalized rather than selective defects. However, reports are increasingly appearing of allelic variation in MHC molecules in many aspects other than their ability to act as restriction elements. K and D loci of H-2 vary in their transcriptional regulation (Chamberlain *et al*, 1988). The sequencing of upstream regulatory regions of HLA alleles has demonstrated variation between alleles as well as loci. This has been shown to be functionally significant in the response to IFN-γ, in which HLA-B7 and HLA-Bw64 contain a 5′ interferon response element that is not present in HLA-B27, B51, B38, A2 or Cw3 (Schmidt *et al*, 1990). B locus alleles have been reported to be susceptible to downregulation by c-*myc*, whereas the A locus is not (Versteeg *et al*, 1989). Alleles vary in their susceptibility to the absence of a peptide transporter in the mutant cell lines 721.174 and 721.134, where some surface expression of A2 occurs but none of B5 (Cerundolo *et al*, 1990; Spies and DeMars, 1991). Marked allelic variation has been reported in efficiency of assembly (Neefjes and Ploegh, 1988; Lie *et al*, 1990; and our unpublished observations) and in the surface half-life of mature class I molecules (Emerson *et al*, 1980). Alleles vary in their susceptibility to the "E3/19K" protein of adenovirus 2 which retains class I MHC molecules in the endoplasmic reticulum (Cox *et al*, 1990; Jeffries and Burgert, 1990). In the transcriptional milieu of a transformed cell, it is conceivable that differential regulation of heavy chain genes, $\beta_2 m$, peptide transporters and chaperone molecules could combine to account for some of the allelic variation we see using the poorly quantitative technique of immunohistochemistry.

Can the Genetic Mechanisms of MHC Class I Loss Provide Clues to Its Aetiology?

The aetiology of MHC loss in colorectal cancer is of considerable interest because, if the loss is due to immunoselective pressure, it implies that colorectal tumours are commonly powerfully immunogenic. If so, the immunological questions raised above, such as the adequacy of stimulatory confactors, lack of T cell help and the immunosuppressive effects of factors such as TGF-β can be ignored. From the discussion above, it can be seen that the genetic basis for the observed loss of MHC class I might point to the correct explanation. If the loss is due to mutations or deletions in the MHC heavy chain genes themselves, this provides strong support for the theory that it is the loss of MHC expression itself that provides a direct selective advantage. If, on the other hand, the changes are consequent on transcriptional regulation, attribution of aetiology is more difficult.

The genetic mechanism of low or absent MHC expression has been identified in a number of cells lines derived from human tumours. In three lines (the Burkitt's lymphoma derived line Daudi, the melanoma line FO-1 [D'Urso *et al*, 1991] and the colorectal line LoVo [Brodsky *et al*, 1979a; Travers *et al*, 1986]), total MHC loss has been shown to be due to deletions and/or mutations in both $\beta_2 m$ genes and promoters. Although a phenotypic advantage dependent on two discrete events is hard to understand unless it can be assumed that the loss of the first copy of the $\beta_2 m$ gene in itself provided partial selective advantage, this sort of defect provides strong evidence for the loss of MHC having arisen through immunoselective pressure.

In another study, small cell lung cancer lines were shown by northern blot analysis to have markedly reduced amounts of HLA class I and β_2m mRNA. (Doyle *et al*, 1985). Blanchet *et al* (1990) found loss of MHC (either focal or total) in 17 of 25 cell lines derived from human tumours. Thirteen of these showed low or absent MHC class I mRNA and in most cases, this could be attributed to the absence of binding of KBF1 to the upstream enhancer region of class I. In a further six lines, lack of transcription of KBF1 itself could be observed.

Similar results were seen in a mouse model (Henseling *et al*, 1990). AKR leukaemias that fail to express H-2K^k can grow in vivo and escape lysis by CTL. Low levels of H-2K^k mRNA are present and can be attributed to low amounts of KBF1 found to be binding to the 5′ enhancer region. Transfected H-2K^k genes, however, are expressed. This is an example of a *cis*-acting mechanism preventing transcription of a normal MHC gene as discussed above.

An additional mechanism has been demonstrated in H-2 class I deficient fibrosarcoma and lung carcinoma lines (Klar and Hammerling, 1989). Class I MHC is not transcribed in these lines but is inducible by IFN-γ. Transfected class I genes are transcribed, and free heavy chains and free β_2m are detectable, but association with β_2m occurs only in response to IFN-γ, implying transcriptional downregulation not only of the class I heavy chain genes but also of another gene(s) necessary for assembly and surface expression. The newly described peptide transporter genes seem to be likely candidates.

The mechanisms of loss in our series are varied. We found loss of all class I alleles in ten cases. In seven, this was seen throughout the section and in a further three focally. In five cases (one focal), both heavy chain and β_2m expression was lost, or was at least below the level of detectability by our method. This strongly implicates a transcriptional alteration as the cause. In two cases (one focal), β_2m expression was lost with the heavy chains still expressed. In two cases (one focal), heavy chain expression was lost, whereas β_2m was retained. In a last case, illustrated in Fig. 1, case 1, HCA2 (staining A locus heavy chain) was retained whereas HC10 (B and C loci) and β_2m were lost. Among allelic loss, four cases showed loss of an A and a B locus product, implicating haplotype loss due to deletion or mitotic disjunction rather than mutation. In several other cases, loss of products of both A loci or both B loci was seen, implying either a regulatory mechanism or sequential mutational events. However, this pattern was also seen in a case of focal loss, strongly suggesting a regulatory mechanism. In addition, we frequently found detectable free heavy chain corresponding to the missing locus, as illustrated in Fig. 1, case 2. Once again, this would suggest regulatory changes. However, the limited experience with the specificity of anti-free heavy chain antibodies with the APAAP technique makes it desirable to confirm these findings with studies on tumour lines. In other cases, we have identified loss of only a single allele, although with the range of antibodies used, it has usually not been possible to confirm that this is in fact a single product loss. We have, however, extended the observations on a cell line previously derived from a colorectal tumour in which the patient's B cells expressed HLA-A1 but the tumour line does not, as detected with both immunofluorescence (Smith *et al*, 1989) and isoelectric focusing. Treatment of the line with IFN-γ and TNF-α did not restore A1 expression. Transfected HLA-A1 genomic DNA was expressed. The underlying genetic mechanism remains to be identified. The overall impression from our series is that transcriptional regulatory mechanisms will prove to be common for both generalized and at least some allelic MHC loss. The finding of free heavy chain in the absence of staining for the mature product suggests that deficient assembly may be common.

These results are consistent with a series of isoelectric focusing studies on primary ex vivo cells from 27 solid human tumours (Wang *et al*, in press), mostly ovarian carcinomas. Many of the tumours showed loss of several allelic products, but this did not appear to be due to haplotype deletion. Inducibility by IFN-γ was variable, both between tumours and between alleles; in most cases, completely absent alleles were not induced by IFN-γ, but in one instance, five of six non-expressed alleles were induced by IFN-γ.

SUMMARY AND CONCLUSIONS

The reason for MHC loss in colorectal tumours remains uncertain. Strong evidence that the downregulation is due to immunoselective pressure would be provided by the finding of deletions or mutations directly involving MHC heavy chain or β_2m genes. However, although in contrast to studies on cell lines (Brodsky *et al*, 1979a; Travers *et al*, 1986; D'Urso *et al*, 1991), our findings are in agreement with other evidence (Doyle *et al*, 1985; Blanchet *et al*, 1990; Henseling *et al*, 1990) that the most common mechanism of downregulation is regulatory, mostly at a transcriptional level. Does this imply that MHC loss in tumours can be incidental? The answer to this question will depend on the nature of the initial lesion identified. The existence of *cis*-acting regulatory mechanisms and dominant negative *trans*-acting mechanisms suggests that a single mutational event could result in transcriptional changes affecting a number of genes. Thus, selective pressure could result in tumour variants whose loss of MHC is due to transcriptional regulatory changes. As these mechanisms are unravelled, it may be possible to draw conclusions about the aetiology of MHC loss in colorectal tumours. Meanwhile, in the absence of demonstrated CTL to colorectal tumours, the case for immunoselective pressure remains unproven.

References

Arce-Gomez B, Jones F, Barnstable C, Solomon E and Bodmer W (1978) The genetic control of HLA-A and B antigens in somatic cell hybrids: requirement for β2-microglobulin. *Tissue Antigens* **11** 96–112

Bjorkman P, Saper M, Samraoui B, Bennett W, Strominger J and Wiley D (1987a) The foreign antigen binding site and T cell recognition regions of class I histocompatibility antigens. *Nature* **329** 512–518

Bjorkman P, Saper M, Samraoui B, Bennett W, Strominger J and Wiley D (1987b) Structure of the human class I histocompatibility antigen, HLA-A$_2$. *Nature* **329** 506–512

Blanchet O, Bourge J, Zinszner H *et al* (1990) Altered binding of regulatory factors to HLA class I enhancer sequence in tumor cell lines lacking class I antigen expression *Human Immunology 1990*, 10th Annual American Society for Histocompatibility and Immunogenetics Meeting Abstracts, p5

Bodmer W (1987) The HLA system: structure and function. *Journal of Clinical Pathology* **40** 948–958

Boucraut J, Hakem R, Gauthier R, Fauchet R and Le Bouteiller P Transfected trophoblast-derived human cells can express a single HLA class I allelic product. *Tissue Antigens* (in press)

Brodsky F, Bodmer W and Parham P (1979a) Characterisation of a monoclonal anti-β2-microglobulin antibody and its use in the genetic and biochemical analysis of major histocompatibility antigens. *European Journal of Immunology* **9** 536–545

Brodsky F, Parham P, Barnstable C, Crumpton M and Bodmer W (1979b) Monoclonal antibodies for analysis of the HLA system. *Immunological Reviews* **47** 3–61

Cerundolo V, Alexander J, Anderson K *et al* (1990) Presentation of viral antigen controlled by a gene in the major histocompatibility complex. *Nature* **345** 449–452

Chamberlain JW, Nolan JA, Conrad PJ *et al* (1988) Tissue-specific and cell surface expression of human major histocompatibility complex class I heavy (HLA-B7) and light (β2-microglobulin) chain genes in transgenic mice. *Proceedings of the National Academy of Sciences of the USA* **85** 7690–7694

Chen E, Karr RW, Frost JP, Gonwa TA and Ginder GD (1986) Gamma interferon and 5-azacytidine cause transcriptional elevation of class I major histocompatibility complex gene expression in K562 leukemia cells in the absence of differentiation. *Molecular and Cellular Biology* **6** 1698–1705

Cordell JL, Falini B, Erber WN *et al* (1984) Immunoenzymatic labelling of monoclonal antibodies using immune complexes of alkaline phosphatase and monoclonal anti-alkaline phosphatase (APAAP complexes). *Journal of Histochemistry and Cytochemistry* **32** 219–229

Cox JH, Yewdell JW, Eisenlohr LC, Johnson PR and Bennink JR (1990) Antigen presentation requires transport of MHC class I molecules from the endoplasmic reticulum. *Science* **247** 715–718

Csiba A, Whitwell HL and Moore M (1984) Distribution of histocompatibility and leucocyte differentiation antigens in normal human colon and in benign and malignant colonic neoplasms. *British Journal of Cancer* **50** 699–709

Degen E and Williams DB (1991) Participation of a novel 88-kD protein in the biogenesis of murine class I histocompatibility molecules. *Journal of Cell Biology* **112** 1099–1115

De Plaen E, Lurquin C, Van Pel A *et al* (1988) Immunogenic (tum–) variants of mouse tumor P815: cloning of the gene of tum– antigen P91A and identification of the tum– mutation. *Proceedings of the National Academy of Sciences of the USA* **85** 2274–2279

de Waal L, van de Meer C, van der Horst A and van der Velde F (1988) A new public antigen shared by all HLA-A locus products except HLA-23-A24-A32 and A25 is probably influenced by the aminoacid residue at position 79 in the α1 domain. *Immunogenetics* **28** 211–213

Doyle A, Martin J, Funa K *et al* (1985) Markedly decreased expression of class I histocompatibility antigens, protein and mRNA in human small-cell lung cancer. *Journal of Experimental Medicine* **161** 1135–1151

D'Urso CM, Wang Z, Cao Y, Tatake R, Zeff RA and Ferrone S (1991) Lack of HLA class 1 antigen expression by cultured melanoma cells FO-1 due to a defect in β2m gene expression. *Journal of Clinical Investigation* **87** 284–292

Emerson SG, Murphy DB and Cone RE (1980) Selective turnover and shedding of H-2K and H-2D antigens is controlled by the major histocompatibility complex. *Journal of Experimental Medicine* **152** 783–795

Engers HD, La Haye T, Sorensen GD, Glasenbrook, AL, Horvath C and Brunner KT (1984) Functional activity in vivo of effector T cell populations. II. Anti-tumour activity exhibited by syngeneic anti-MoMuLV-specific cytolytic T cell clones. *Journal of Immunology* **133** 1664–1670

Fearon ER and Vogelstein B (1990) A genetic model for colorectal tumorigenesis. *Cell* **61** 759–767

Fearon ER, Pardoll DM, Itaya T *et al* (1990) Interleukin-2 production by tumour cells bypasses T helper function in the generation of an antitumour response. *Cell* **60** 397–403

Fleming K, McMichael A, Morton J, Woods J and McGee J (1981) Distribution of HLA-class I antigens in normal human tissue and in mammary cancer. *Journal of Clinical Pathology* **34** 779

Gattoni-Celli S, Willett CG, Rhoads DB *et al* (1988) Partial suppression of anchorage-independent growth and tumorigenicity in immunodeficient mice by transfection of the H-2 class I gene $H-2L^d$ into a human colon cancer cell line (HCT). *Proceedings of the National Academy of Sciences of the USA* **85** 8543–8547

Glynne R, Powis SH, Beck S, Kelly A, Kerr L-A and Trosdale J (1991) A proteasome-related gene between the two ABC transporter loci in the class II region of the human MHC. *Nature* (in press)

Goelz SE, Vogelstein B, Hamilton SR and Feinberg AP (1985) Hypomethylation of DNA from benign and malignant human colon neoplasms. *Science* **228** 187–190

Hämmerling G, Klar D, Plum W, Momburg F and Moldenhauer G (1987) The influence of major histocompatibility complex class I antigens on tumor growth and metastasis. *Biochimica et Biophysica Acta* **25** 245–259

Henseling U, Schmidt W, Scholer HR, Gruss P and Hatzopoulos AK (1990) A transcription factor interacting with the class 1 gene enhancer is inactive in tumorigenic cell lines which suppress major histocompatibiblity class I genes. *Molecular and Cellular Biology* **10** 4100–4109

Herin M, Lemoine C, Weynants P *et al* (1987) Production of stable cytolytic T-cell clones directed against autologous human melanomas. *International Journal of Cancer* **39** 390–396

Jeffries WA and Burgert H-G (1990) E3/19K from adenovirus 2 is an immunosubversive protein that binds to a structural motif regulating the intracellular transport of major histocompatibility complex class I proteins. *Journal of Experimental Medicine* **171** 1653–1664

Kabawat S, Bast RJ, Welch W, Knapp R and Bhan A (1983) Expression of major histocompatibility antigens and nature of inflammatory cellular infiltrate in ovarian neoplasms. *International Journal of Cancer* **32** 547

Kelly A, Powis SH, Glynne R, Radley E, Beck S and Trowsdale J (1991) Second proteasome-related gene in the human MHC class II region. *Nature* **353** 667–668

Klar D and Hammerling GL (1989) Induction of assembly of MHC class I heavy chains with β2-microglobulin by interferon-gamma. *EMBO Journal* **8** 475–481

Knuth A, Wolfel T, Klehmann E, Boon T and Meyer zum Büschenfelde K-H (1989) Cytolytic T-cell clones against an autologous human melanoma: specificity study and definition of three antigens by immunoselection. *Proceedings of the National Academy of Sciences of the USA* **86** 2804–2808

Krangel M, Orr H and Strominger J (1979) Assembly and maturation of HLA-A and HLA-B antigens in vivo. *Cell* **18** 979–991

Krangel M, Pious D and Strominger J (1982) Human histocompatibility antigen mutants immunoselected in vitro: biochemical analysis of a mutant which synthesizes an altered HLA-A2 heavy chain. *Journal of Biological Chemistry* **257** 5296–5305

Lancet D, Parham P and Strominger J (1979) Heavy chain of HLA-A and HLA-B antigens in conformationally labile: a possible role for β2-microglobulin. *Proceedings of the National Academy of Sciences of the USA* **76** 3844–3848

Lie WR, Myers NB, Gorka J, Rubocki RJ, Connolly JM and Hansen TH (1990) Peptide ligand-induced conformation and surface expression of the Ld class I MHC molecule. *Nature* **344** 439–441

Lurquin C, Van Pel A, Mariame B *et al* (1989) Structure of the gene coding for tum– antigen p91A: a peptide encoded by the mutated exon is recognised with Ld by cytolytic T cells. *Cell* **58** 293–303

Maryanski JL and Boon T (1982) Immunogenic variants obtained by mutagenesis of mouse mastocytoma P815. IV. Analysis of variant specific antigens by selection of antigen-loss variants with cytolytic T-cell clones. *European Journal of Immunology* **12** 406–412

McMichael A, Parham P, Rust N and Brodsky F (1980) A monoclonal antibody that recognizes an antigenic determinant shared by HLA-A2 and B17. *Human Immunology* **1** 121–129

Möller P, Herrmann B, Moldenhauer G and Momburg F (1987) Defective expression of MHC class-I antigens is frequent in B-cell lymphomas of high grade malignancy. *International Journal of Cancer* **40** 32–39

Momburg F, Degener T, Bacchus L, Moldenhauer G, Hämmerling G and Möller P (1986) Loss of HLA-A, B, C and de novo expression of HLA-D in colorectal cancer. *International Journal of Cancer* **37** 179

Momburg F, Ziegler A, Harpprecht J, Moller A, Moldenhauer G and Hämmerling G (1989) Selective loss of HLA-A or HLA-B antigen expression in colon carcinoma. *Journal of Immunology* **142** 352–358

Natali P, Nicotra M, Bigotti A *et al* (1989) Selective changes in expression of HLA class I polymorphic determinant in human solid tumours. *Proceedings of the National Academy of Sciences of the USA* **86** 6719–6723

Neefjes JJ and Ploegh HL (1988) Allele and locus-specific differences in cell surface expression and the association of HLA class I heavy chain with β2-microglobulin: differential effects of inhibition of glycosylation on class I subunit association. *European Journal of Immunology* **18** 801–810

Ploegh H, Orr H and Strominger J (1981) Major histocompatibility antigens: the human (HLA-A, B, C) and murine (H-2K, H-2D) class I molecules. *Cell* **24** 287–299

Rees R, Buckle A, Gelsthorpe K *et al* (1988) Loss of polymorphic A and B locus HLA antigens in colon carcinoma. *British Journal of Cancer* **57** 374–377

Rosa F, Fellous M, Dron M, Tovey M and Revel M (1983) Prescence of an abnormal β2-microglobulin mRNA in Daudi cells: induction by interferon. *Immunogenetics* **17** 125–131

Schmidt H, Gekeler V, Haas H *et al* (1990) Differential regulation of HLA class I genes by interferon. *Immunogenetics* **31** 245–252

Silverman AL, Park J-G, Hamilton SR, Gadzar AF, Luk GD and Baylin SB (1989) Abnormal methylation of the calcitonin gene in human colonic neoplasms. *Cancer Research* **49** 3468–3473

Singer DS and Maguire JE (1990) Regulation of the expression of class I MHC genes. *Critical Reviews in Immunology* **10** 235–257

Slamon DJ and Cline MJ (1984) Expression of cellular oncogenes during embryonic and fetal development of the mouse. *Proceedings of the National Academy of Sciences of the USA* **81** 7141–7145

Slavin SF, Lackman RD, Ferrone S, Kiely PE and Mastrangelo MJ (1986) Cellular immune response to human sarcomas: cytotoxic T cell clones reactive with autologous sarcomas. I. Development, phenotype and specificity. *Journal of Immunology* **137** 3042–3048

Smith M, Bodmer W and Bodmer J (1988) Selective loss of HLA-A, B, C locus products in colorectal adenocarcinoma. *Lancet* **i** 823–824

Smith M, Marsh S, Bodmer J, Gelsthorpe K and Bodmer W (1989) Loss of HLA-A, B, C allele products and lymphocyte function-associated antigen 3 in colorectal neoplasia. *Proceedings of the National Academy of Sciences of the USA* **86** 5557–5561

Spies T and DeMars R (1991) Restored expression of major histocompatibility class I molecules by gene transfer of a putative peptide transporter. *Nature* **351** 323–324

Stam NJ, Spits H and Ploegh HL (1986) Monoclonal antibodies raised against denatured HLA-B locus heavy chains permit biochemical characterization of certain HLA-C locus products. *Journal of Immunology* **137** 2299–2306

Stam N, Vroom T, Peters P, Pastoors E and Ploegh H (1990) HLA-A and HLA-B specific monoclonal antibodies reactive with free heavy chains in western blots, in formalin-fixed paraffin-embedded tissue sections and in cryo-immuno-electron microscopy. *International Immunology* **2** 113–125

Stein B, Momburg F, Schwarz V, Schlag P, Moldenhauer G and Möller P (1988) Reduction or loss of HLA-A, B, C antigens in colorectal carcinoma appears not to influence survival. *British Journal of Cancer* **57** 364–368

Sunday ME, Isselbacher KJ, Gattoni CS and Willett CG (1989) Altered growth of a human neuroendocrine carcinoma line after transfection of a major histocompatibility complex class I gene. *Proceedings of the National Academy of Sciences of the USA* **86** 4700–4704

Tomita Y, Matsumoto Y, Nishiyama T and Fujiwara M (1990a) Reduction of major histocompatibility complex class I antigens on invasive and high grade transitional cell carcinoma. *Journal of Pathology* **162** 157–164

Tomita Y, Nishiyama T, Fujiwara M and Sato S (1990b) Immunohistochemical detection of major histocompatibility complex antigens and quantitative analysis of tumour infiltrating mononuclear cells in renal cell cancer. *British Journal of Cancer* **62** 354–359

Torre-Amione G, Beaucham RD, Koeppen H *et al* (1990) A highly immunogenic tumor transfected with a murine transforming growth factor type beta-1 cDNA escapes immune surveillance. *Proceedings of the National Academy of Sciences of the USA* **87** 1486–1490

Townsend A, Bastin J, Bodmer H *et al* (1989a) Recognition of influenza virus proteins by cytotoxic T lymphocytes. *Philosophical Transactions of the Royal Society of London Biology* **323** 527–533

Townsend A, Öhlén C, Bastin J, Ljunggren H, Foster L and Kärre K (1989b) Association of class I major histocompatibility heavy and light chains induced by viral peptides. *Nature* **340** 443–446

Travers P, Arklie J, Trowsdale J, Patillo R and Bodmer W (1986) Lack of expression of HLA-A, B, C antigens in choriosarcoma and other human tumour cell lines. *International Journal of Gynaecology and Obstetrics* **24** 301–307

Trowsdale J, Hanson I, Mockridge I, Beck S, Townsend A and Kelly A (1990) Sequences encoded in the class II region of the MHC related to the "ABC" superfamily of transporters. *Nature* **348** 741–743

Turbitt M and Mackie R (1981) Loss of β2-microglobulin from the cell surface of cutaneous malignant and premalignant lesions. *British Journal of Dermatology* **104** 507–513

Van den Eynde B, Lethe B, Van Pel A, De Plaen E and Boon T (1991) The gene coding for the major tumor rejection antigen of tumor P815 is identical to the normal gene of syngeneic DBA/2 mice. *Journal of Experimental Medicine* **173** 1373–1384

Van den Ingh H, Ruiter D, Griffioen G, van Muijen G and Ferrone S (1987) HLA antigens in colorectal tumours—low expression of HLA class I antigens in mucinous colorectal carcinomas. *British Journal of Cancer* **55** 125–130

Versteeg R, Kruse-Wolters M, Plomp AC *et al* (1989) Supression of class I human histocompatibility leukocyte antigen by c-*myc* is locus specific. *Journal of Experimental Medicine* **170** 621–635

Wang P, Vanky F, Li S-L, Vegh Z, Persson U and Klein E Expression of MHC class I antigens on human carcinomas and sarcomas analysed by iso-electric focusing. *International Journal of Cancer* (in press)

Whitwell H, Hughes H, Moore M and Ahmed A (1984) Expression of major histocompatibility antigens and leukocyte infiltration in benign and malignant human breast disease. *British Journal of Cancer* **49** 161–168

The authors are responsible for the accuracy of the references.

T Cell Immune Response to Cancer in Humans and Its Relevance for Immunodiagnosis and Therapy

R T D OLIVER • A M E NOURI
Department of Medical Oncology, The Royal London Hospital Medical College, Turner Street, London E1 2AD

INTRODUCTION

The idea that patients' immunity can be harnessed to resist cancer was first considered at the end of the 19th century, when the science of immunity to infectious disease was first established (Currie, 1972). After nearly a century of waxing and waning enthusiasm, there is still considerable uncertainty as to its relevance in the day to day management of cancer patients. Most of the early efforts only helped to clarify the basis of allogeneic transplantation rejection

TABLE 1. Cancer in immunosuppressed transplants[a]

	Increase	Proportion of cancer (%)
Kaposi sarcoma	x400	5.7
Lymphoma	x90	13
Vulva/perineum	x100	3
Skin	x29	38
Cervix	x14	16
Liver	x30	10
Breast	na	10
Prostate	na	2

na = not available
[a]Penn (1988)

(Gorer, 1937), a paradox, as today the principal antigens defined by this process are proving to be the key to understanding tumour rejection (Oliver *et al*, 1989b). Once the genetic basis of the major histocompatibility complex had been worked out in experimental animals (Snell and Higgins, 1951), it was then possible to demonstrate that rejection of syngeneic tumours was also mediated by immune response (Gross, 1943) and that immune memory rested in T lymphocytes (Mitchison, 1953a), as did memory for graft rejection (Mitchison, 1953b). This paper reviews evidence that T cell immune response is relevant to the resistance of cancer in humans, considers laboratory techniques for defining the degree to which the tumour has escaped from immune surveillance and discusses ways in which this observation can be exploited to improve survival in all types of cancer.

CLINICAL CLUES

Tumours in Immunosuppressed Individuals

It is a basic tenet of medical science that in order to prove the relevance of a particular process, it is necessary to investigate first the effects of suppression and then the effects of overstimulation of the system. There can be little doubt that suppression of the immune response increases the incidence of some cancers (Table 1) and that the more profound the immunosuppression the more

TABLE 2. Development of lymphoma after transplantation[a]

Method of immunosuppression	Months to onset	Proportion of patients with cancer (%)
Azothioprine based	48	11
+ cyclosporin	15	23
+ a – OKT3	7	64

[a]Penn (1988)

rapid the development (Table 2). However, many of these cancer varieties are not commonly encountered in immunocompetent subjects (Penn, 1988, 1990), and this has been a major reason for the long held scepticism about the general relevance of immune surveillance to cancer development.

Most patients on immunosuppressive drugs will be under constant medical surveillance and will undoubtedly have been encouraged to stop smoking. Moreover, renal transplant recipients, the largest single group of patients to receive immunosuppressive drugs, will have had periods of strict protein restriction while on dialysis. Saturated animal fats are a possible aetiological factor for colon and breast cancer. It is therefore perhaps not surprising that the three most common cancers (breast, colon and lung) may be less frequent in patients on immunosuppressive drugs than some unusual cancers whose cause is not as well understood. At age 35, the average for transplant patients, the expected annual incidence of cancer in the general population is less than 20–30 per 100 000, which is substantially less than the 1 per 200 seen annually during 5 years of follow-up reported in one study of kidney transplant patients (Vogt *et al*, 1990) and substantially more than that seen in patients with renal failure treated with dialysis alone (Port *et al*, 1989).

A possibly more significant indicator of the importance of immune surveillance, although less well documented, is that cancers in immunosuppressed patients are at presentation often more advanced than those in adults with a normal immune response, although not necessarily less differentiated. Supporting evidence for this suggestion comes from the observation that tumours arising in immunosuppressed individuals have less frequent loss of HLA class I and II antigens (List *et al*, 1991). This leads to the paradox that survival may not necessarily be any worse than that with spontaneous tumours. The poor survival of patients with human immunodeficiency virus (HIV) infection in whom lymphomas develop (Roithmann *et al*, 1991) may be partly explained by the increased susceptibility to fulminating AIDS related infections due to immunosuppressive chemotherapy (Roithmann *et al*, 1991). However, testis cancer in HIV infected individuals presents in a more advanced stage than normal both pathologically (Tessler and Catanese, 1987) and clinically (Damstrup *et al*, 1990), but the cure rate is not affected.

Spontaneous Regression

The second piece of evidence for the existence of immune resistance factors to cancer comes from the many reports of so called "spontaneous" regression of cancer (Table 3) (Challis and Stam, 1990). Although melanoma, kidney tumours and lymphoma predominate, spontaneous regression has been reported for almost every type of tumour. Nevertheless, common cancers such as those of lung, bowel and breast seem less likely to undergo spontaneous regression than do some of the rarer cancers.

Although unexplained "spontaneous" regressions are relatively rare, as Table 4 demonstrates, the more carefully one looks the more frequently one

TABLE 3. Spontaneous regression of cancer[a]

	No. of cases
Leukaemia/lymphoma	121
Melanoma	69
Renal cell cancer	68
Neuroblastoma	41
GI cancer	34
Retinoblastoma	33
Lung and bronchus	25
Breast	22
Testis	16
Others	75
Total	504

[a]Challis and Stam (1990)

sees it. Before our studies in kidney cancer, it was thought that fewer than 1 in 500 underwent spontaneous regression (Possinger *et al*, 1988). This was certainly so if patients once diagnosed as terminal were just sent home to die. The more often X ray examinations are repeated the higher the frequency of spontaneous regression observed. In our study of kidney cancer, all patients were checked with X rays every month without receiving treatment. Regression was detected in more than 1 in 20 patients (Oliver *et al*, 1989a).

The next section will illustrate a few of these anecdotal observations to demonstrate the spectrum of clinical evidence supporting the concept of tumour resistance mechanisms, although of course not proving that it is the immune system per se that is involved.

The most dramatic example was in a patient who presented with growing lung metastases after nephrectomy (Fig. 1, top) and failed hormone treatment. Over a period of 12 months, the tumours disappeared without any treatment (Fig. 1, bottom). Her husband was an alcoholic, who regularly attacked her. After counselling and support, she remained well for 4 years. However, her husband's alcoholism and violence then recurred and so did her tumour. She left her husband, the new metastasis was excised and she has now remained free of disease for 3 years.

The next two cases illustrate other aspects of the body's resistance to cancer that can only be observed when the cancer can be seen directly. The first case (Fig. 2), however, shows how growing and regressing melanomas can co-exist (Bodenham, 1968). This provides a very graphic demonstration of the fact that when the number of cell divisions in a cancer mass is counted and at the same time its rate of growth is measured by serial measurement, it will be apparent that all tumours have a substantial proportion of cells dying. In some patients, 90% of extra cells produced by cell division are lost (Oliver, 1982).

The final case (Fig. 3) shows how cancer can take hold at a site where previous ultraviolet radiation has damaged tissue Langerhans cells (Azizi *et al*,

TABLE 4. Comparison of spontaneous regression in testis tumour, melanoma and renal cell cancer

	Primary tumour regression in metastatic cases		Metastases regression (CR + PR)	
	presumed complete regression (CR)	apparent "partial" regression (PR)	literature series	author's series
Testis seminoma	8% (52)[a]	10% (52)	0.48% (827)	1/52
Malignant teratoma	2% (108)	4% (108)	0.48% (827)	0/180
Melanoma	5.4% (4,344)	15% (563)	0.22% (4541)	1/45
Renal cell carcinoma	na	na	0.35% (1447)	5/73

For references, see Oliver (1990b)
na = not available
[a]Figures in parentheses are numbers of cases studies

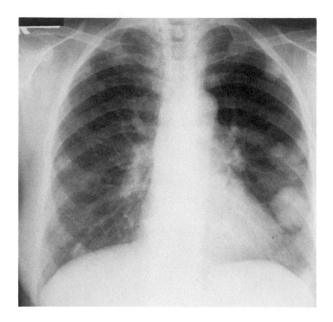

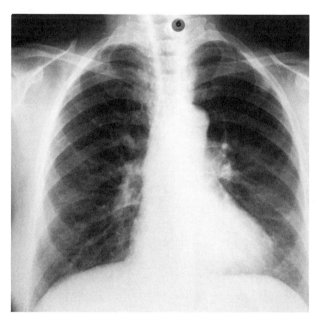

Fig. 1. Chest X-ray of patient before (*top*) and after (*bottom*) unexplained "spontaneous" regression

1987), creating an "Achilles heel" in the body enabling tumour cells to escape rejection until there was a breakdown in the patient's resistance mechanisms elsewhere. This patient developed a melanoma at a site where he had had severe sunburn 2 years previously while convalescing from glandular fever. Despite multiple surgery and radiation, his disease kept recurring in this one

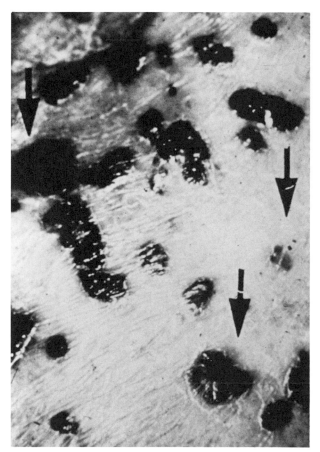

Fig. 2. Multiple cutaneous metastases from melanoma showing coincident progressing and regressing lesions

area. Two years before his death, a lesion developed on his right tibia after a football injury, suggesting that melanoma cells may have been circulating in his bloodstream but were eliminated until tissue damage created the environment for cells to settle. No other metastases were discovered until a cerebral haemorrhage, from which he died within 2 hours, was traced to a single brain metastasis.

These anecdotes are not scientific proof for the existence of cancer resistance in humans, but because they come from tumours that are easily visualized sequentially, they give a visual impression of the extremes in the spectrum of tumour behaviour, illustrating the immune surveillance that is probably occurring in a proportion of patients with all types of cancer.

Tumour Infiltrating Lymphocytes

The third line of evidence for the existence of immune surveillance against cancer comes from data correlating lymphoid cell infiltration with prognosis.

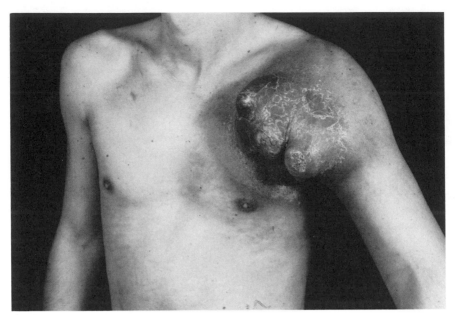

Fig. 3. Recurrent melanoma at site of previous major ultraviolet burn

Although first suggested as prognostic factor by MacCarty in 1922, there has been considerable controversy over its significance (Klein *et al*, 1980). As Fig. 4 demonstrates, the action of this prognostic factor is only apparent after 5–10 years of follow-up (Yoshimoto *et al*, 1989), which may explain why some authors have not provided such conclusive evidence for correlation between degree of infiltration and survival. The advent of therapeutic interleukin-2 (IL-2) has aroused considerable interest in tumour infiltrating lymphocytes (TIL), because IL-2 can be used to clone these cells from tumours, expand them in vitro and return them to the patient to induce regression of metastases (Rosenberg *et al*, 1986; Topalian *et al*, 1988). For melanoma (the tumour most thoroughly investigated), about 40% of patients have HLA restricted CD8 positive cytotoxic T cells (Itoh *et al*, 1988). These T cells have been labelled with a neomycin resistance gene and after infusion into the patients were shown to circulate in blood for up to 200 days and were found in excised partially rejected tumours for up to 70 days (Rosenberg *et al*, 1990). The most convincing confirmation that these T cells are specific comes from studies using a polymerase chain reaction based technique to type the melanoma TIL for T cell receptor α-chain usage. These demonstrated restricted oligoclonal representation (Nitta *et al*, 1990; Morita *et al*, 1991).

IMMUNOLOGICAL ESCAPE MECHANISMS

For successful anti-HLA cell mediated immunity, it is necessary for HLA class II antigens to present antigens to CD4 helper T cells and for class I HLA

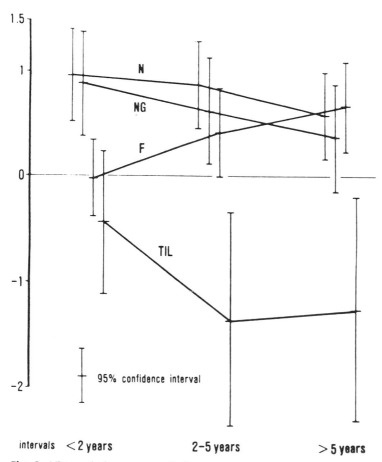

Fig. 4. Histopathology prognostic factors regression analysis in breast cancer (n = 480). N = lymph node +, NG = nuclear grade, F = fat invasion, TIL = TIL index. (Yoshimoto *et al*, 1989)

molecules to induce CD8+ cytotoxic T cells. There is increasing evidence that defects of HLA class I and class II antigen expression in tumour cells occur. This may explain the inability of IL-2 to induce class I restricted cytotoxic T lymphocytes (CTL) from TIL in most tumours other than melanoma.

HLA Class II Antigen Defects in Melanoma and Acute Myeloid Leukaemia

HLA class II antigens are not usually detectable in normal skin, and it has long been known (Natali *et al*, 1987) that class II antigens are switched on more frequently in the more malignant melanomas (Table 5). This is paradoxical, given the observation in autoimmune disease that inappropriate expression of class II antigens may lead to presentation to T lymphocytes of previously non-immunogenetic organ specific antigens and induction of the autoimmune process (Bottazo *et al*, 1983). Alexander *et al* (1989) have provided a possible explanation for this paradox by demonstrating that a melanoma cell grown from a metastasis failed to function, as measured by its ability to present tetanus

TABLE 5. Expression of HLA class II on benign and malignant lesions of melanocyte origin[a]

	No. tested	No. positive
Benign	345	21 (6%)
Primary	601	297 (49%)
Malignant/metastases	641	405 (63%)

[a]Natali *et al* (1987)

TABLE 6. Failure of metastatic melanoma DR antigen to present tetanus toxoid to tetanus toxoid immune T cell clone[a]

Antigen presenting cell type	Anti-tetanus JFTT-7	T cell clone CJTT-6
Tetanus toxoid (TT) alone	97[b]	210
TT + JF non-T cells	11,607	281
TT + CJ non-T cells	107	14,444
TT + JF melanoma (1°)	25,031	164
TT + CJ melanoma (MET)	107	176

MET = metastatic
[a]Alexander *et al* (1989)
[b]cpm after 24 hr thymidine incorporation begun 24 hr after exposure to TT

TABLE 7. Cold target cell inhibition experiments demonstrating specificity of autologous T lymphocyte cytoxicity in AML[a]

Patient no.	Target cell mixtures			
	autologous blasts-^{51}Cr (1 x 10^4)	autologous blasts-^{51}Cr (1 x 10^4)+ cold autologous blasts (1 x 10^4)	autologous blasts-^{51}Cr (1 x 10^4)+ cold autologous remission lymphocytes (1 x 10^4)	autologous blasts-^{51}Cr (1 x 10^4)+ cold allogeneic blasts (1 x 10^4)
1	34	5	36	31, 34, 37
2	21	1	18	(23)[e], 19
3	2	0	6	12, 18
4	43	30[b]	41[b]	35[b,f]
		6[c]	39[c]	36[c,f]
		0[d]	40[d]	33[d,f]

Figures indicate specific ^{51}Cr release caused by in vitro primed remission lymphocytes mixed 20:1 with ^{51}Cr labelled targets
[a]Modified from Oliver and Lee (1979)
[b]Cold targets 1 x 10^4
[c]Cold targets 1 x 10^4
[d]Cold targets 4 x 10^4
[e]Cold tagets = Daudi
[f]Cold targets - allogeneic phytohaemagglutinin blasts

toxoid to autologous T cell clones, whereas a similar line from a primary tumour in a patient without metastases functioned as well as autologous B cells in this same assay (Table 6). The defect in presentation could be corrected by transfection into the malignant cell of a normal copy of the defective class II gene (Alexander *et al*, 1991), although it was not possible to determine whether the transfected cell line had altered metastatic capacity.

Most studies of TIL cells from adult solid tumours have failed to generate HLA class I restricted CTL, and possible reasons for this will be discussed in the next three sections. However, one malignancy that has not been studied adequately where HLA class I restricted CTL cells might be present is acute myeloid leukaemia (AML). As with several solid tumours, the level of lymphocyte infiltration in AML patient's peripheral blood at presentation correlates with prognosis (Tupitsyn *et al*, 1990). Furthermore, several studies have demonstrated that AML tumour cells, like melanoma cells, overexpress class II antigens (Lecchi *et al*, 1989), suggesting that they too could have some cells with non-functioning class II antigens (Alexander *et al*, 1989). Early experiments demonstrated that 40% of patients with AML in remission had T cells in the peripheral blood that although not directly cytotoxic for autologous blasts, could become so if the blasts were presented in association with third party allogeneic class II stimulator cells (Lee and Oliver, 1978). In a small series of cold target inhibition studies, it was possible to show that inhibition of cytotoxicity occurred only with autologous and not allogeneic leukaemic blasts or autologous phytohaemagglutinin transformed lymphoblasts (Table 7), suggesting that it might have been class I restricted killing (Oliver and Lee, 1979).

The data from bone marrow transplant studies showing that graft versus leukaemia rejection occurs more frequently after HLA matched allografts than autografts (Kersey *et al*, 1987) and allogeneic leukocyte transfusions (Ford *et al*, 1980) could be in vivo correlates of this in vitro observation. Recently, an attempt has been made to use IL-2 to propagate AML TIL. This was successful in a proportion of patients, particularly those with the M4 type of AML (Table 8), and experiments are in progress to study their cytotoxic potential against autologous leukaemic blasts.

Thymic Hormones

The thymus atrophies at puberty, and levels of thymic hormones decline from then on (Fabris *et al*, 1984), although the decline is most marked after the age of 60, when the common solid adult cancers begin to reach their peak incidence. Diffusion chamber studies in 1964 first established the critical importance of the thymus as an endocrine organ (Law *et al*, 1964). Subsequent studies in mice demonstrate that thymic hormone can convert broadly autoreactive NK/LAK type lymphocytes from athymic and surgically thymectomized animals into more specific CTL in synergy with IL-2 (Trainin *et al*, 1973; Wagner *et al*, 1980; Mastino *et al*, 1991). There have been no such studies in humans. Since melanoma and AML patients, who provided the best

TABLE 8. Influence of acute leukaemic cell subtype on success of lymphocyte expansion[a]

Leukaemia 4type	No. of cases	Successful expansion	
		+IL-2	−IL-2
ALL	2	1	0
AML (M1)	4	0	0
AML (M2)	1	1	0
AML (M4)	4	3	0
AML (M5)	2	2	0
AML (EM[b])	1	1	0

[a]Nouri *et al* (unpublished)
[b]EM = extramedullary

evidence for specific HLA restricted anti-tumour CTL, were 10–20 years younger than the average patient with adult solid cancer, more studies in this area are clearly indicated. However, recent reports have suggested that use of this active thymic hormone (thymic humoral factor γ-2, an octopeptide) accelerates recovery from persistent virus infection and is associated with increased levels of T cell (Handzel *et al*, 1990).

HLA Class I Antigen Defects

Intrinsic T cell defects including lack of thymic hormone may partly explain why TIL from adult solid tumours rarely demonstrate major histocompatibility complex (MHC) restricted killing, but a more significant finding is that a substantial proportion of tumour cells from all tumour types studied have variable degrees of reduced expression of HLA class I antigen (reviewed in Oliver *et al*, 1989b). Normal expression is of course a prerequisite for HLA restricted T cell mediated cytotoxicity to occur. Table 9 summarizes our results in bladder cancer. Although global loss of all class I antigen is rare, selective loss of individual polymorphic determinants and generally reduced levels of expression com-

TABLE 9. Numerical representation of MHC and adhesive molecules on bladder tumours

	Normal	Low	Selective loss	Complete loss
HLA-ABC	23/44 (52%)	144/44 (31%)	1/18 (5%)	6/44 (13%)
Free heavy chain	6/41 (15%)	17/41 (41%)	na na	18/41 (44%)
β_2m	26/43 (60%)	16/43 (38%)	na na	1/43 (2%)
LFA-3	26/37 (70%)	8/37 (22%)	na na	3/37 (8%)

na = not applicable

pared with non-malignant cells are more frequent. Fewer than 20% of patients had normal expression. These studies also demonstrated that it was more difficult to grow TIL from the tumours with decreased class I expression (Nouri et al, 1990 and in press).

Shedding of Tumour and HLA Antigens as an Immune Escape Mechanism

One observation of interest to emerge from the study of HLA antigen loss in lymphomas was the finding that tumours showing HLA loss had higher circulating levels of β_2-microglobulin (Swan et al, 1988), suggesting that the HLA loss seen in these tumours may be due not to switching off of the HLA class I gene but to enhanced turnover and shedding from the cell membrane. This would make it more difficult to detect with standard immunofluorescence techniques, since the incubation time for the assay is sufficient for the cells to cap the antigen-antibody complex off the cell surface. Currie and Alexander (1974) demonstrated that the higher the rate of shedding of tumour antigen from animal tumours the more malignant the tumour behaviour in vivo. Studies in our own laboratory (Lee SK and Oliver RTD, unpublished) have demonstrated that a similar phenomena may be occurring in AML, although there may be an additional factor in that pretreatment but not remission serum contained a paracrine factor that accelerated the rate of shedding (Fig. 5). Recent observations in myeloma demonstrate that exogenously produced IL-6 (possibly from marrow stroma) can accelerate tumour growth (Huber et al, 1991) and that in some breast cancer patients, the stroma produce excess amounts of fibroblast growth factors (Winstanley et al, 1961) are two further examples of this phenomenon.

β-hCG, ICAM-1 and Other Tumour Cell Membrane Changes

HLA antigens are not the only cell membrane antigens that are lost during malignant transformation. There has long been interest in altered carbohydrate blood group antigens on bladder cancers (Feizi, 1985) and leukaemias, where decreased expression has been shown to be due to alterations in serum levels of glycosyltransferase enzymes (Kuhns et al, 1980). Although these changes may not necessarily affect tumour immunogenicity, they could affect the fluidity of the membrane, leading to alteration of antigen shedding rate.

One other set of antigens that are undoubtedly of importance for effective T cell mediated cytotoxicity are cell adhesion molecules such as LFA-3 and ICAM-1. The importance of these antigens has been well documented in studies of T cell cytoxicity against Epstein-Barr virus infected cells, and several authors have noted that some malignant tumours have such losses, usually, but not always, in association with class I loss. Vanky et al (1990) have demonstrated clear evidence that such loss synergizes with HLA class I loss to enhance malignant behaviour (Table 10).

There has long been speculation that an understanding of how the semi-

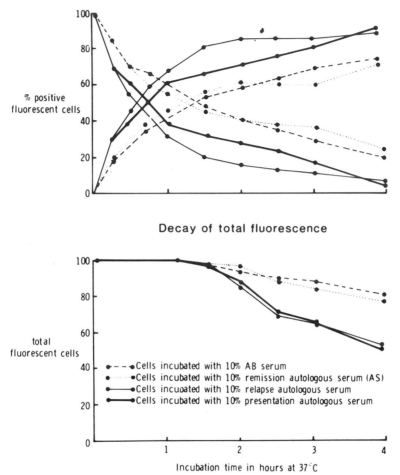

Indirect immunofluorescence of rabbit anti human β₂microglobulin

Decay of total fluorescence

Incubation time in hours at 37°C

Fig. 5. Changes in distribution of β₂-microglobin in acute myeloid leukaemia blast cells after incubation with remission and relapse autologous serum

TABLE 10. Effect of HLA class I and ICAM-1 loss on autologous T cell immune response and metastases[a]

	Class I+ ICAM 1+	Only one of them present	Class I− ICAM 1−
Auto-tumour reactivities	6/7 (86%)[b]	0/11	0/7
Metastatic state	1/7 (14%)	6/11 (55%)	4/7(57%)

[a]Modified from Vanky *et al* (1990)
[b]Positives/number tested

allogeneic placenta evades immune rejection might help to explain tumour escape from immune surveillance. Possibly related to this is the accelerated growth sometimes seen in breast tumours that arise during pregnancy compared with similar tumours arising in non-pregnant women (Clark and Chua, 1989).

Further interest in the mechanism of placental escape from immune rejection has arisen from the observation that a minority of tumours from several sites such as bladder, stomach and lung switch on β human chorionic gonadotrophin (β-hCG) in association with accelerated tumour growth, metastasis and possible resistance to treatment (reviewed in Iles *et al*, 1989; Oliver *et al*, 1989b).

In bladder cancer, the β-hCG producing tumours also had reduced HLA class I expression (Oliver *et al*, 1989b; Nouri *et al*, 1990). The World Health Organization has been investigating the use of a vaccine against β-hCG as a contraceptive because it causes the mother to reject the β-hCG bearing trophoblast of the fetus (Stevens and Crystal, 1973). This vaccine might also be considered for the treatment of β-hCG producing bladder cancers.

APPROACHES TO IMMUNOTHERAPY

Non-specific Immunotherapy

There is little doubt that superficial bladder tumours (both pTa and pTi) are the human tumours that have shown the most clear-cut evidence of being controlled by stimulation of immune response. Induction of non-specific immune stimulation in the bladder lining by instilling BCG vaccine into the bladder produced complete tumour rejection in more than two-thirds of patients (reviewed in Oliver, in press). Failure of immunological response as measured by a lack of production of IL-2 (Fleishman *et al*, 1989) and failure of induction of HLA class II on tumour cell (Prescott *et al*, 1989) correlated with poor prognosis as measured by tumour response.

Cytokines, Interleukin-2 and Interferon-α

Interleukin-2 is a cytokine, which acts as a short range messenger regulating the activity of cells involved in immune response (Balkwill, 1989). Interleukin-2 is specifically produced by CD4+ T lymphocytes when they recognize antigen, and it raises lymphocyte concentrations at the site of an active immune response by inducing mitosis in CD4 and CD8 T cells (Taniguchi *et al*, 1986). This cytokine has been under assessment in a phase 1/2 setting but has been seriously evaluated only in kidney cancer and melanoma. There is little doubt that it can produce durable complete remission (Fig. 6 and Table 11). There is a general impression, borne out by study of cumulative series in the literature, that complete remissions are more common and occur in patients with more advanced disease than those seen after interferon-α (IFN-α)

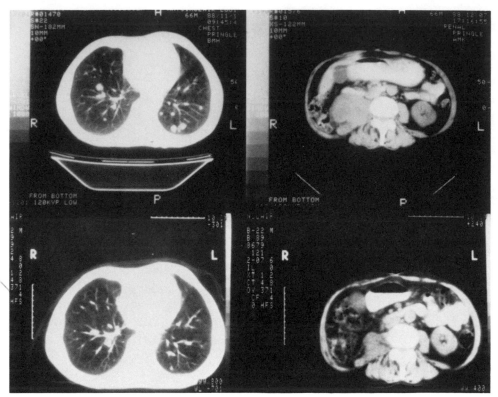

Fig. 6. Lung metastases from renal cell cancer before (a) and after (b) IL-2, and recurrence in renal bed of renal cell cancer before (c) and after (d) IL-2

(Tables 12 and 13). The observation that transient autoimmune thyroiditis develops in 14% of patients on interferon, 21% of patients on IL-2 and 40% of patients on combined IL-2 and interferon supports the view that immunological response is relevant to these tumour responses (Pichert *et al*, 1990), and

TABLE 11. Metastatic renal cell cancer and complete response to BCG, IFN-a, IL-2 and IL-2 plus IFN-a[a]

	All cases		Lung only metastases post-nephrectomy	
	no. of cases	CR	no. of cases	CR
BCG	19	5%	7	14%
IFN-α	81	3%	17	12%
IL-2	11	9%	4	25%
IL-2 + IFN-α	16	0%	3	—
Total	127	3%	31	13%

CR = complete remission
[a]Oliver RTD. personal observations

TABLE 12. Impact of schedule and dose on response of metastatic renal cell carcinoma to IFN-a[a]

Frequency of treatment	$<3 \text{ mu/m}^2$ CR+PR	$3\text{-}10 \text{ mu/m}^2$ CR+PR	$>10 \text{ mu/m}^2$ CR+PR
>5/week	4%+14% (n = 153)	2%+16% (n = 203)	2%+13% (n = 494)
<5/week	2%+8% (n = 51	0%+13% (n = 54)	0%+13% (n = 147)
<5/wk + q3 V week			3%+22% (n = 207)

CR = complete remission; PC = partial remission; q3 = repeated every 3 weeks; V = vinblastine
[a]Modified from Horoszewicz and Murphy (1989)

there is some evidence that the development of thyroiditis correlates with duration of response (Atkins *et al*, 1988).

The critical issue for both interferon and IL-2 is the dose schedule, which is increasingly accepted as not following the rules developed for chemotherapy studies. As can be seen from studies of interferon alone, IL-2 alone and interferon and IL-2 in combination (Tables 12 and 13), high dosage causes increased toxicity and shows no clear-cut benefit. However, the interferon data suggest that it may be important to give treatment for a continuous period, which has been routine with IL-2. Evidence from animal IL-2 dose-response studies (Cheever *et al*, 1985) supports the low dose approach, since the area under the curve (more enhanced by subcutaneous injection) may relate better to the biological effect than the peak dose (more marked with intravenous bolus dosage). There is also evidence from in vitro studies that prolongation of stimulus beyond 4 days leads to downregulation of expression of high affinity IL-2 receptors (Gullberg and Smith, 1989). This, taken with the evidence that there may be a bell shaped dose-response curve, ie high dose inhibition of response, in experimental animal models (Talmadge *et al*, 1987), provides ample justification for more extensive exploration of the intermittent lower dose subcutaneous regimens.

Interleukin-2 (a T cell mitogen; Taniguchi *et al*, 1986) and IFN-α (which augments HLA class I expression; Lindahl *et al*, 1974) have differing sites of action on immune response, and there is strong evidence from animal studies

TABLE 13. Pooled results of IL-2 +/- LAK for renal cancer [a]

	Single agent IL-2	IL-2 + IFN-α	IL-2 + +LAK cells
Low dose IL-2 (outpatient)	3 + 2/56 (20%)	4 + 27/145 (21%)	na
High dose IL-2 (inpatient)	15 + 33/328 (13%)	4 + 17/105 (20%)	17 + 37/302 (18%)

na = not available
[a]For references, see Oliver (1991)

that IL-2 and IFN-α are additive when used in combination (Igo et al, 1988; Rosenberg et al, 1988). However, to date, the results from clinical trials are conflicting. Although some of the earlier studies showed response rates in excess of 30% (compared with 15% for either agent alone), a recent review of more than 200 patients (Table 13) showed overall responses of 21% (compared with 14% for IL-2 alone and 14% for IFN-α alone). The only formalized randomized trial showed a worse response for the combination treatment than for the single agent treatment (Atkins, 1991). Most of these studies were small pilot studies, and few provided extensive dose-response escalation. The only one to do so showed a bell shaped dose response with lower responses at high doses than at intermediate doses (Rosenberg et al, 1989). Perhaps the optimum dosing schedule has yet to be defined. Testing of even lower doses may be needed, since animal studies have shown some evidence that the optimum dose for cytokines in combination is one log lower than the optimum dose of single agents (McHeyzer-Williams, 1989).

Given the current economic climate with controlled access even for heart transplants, which are considerably more successful, the level of activity seen in the renal cell cancer cytokine studies is barely sufficient to justify its routine use in renal cancer, let alone encourage its evaluation in other tumour types. However, if it were possible either by use of clinical criteria (Maladazyz and de Kernian, 1986) or by immunological testing, for example demonstrating that HLA class I antigen expression on tumour was normal, and study of levels of IL-2 (Lissoni et al, 1991) or IL-2 receptor in blood (Carteni et al, in press) to define subgroups with a high prediction of response, there would be a better case to encourage more widespread study of its use in other cancers. There is already some evidence from the study of renal cell cancer that such a selection maximizes the frequency of response when compared to the frequency of spontaneous regression (Oliver et al, 1989a).

Other Cytokines

Several other cytokines have been investigated in clinical trials, although only two of them, IFN-γ and tumour necrosis factor (TNF), have been examined as thoroughly as IFN-α and IL-2. Neither has demonstrated a major benefit in malignant disease, although IFN-γ has shown considerable promise, leading to a licence for its use in treatment of chronic granulomatous disease (Eckowitz, 1991), and TNF has proven particularly effective at controlling ascites (Raeth et al, 1991). It is paradoxical that IFN-γ should prove so ineffective in cancer, given its particularly marked effect in upregulating class II antigens (putatively involved as an intermediary in development of autoimmune disease; Bottazzo et al, 1983). Some experimental studies have demonstrated that tumour growth and metastatic spread can be enhanced with IFN-γ (Kelly et al, in press). As there is some evidence that there are immune suppressor genes controlled by the class II region (Zaitseva and Brondz, 1990), it is perhaps not surprising that dose may be critical in determining responses.

Viral Vaccines and Cancer Prevention

In humans, associations with cancer development have been unequivocally established for three viruses—hepatitis B in hepatoma, Epstein-Barr virus in Burkitt's lymphomas and human papillomavirus (HPV) in cancer of the cervix. These cannot on their own lead to the complete development of terminal cancer, and their principal role is believed to be to provide an initiating proliferative signal that keeps the target tissue dividing faster than normal, thus reducing DNA repair time (Yang et al, 1982) and increasing the cells' susceptibility to background mutagenic activity.

Today, the race is on to establish whether by eliminating one of these viruses the associated cancer will disappear. The most likely one to produce information is hepatitis B virus, because a hepatitis B vaccine is now being routinely used in the third world (Whittle et al, 1991), where liver cancer is one of the commonest malignancies. However, it is likely to be at least 10–20 years before we will know whether vaccination does protect. Unfortunately, chronic hepatitis B infection develops in about 3% of people vaccinated (Whittle et al, 1991).

The majority of bladder cancer patients present with papillary rather than solid tumours. These usually do not show all of the characteristics of malignant tumours but tend to behave more like warts in that they come and go unpredictably and may continue to behave in this way for variable periods, sometimes as long as 10–20 years, before progressing to invasive and metastatic cancer (Oliver, 1990c).

Warts are caused by papillomaviruses (Pfister et al, 1986), a group that includes the common verruca virus that most children get these days from swimming in public swimming pools. This group of viruses has been associated with tumours in many animal species. In all of these species, there are many subtypes, and although the associated tumours show a varying degree of malignancy, the majority are benign. The complexity of the relationship of the virus subtype to the degree of malignancy is best illustrated by the classic studies with the Shope papillomavirus in rabbits. These studies demonstrated that it was possible to have benign or malignant tumours from the same virus depending on the genetic resistance of the individual recipient or the amount of carcinogen treatment that was given to individual animals with a benign tumour. These studies have also demonstrated that it was possible to use vaccination to control infection. In humans, the most convincing evidence for involvement of immune response in controlling warts comes from a classic controlled study demonstrating rejection of warts by hypnosis (Spanos et al, 1990), presumed to be due to stimulation of the areas of the brain involved in regulation of immune response.

In humans, superficial bladder cancers are as yet not proven to be caused by a specific papillomavirus. However, there have been several anecdotal reports of association with a variety of different types of papillomaviruses (Oliver et al, 1989b; Querci della Rovera et al, 1989). This is perhaps not surprising, given the variable morphology of these tumours (Oliver, 1990c). There is clearly a need to do more detailed human papillomavirus DNA studies in early bladder cancer samples, since a vaccination programme in patients with premalignant lesions would be justified if a papillomavirus antigen common to both cervical and bladder cancer were found.

Evidence has been accumulating that the mumps virus in association with diminished immune response, which allows persistence of chronic mumps virus infection and results in testicular atrophy, may be an initiating factor in testis cancer (Beard *et al*, 1977; Oliver, 1990a,b). Vaccination against mumps virus has now become routine in the UK for all preschool children. At least 25 years' follow-up of more than 5000 children (the lifetime risk of testis cancer is 1:500) would be necessary to prove whether vaccination did protect against the development of testis cancer, although the number would be smaller for individuals with cryptorchidism, who have a 1:50 lifetime risk.

RELEVANCE OF HOST RESISTANCE FACTORS TO OTHER MODALITIES OF CANCER TREATMENT

There is little doubt that of the two host factors responsible for resistance to cancer, DNA repair enzyme function has a more significant role than immune response. This is because there are few identified adults with DNA repair enzyme defects who have not developed some form of tumour, whereas only a minority of subjects who are immunosuppressed (by treatment with immunosuppressive drugs, infection with an immunosuppressive virus or inheritance of a genetic immunodeficiency syndrome) develop tumours. However, given the greater availability of reagents for reversing immunodeficiency and the unlikelihood that replacement of deficient DNA repair enzymes will undo an established tumour, for the immediate future, exploration of approaches to harness immune resistance seems likely to be more productive.

Combination of Immunotherapy with Radiotherapy and Surgery

Duration of anaesthesia for surgery (Hattori *et al*, 1980) and radiation, particularly if fractionated over long periods (Sternswald *et al*, 1978), influences the degree of immunosuppression after treatment. Thus, it is surprising that combination of immunotherapy with conventional treatments for all tumour types has been studied very little.

Studies in animals have demonstrated clearly that the degree of immunosuppression correlates with the duration of anaesthesia (Oliver *et al*, in press), and in humans, there is an additional factor, ie blood transfusion, that in renal transplant recipients improves chances of survival of HLA incompatible grafts (Opelz and Terasaki, 1974). By contrast, and providing additional support for the relevance of immune surveillance, whole blood transfusion of cancer patients increases the chance of recurrence of colon, breast and lung cancer patients after radical surgery (Meryman, 1989), whereas one study has demonstrated no such effect from use of packed red cells (March *et al*,

1990). Further investigation is clearly justified, since use of leukocyte depleted blood is likely to be more cost effective than cytokine treatment.

There have been few large scale formal randomized trials combining immunotherapy and surgery with 5–10 years follow-up, although the results of a trial of BCG/tumour cell vaccine therapy after surgery for colon tumours are perhaps the most convincing evidence for benefit (Hoover et al, 1985). The absence of benefit in the subgroup of rectal cancer patients who received prophylactic radiotherapy during the period of vaccination demonstrates that the question of timing may be critical. An additional factor in this study influencing benefit from treatment was the presence of inducible class II antigens on the tumour cells used as vaccine (Ransom et al, 1991).

Little work has been done on combining cytokines with surgery, but the data of Ramani et al (1986) in experimental animals suggest that there may be a window of opportunity for reducing the frequency of take of tumour cells that escape into the bloodstream during operative manipulation. Pilot studies, done because it was uncertain whether cytokine treatment might delay postoperative healing, have demonstrated no unexpected difficulties when either IFN-α (Cockerell et al, 1991) or IL-2 (Oliver RTD, unpublished) is given during the preoperative week.

There has been even less effort to evaluate radiotherapy in combination with immunotherapy, despite evidence of synergy with both interferon and IL-2 in animal studies. The only randomized clinical study involved only 43 patients with squamous cell lung cancer after radical radiotherapy. One year survival was 30% in the 20 who received BCG, compared with 17% in 23 control patients (Pines, 1976).

Combination of Immunological Treatments with Chemotherapy

Considerable numbers of studies have investigated chemotherapy in combination with immunotherapy, although few have provided evidence of major benefit. The most substantial have been the studies investigating levamisole in combination with 5-flurouracil in colon cancer (Table 14) (Windle et al, 1987; Moertel et al, 1990). These studies illustrate an important issue of such trials, ie that the benefit of immunotherapy occurs late. This might have been predicted from the data of Yoshimoto et al (1989) discussed earlier which demonstrated that TIL cell infiltration was only prognostic for late relapse (see Fig. 4). On the basis of these observations, the US National Institutes of Health consensus conference, summarized in the *Journal of the American Medical Association* (National Institutes of Health 1991), has recommended that this should become standard treatment, which is possibly a little premature given that in the early stage cases, ie stage B, no benefit was demonstrable.

The possibility that there might be more widespread benefit from use of cytokine treatments in combination with chemotherapy comes from the studies of Logothetis et al (1991), who demonstrated durable responses with chemotherapy in combination with IFN-α in patients in whom chemotherapy alone had failed.

TABLE 14. Impact of 5-FU/levamisole on 2 and 5 year survival of stage C colorectal carcinoma

Adjuvant trial	No. of cases	Survival	
		2 year	5 year
Moertel *et al* (1990)			
Observation	315	76%	52%
Levamisole	310	75%	58%
Levamisole/5-FU	304	80%	75%
Windle *et al* (1987)			
Observation	49	85%	65%
Levamisole	45	80%	65%
Levamisole/5-FU	47	84%	82%

5-FU = 5-fluorouracil

Combination of Biological Treatment with Hormone Therapy

Studies of biological treatment in combination with hormone therapy are even rarer than those of combination with other modalities of cancer treatment. The only positive study (Table 15) was a Japanese study involving only 31 patients (Kosaka *et al*, 1985). However, it identified one issue that may be extremely important for defining the optimum way of identifying synergy between endocrine and immunological treatment. The critical issue was that these authors treated only patients whose tumours had shown a major response to hormone treatment before they were randomized to immunotherapy or control. As hormone sensitivity is a marker of differentiation, this would have been a way of selecting the most differentiated tumours, which the experience with BCG treatment in bladder cancer has demonstrated is critical in achieving response to biological treatment.

A further factor that makes study of hormone and immunotherapy worth further exploration is the fact that castration induces regeneration of the thymus and lymphocytosis (Grossman, 1985). Recent studies in rats have confirmed that this also occurs when synthetic gonadotrophin releasing hormones are used (Fitzpatrick *et al*, 1985). Retrospective analysis of prostatic cancer patients receiving the gonadotrophin releasing hormone analogue confirmed

TABLE 15. Influence of immunotherapy (lentinin) on progression free survival of breast cancer responders to hormone therapy[a]

	No. of cases	Progression free survival at 3 years[b]
Controls	16	13% (2)
Lentinin	15	46% (7)

[a]Kosaka *et al* (1985)
[b]χ^2 4.2, p <0.05

that lymphocyte levels rise during the first 4 weeks of treatment, and some patients even show reduced numbers of lymphocytes during the surge in testosterone levels that occurs in the first week after treatment is initiated (Joseph J and Oliver RTD, unpublished).

Immunoprevention of Cancer

Currently, screening techniques for early detection of cervical and breast cancer are being applied widely. Although the approach is relatively economic when assessed on the basis of cost of the test per cancer detected, these figures do not take into consideration the considerable false positive rate, which generates considerable anxiety in healthy individuals, as well as the need for costly reassessments and possible surgical intervention in considerably more individuals than have gained benefit from detection of proven cancer (Mant and Fowler, 1990). Furthermore, the incidence of cancer in the screened population is often higher than in the unscreened population, suggesting that some tumours may be detected by screening that might otherwise have undergone spontaneous regression. Attempts to achieve early diagnosis of prostate cancer by means of annual digital examination (Crawford *et al*, 1991) and ovarian cancer by ultrasound and tumour marker assays (Jacobs *et al*, 1988) have produced equally large numbers of false positives requiring expensive investigations. Many latent foci of prostatic cancer detected at necropsy in patients dying without a diagnosis of cancer (Breslow *et al*, 1977) would also be detected.

Were it possible to develop low cost population based (or high risk group) intervention to boost immune resistance, it is possible that the gain would be more substantial than with any screening programme, since it would not have to be organ specific. In earlier sections, evidence was presented that immune rejection of cancer and precancer is likely to be most efficient with the well differentiated early stages, particularly in the virally induced tumours before immunoselection has led to emergence of clones that have downregulated or mutated HLA class I antigens. Two preliminary studies support this view. In the first study, immunotherapy was given to a randomized group of workers who had a high risk of cancer because they were exposed to high level chemical pollution in a poison gas factory. After a 5 year follow-up, cancer developed in 17 of 146 controls and 7 of 146 individuals treated with nocardia rubra cell wall skeleton (Yamakido *et al*, 1990). The second study, from Korea, demonstrated in a case control study (Table 16) that regular ginseng consumption increased resistance to cancer (Yun and Choi, 1990). Recent animal studies have demonstrated that d-limonene, a component of the oil from the gland in orange peel, may have a similar effect (Elegbede *et al*, 1986).

CONCLUSIONS

The tumours that develop after immunosuppressive drug treatment provide unequivocal evidence that immune surveillance is relevant to cancer resistance for an increasing proportion of cancer sites, particularly those with evidence

TABLE 16. Ginseng consumption and cancer risk[a]

Frequency of ginseng intake	Males			Females		
	hospital cancer cases	hospital non-cancer controls	odds ratio (95% CI)	hospital cancer cases	hospital non-cancer cases	odds ratio (95% CI)
None	117	56	1.00	226	175	100
1–3 times/year	132	108	0.58 (0.38–0.90)	111	106	0.81 (0.57/1.15)
4–11 times/year	104	115	0.43 (0.28–0.67)	75	103	0.56 (0.39–0.82)
Once/month or more	83	157	0.25 (0.16–0.39)	57	85	0.52 (0.35–0.78)
Total	436	436		469	469	
Linear trend test (1 df)		45.59 (p<0.00001)			3.98 (p<0.05)	
χ² homogeneity test (3 df)		47.28 (p<0.00001)			16.53 (p<0.001)	4

[a]Modified from Yun and Choi (1990)

for viral involvement in the initiation process. It may well be that this group of tumours will demonstrate the most dramatic benefit from immunotherapy, because the tumours that develop, although they tend to become widespread early, also tend to remain well differentiated and not have reduced HLA class I and II antigens or adhesion molecule expression. These characteristics are increasingly recognized as a means of escape from immune surveillance in cancers arising spontaneously in non-immunosuppressed individuals.

The data that single agent cytokines, interferon and IL-2 produce durable complete remission in a minority of patients with progressive renal cell cancer (predominantly early small volume lung metastases) is the most convincing evidence that manipulation of immune response can produce tumour rejection, although the late follow-up studies from superficial bladder tumours and colon cancer reviewed from the 1970s demonstrate that immunotherapy can indeed improve long term survival advantage for all types of tumours by 10–15%. However, to realize this will require considerable investment of resources in long term studies. Because the beneficial effects of immunostimulation have been more marked in early and premalignant stages of cancer development, there is increasing interest in the idea that low cost population based intervention could yield greater benefit than current cancer screening programmes.

The possibility of using viral vaccines to control tumours with a viral factor in their aetiology is attractive but may prove economically non-viable because of the large number of individuals who will need to be vaccinated without benefit and the long period of follow-up necessary to prove the benefit. The only possible candidates are those viruses that cause additional morbidity other than cancer, as is the case with hepatitis B virus associated with hepatoma and mumps virus associated with testis cancer. However, it will take at least 20 years before any effect of these two vaccines on the incidence of associated tumours will be known.

SUMMARY

Review of the relationship between the degree of immunosuppression and malignancy in patients on immunosuppressive drugs or immunosuppressed by HIV infection, postoperative blood transfusion or pregnancy provides the most convincing evidence of the importance of intact T cell immunity in resistance to cancer. Defective HLA class I and II antigen expression on tumours arising in non-immunosuppressed individuals and correlation of these changes with increased malignancy and diminished TIL provide the most convincing evidence that one factor necessary to ensure survival of most spontaneous tumours is mutation that enables tumour cells to escape rejection by cytotoxic T cells. These changes are less frequent in tumours in immunosuppressed patients, and preliminary data suggest that use of cytokine therapy is more successful in these tumours and the one in five spontaneous tumours demonstrating normal expression of HLA antigens and high levels of T cell infiltration. These observations suggest that future use of this therapy should be focused on these cases.

All modalities of cancer therapy except hormone therapy (ie surgery, radiotherapy and chemotherapy) suppress immune responses. Defects of HLA antigen expression are less marked in early cancer. Combinations of immunotherapy with conventional treatment at presentation, including hormone therapy in view of data demonstrating regeneration of the thymus after castration, needs further investigation.

Preliminary results from randomized trials involving nearly 300 individuals accidentally exposed to carcinogens demonstrated nearly 60% reduction of incidence of malignancy at 5 years in the arm receiving non-specific immunotherapy. If confirmed, such an approach might be more cost-effective as an approach for cancer prevention than organ specific cancer screening or vaccination against cancer associated viruses such as hepatitis B or papillomaviruses.

Acknowledgements

This work was supported by grants from the Imperial Cancer Research Fund, Grand Metropolitan Charitable Trust, Stadium, Mercury Trust and the Barclay Foundation. The author gratefully acknowledges the helpful comments of Dr Frances Balkwill, Dr Mike Owen and Dr Peter Beverley and the help of Deborah Goodhart and Ruth Jackson with the preparation of the manuscript.

References

Alexander MA, Bennicelli J and Guerry D (1989) Defective antigen presentation by human melanoma cell lines cultured from advanced, but not biologically early, disease. *Journal of Immunology* **142** 4070–4078

Alexander MA, Lee W and Guerry D (1991) Retroviral vectro transfection of a class II positive human metastatic melanoma cell line with a matched HLA-DR B1 gene restores its capacity to present antigen. *Proceedings of the American Association for Cancer Research* **32** 1413 [**Abstract**]

Atkins MB, Mier JW, Parkinson DR *et al* (1988) Hypothyroidism after treatment with interleukin-2 and lymphokine activated killer cells. *New England Journal of Medicine* **318** 1557–1563

Atkins MB, Sparano J, Fisher RI *et al* (1991) Randomized phase II trial of high dose IL-2 either alone or in combination with interferon alpha 2B (IFN) in advanced renal cell carcinoma (RCCA). *Proceedings of the American Society of Clinical Oncology* **10** 526 [**Abstract**]

Azizi E, Bucana C, Goldberg L and Kripke LM (1987) Perturbation of epidermal Langerhan cells in basal cell carcinomas. *American Journal of Dermatopathology* **9** 6465-6473

Bagenal FS, Easton DF, Harris E, Chilvers CE and McElwain T (1990) Survival of breast cancer patients attending Bristol Cancer Help Centre. *Lancet* **335** 606–610

Balkwill FR (ed) (1989) Understanding and exploiting the cytokine network, In: *Cytokines in cancer therapy,* pp 207–235, Oxford University Press, Oxford

Beard CM, Benson RC and Kelalis PP (1977) The incidence and outcome of mumps orchitis in Rochester, Minnesota 1935-1974. *Mayo Clinic Proceedings* **52** 3–7

Bernstein L, Ross RK, Lobo RA *et al* (1987) The effects of moderate physical activity on the menstrual cycle patterns in adolescence: implications for breast cancer prevention. *British Journal of Cancer* **55** 681–685

Bodenham (1968) A study of 650 observed malignant melanomas in the South-West region. *Annals of the Royal College of Surgeons* **43** 218

Bottazzo GF, Pujol-Borrell R and Hanafusa T (1983) Role of aberrant HLA-DR expression and antigen presentation in the induction of endocrine autoimmunity. *Lancet* **ii** 1115–1119

Breslow N, Chan CW, Dhom G *et al* (1977) Latent carcinoma of prostate at autopsy in seven areas. *International Journal of Cancer* **20** 680–688

Carteni B, Tucci A, Spada OA *et al* High serum levels of soluble interleukin-2 receptor in patients with ovarian cancer. *British Journal of Cancer* (in press)

Challis GB and Stam HJ (1990) The spontaneous regression of cancer: a review of cases 1900–1987. *Acta Oncologica* **29** 545–550

Cheever MA, Thompson JA, Kern D and Greenberg PD (1985) Interleukin-2 (IL-2) administered in vivo: influence of IL-2 route and timing on T cell growth. *Journal of Immunology* **134** 3895

Clark RM and Chua T (1989) Breast cancer and pregnancy: the ultimate challenge. *Clinical Oncology* **1** 11–18

Cockerell OC, Oliver RTD and Nethersall A (1991) Nephrectomy combined with perioperative alpha-interferon in the treatment of advanced local and minimally metastatic renal cell cancer. *Urology International* **46** 46–49

Crawford ED, Moon T, Stone NN *et al* (1991) Prostate cancer awareness week: results of screening. *Proceedings of the American Society of Clinical Oncology 1991* 167 [**Abstract 531**]

Currie GA (1972) Eighty years of immunotherapy. *British Journal of Cancer* **26** 141

Currie GA and Alexander P (1974) Spontaneous shedding of TSTA by viable sarcoma cells; its possible role in facilitating metastatic spread. *British Journal of Cancer* **29** 72

Damstrup L, Daagaard G, Gerstoft J and Rorth M (1990) Effects of antineoplastic treatment of HIV-positive patients with testicular cancer. *European Journal of Cancer and Clinical Oncology* **25** 983–986

Eckowitz RAB (1991) A controlled trial of interferon gamma to prevent infection in chronic granulomatous disease. *New England Journal of Medicine* **324** 509–515

Elegbede JA, Elson CE, Tanner MA, Qureshi AA and Gould MN (1986) Regression of rat primary tumours following dietary d-limonene. *Journal of the National Cancer Institute* **76** 323–325

Eysenck H J (1988) Personality, stress and cancer: prediction and prophylaxis. *British Journal of Medical Psychology* **61** 57–75

Feizi T (1985) Carbohydrate antigens in human cancer. *Cancer Surveys* **4** 243–269

Fink JM (1988) *Third Opinion An International Guide to Alternative Therapy Centers for the Treatment and Prevention of Cancer*, Avery Publishing Group Inc, New York

Fitzpatrick FTA, Kendall MD, Wheeler MJ *et al* (1985) Reappearance of thymus of ageing rats after orchidectomy. *Journal of Enodocrinology* **106** R17–R19

Fleishman JD, Toosi Z, Ellner DB *et al* (1989) Urinary interleukins in patients receiving intravesical bacillus Calmette-Guérin therapy for superficial bladder cancer. *Cancer* **64** 1447–1454

Ford JM, Cullen MH, Oliver RTD and Lister TA (1980) Granulocyte transfusions: possible prolongation of marrow remission in leukemia. *New England Journal of Medicine* **302** 583–584

Frish RE, Wyshak G, Albright NL *et al* (1985) Lower prevalence of breast cancer and cancers of the reproductive system among former college athletes compared to non-athletes. *British Journal of Cancer* **52** 885–891

Gorer PA (1937) The genetic and antigenic basis of tumour transplantation. *Journal of Pathology and Bacteriology* **44** 691

Gross L (1943) Intradermal immunisation of C3H mice against a sarcoma that originated in an animal of the same line. *Cancer Research* **3** 326

Grossman CJ (1985) Interactions between the gonadal steroids and the immune system. *Science* **227** 257–261

Gullberg M and Smith KA (1986) Regulation of T cell autocrine growth. *Journal of Experimental Medicine* **163** 270–284

Hajto T, Hostanska K, Frei K, Rordorf C and Gabius H (1990) Increased secretion of tumor necrosis factor alpha, interleukin 1 and interleukin 6 by human mononuclear cells exposed to beta-galactoside-specific lectin from clinically applied mistletoe extract. *Cancer Research* **50** 3322– 326

Handzel ZT, Burstein Y, Buchner V, Pecht M and Trainin N (1990) Immunomodulation of T-cell deficiency in humans by thymic humoral factor: from crude extract to synthetic THF-γ2. *Journal of Biological Response Modifiers* **9** 269–278

Hattori T, Hamai V and Takyama W (1980) Enhancing effect of thoracotomy on tumour growth rates. *Gann* **71** 280

Hoover HC, Surdyke MD, Dangel RB, Peters LC and Hanna MG (1985) Prospectively randomized trial of adjuvant active-specific immunotherapy for human colorectal cancer. *Cancer* **55** 1236–1243

Horoszewicz JS and Murphy GP (1989) An assessment of interferon in urological cancer. *Journal of Urology* **142** 1173–1178

Huber H, Nachbaur DM, Krainer M *et al* (1991) Prognostic relevance of interleukin-6 in multiple myeloma. *Proceedings of the American Association for Cancer Research* **32** 192 **[Abstract 1148]**

Hung CY, Lefkowitz SS, Geber WF *et al* (1973) Interferon inhibition by narcotic analgesics. *Proceedings of the Society of Biology and Medicine* **142** 106–111

Igo M, Sakurai M, Tamura T *et al* (1988) In vivo activity of multiple injections of recombinant interleukin-2, alone and in combination with three different types of recombinant interferons on various syngeneic murine tumour. *Cancer Research* **48** 260–264

Iles RK, Jenkins BJ, Oliver RTD *et al* (1989) Beta human chorionic gonadotrophin in serum and urine: a marker for metastatic urothelial cancer. *British Journal of Urology* **64** 241–244

Itoh K, Platsoucas CD and Balch CM (1988) Autologous tumour specific cytotoxic T lymphocytes in the infiltrate of human metastatic melanomas: activation by interleukin-2 and autologous tumour cells and involvement of the T cell receptor. *Journal of Experimental Medicine* **168** 1419

Jacobs I, Stabile I, Bridges J *et al* (1988) Multimodal approach to screening for ovarian cancer. *Lancet* **i** 268–271

Kelly SA, Gschmeissner S, East N and Balkwill FR Enhancement of metastatic potential by interferon gamma. *Cancer Research* (in press)

Kersey JH, Weisdorf D, Nesbit ME *et al* (1987) Autologous or allogeneic bone marrow transplantation for refractory acute leukaemia. *New England Journal of Medicine* **317** 461–467

Kjaer M (1989) Misteltoe (iscador) therapy in stage IV renal adenocarcinoma: a phase II study in patients with measurable lung metastases. *Acta Oncologica* **28** 489–494

Klein, Vanky F, Galili B and Vose BM (1980) Separation and characteristics of tumor-infiltrating lymphocytes in man. *Contemporary Topics in Immunobiology* **10** 79–107

Kosaka A, Hattori Y, Imaizumi A and Yamashita A (1985) Synergistic effect of lentinan and surgical endocrine therapy on the growth of DMBa-induced mammary tumors of rats and of recurrent human breast cancer: rationale of biological response modifiers in cancer. *Excerpta Medica International Conference Symposium No 690* 138–149

Kuhns WJ, Oliver RTD, Watkins WM and Greenwell P (1980) Leukemia-induced alterations of serum glycosyltransferase enzymes. *Cancer Research* **40** 268–275

Law LW, Trainin N, Levey RH and Barth WF (1964) Humoral thymic factor in mice: further evidence. *Science* **143** 1049–1051

Lecchi M, Lovisone E, Genetta C *et al* (1989) γ-IFN induces a differential expression of HLA-DR, DQ and DP antigens on peripheral blood myeloid leukaemic blasts at various stages of differentiation. *Leukemia Research* 133 221–226

Lee SK and Oliver RTD (1978) Autologous leukemia-specific T-cell-mediated lymphocytoxicity in patients with acute leukemia. *Journal of Experimental Medicine* 147 912–922

Lindahl P, Leary P and Gresser I (1974) Enhancement of the expression of histocompatibility antigens of mouse lymphoid cells by interferon in vitro. *European Journal of Immunology* 4 779–784

Lissoni P, Tancini G, Rovelli F, Cattaneo G, Archili C and Barni S (1990) Serum interleukin-2 levels in relation to the neuroendocrine status in cancer patients. *British Journal of Cancer* 62 838–839

Lissoni P, Barni S, Rovelli F and Tancini G (1991) Lower survival in metastatic cancer patients with reduced interleukin-2 blood concentrations. *Oncology* 48 125–127

List AF, Grogan TM, Spier TP and Miller TP (1991) Tumor-infiltrating T-lymphocyte (T-TIL) response is deficient in B-cell NHL arising in immunocompromised (IC) hosts. *Proceedings of the American Society of Clinical Oncology* 10 [Abstract 940]

Logothetis CJ, Mosson E, Sella A *et al* (1991) 5-fluorouracil and recombinant interferon alpha 2a in metastatic chemotherapy refractory urothelial tumours. *Journal of the National Cancer Institute* 83 285–288

MacCarty WC (1922) Factors which influence longevity in cancer. *Annals of Surgery* 76 9–12

McHeyzer-Williams MG (1989) Combinations of interleukins 2,4 and 5 regulate the secretion of murine immunoglobin isotypes. *European Journal of Immunology* 19 2025–2030

Maladazyz JD and de Kernion JB (1986) Prognostic factors in metastatic renal carcinoma. *Journal of Urology* 136 376–379

Mant D and Fowler G (1990) Mass screening: theory and ethics. *British Medical Journal* 300 916–918

Marsh J, Donna PT and Hamer-Hodges DW (1990) Association between transfusion with plasma and the recurrence of colorectal carcinoma. *British Journal of Surgery* 77 623–626

Mastino A, Favalli C, Grellie S, Innocenti F and Garaci E (1991) Thymosin-alpha-1 potentiates interleukin 2-induced cytotoxic activity in mice cell. *Immunology* 133 196–205

Meryman HT (1989) Transfusion-induced alloimmunization and immunosuppression and the effects of leukocyte depletion. *Transfusion Medical Reviews* 3 180–193

Mitchison NA (1953a) Passive transfer of transplantation immunity. *Proceedings of the Royal Society Series B* 142 72–87

Mitchison NA (1953b) Passive transfer of transplantation immunity. *Nature* 171 267

Moertel CG, Fleming TR, Rubin J *et al* (1982) A clinical trial of amygdalin (laetrile) in the treatment of human cancer. *New England Journal of Medicine* 306 201–206

Moertel CG, Fleming TR, MacDonald JS *et al* (1990) Levamisole and fluorouracil for adjuvant therapy of resected colon carcinoma. *New England Journal of Medicine* 322 352–358

Morita T, Salmeron MA, von Eschenbach AC *et al* (1991) Oligoclonal expansion of human tumor-infiltrating lymphocytes (TILs). *Proceedings of the American Association for Cancer Research* 32 [Abstract 1402]

Natali P, Bigotti A and Cavaliere R (1987) HLA class II antigens synthesized by melanoma cells. *Cancer Review* 9 1–33

National Institutes of Health Consensus Conference (1991) Adjuvant therapy for patients with colon and rectal cancers. *Journal of the American Medical Association* 264 1444–1450

Nitta T, Oksenber JR, Rao NA and Steinman L (1990) Predominant expression of T cell receptor Va 7 tumour infiltrating lymphocytes of uveal melanoma. *Science* 249 672

Nouri AME, Smith MEF, Crosby D and Oliver RTD (1990) Selective and non-selective loss of immunoregulatory molecules (HLA-A,B,C antigens and FA-3) in transitional cell carcinoma. *British Journal of Cancer* 62 603–606

Nouri AME, Dos Santos AVL and Oliver RTD Class I antigen expression and IL-2 induced expansion of tumour infiltrating lymphocytes from bladder tumour biopsies. *British Journal of Cancer* (in press)

Oliver RTD (1982) Biology of host/tumour cell interaction, In: Chisholm GD and Williams DI (eds). *Scientific Foundations of Urology*, p 624, William Heinemann, London

Oliver RTD (1989) Psychological support for cancer patients. *Lancet* ii 1209

Oliver RTD (1990a) Atrophy, hormones, genes and viruses in aetiology germ cell tumours. *Cancer Surveys* 9 263–286

Oliver RTD (1990b) Clues from natural history and results of treatment supporting the monoclonal origin of germ cell tumours. *Cancer Surveys* 9 no 2, pp 333–368

Oliver RTD (1990c) Medical management of bladder cancer with an emphasis on the role of immune modulators and chemotherapy, In: RTD Oliver (ed). *Urological and Genital Cancer,* pp 115–126, Blackwell, Oxford

Oliver RTD (1991) Topical BCG for recurrent superficial bladder cancer. *Lancet* 337 821

Oliver RTD Interleukin-2 plus or minus alpha interferon for renal cell cancer. *Urology Topics* (in press)

Oliver RTD, Nethersell ABW and Bottomley JM (1989a) Unexplained spontaneous regression and alpha-interferon as treatment for metastatic renal carcinoma. *British Journal of Urology* 63 128–131

Oliver RTD and Lee SK (1979) Self-restricted cytotoxicity against acute myeloid leukemia cells, In: Reithmuller C (ed). *Natural and Induced Cell-Mediated Cytotoxicity,* pp 183–189, Academic Press, New York

Oliver RTD, Nouri AME, Crosby D *et al* (1989b) Biological significance of beta hCG, HLA and other membrane antigen expression on bladder tumours and their relationship to tumour infiltrating lymphocytes (TIL). *Journal of Immunogenetics* 16 381

Oliver RTD, Riddle P and Blandy JP Operative factors and tumour membrane antigen changes in escape from immune surveillance, In: Smith P (ed). *EORTC Genitourinary Group Monograph 10,* John Wiley, New York (in press)

Opelz G and Terasaki PI (1974) Poor kidney-transplant survival in recipients with frozen-blood transfusions or no transfusion. *Lancet* ii 696–698

Penn I (1988) Tumors of the immunocompromised patient. *Annual Review of Medicine* 39 63–73

Penn I (1990) Cancers complicating organ transplantation. *New England Journal of Medicine* 323 1967–1968

Pfister H, Krubke J, Dietrick W, Iftner T and Fuchs PG (1986) Classification of the papilloma viruses—mapping the genome. *Papilloma Viruses,* Ciba Foundation Symposium, 120 pp 3–22, Wiley, Chichester

Phillips DP and King EW (1988) Death takes a holiday: mortality surrounding major or social occasions. *Lancet* ii 728–732

Pichert G, Jost LM, Zobeli L, Odermatt B, Pedio G and Stahel RA (1990) Thyroiditis after treatment with interleukin-2 and interferon alpha-2a. *British Journal of Cancer* 62 100–104

Pines A (1976) A 5-year controlled study of BCG and radiotherapy for inoperable lung cancer. *Lancet* i 380–385

Possinger K, Wagner H, Beck R and Staebler A (1988) Renal cell carcinoma. *Controversies in Oncology* 30 195–207

Port F, Ragheb NE, Schwartz AG and Hawthorne VM (1989) Neoplasms in dialysis patients: a population-based study. *American Journal of Kidney Disease* 14 119

Prescott S, James K, Busuttil J *et al* (1989) HLA DR expression by high grade superficial bladder cancer treated with BCG. *British Journal of Urology* 63 264–269

Querci della Rovere G, Oliver RTD, McCance DJ and Castro JE (1989) Development of bladder tumour containing HPV type 11 DNA after renal transplantation. *British Journal of Urology* 62 36–38

Raeth U, Schmid H, Karch U, Kempeni J, Schlick E and Kaufmann M (1991) Phase II trial of recombinant human tumor necrosis factor-alpha (rHuTNF) in patients with malignant ascites from ovarian carcinomas and non-ovarian tumors with intraperitoneal spread. *Pro-*

ceedings of the American Society of Clinical Oncology **10** 610 [**Abstract 187**]

Ramani P, Hart IR and Balkwill FR (1986) The effect of interferon on experimental metastases in immunocompetent and immunodeficient mice. *International Journal of Cancer* **37** 563–568

Ramirez AJ, Craig TKJ, Watson JP *et al* (1989) Stress and relapse in breast cancer. *British Medical Journal* **298** 291–293

Ransom JH, Pelle B and Hanna MG (1991) Expression of class II major histocompatibility complex molecules correlates with human colon tumor vaccine efficacy. *Proceedings of the American Association for Cancer Research* **32** [**Abstract 1516**]

Roithmann S, Toledano M and Tourani JM (1991) HIV-associated non-Hodgkin's lymphomas: clinical characteristics and outcome: the experience of the French registry of HIV-associated tumors. *Annals of Oncology* **2** 289–295

Rosenberg SA, Spiess P and Lafreniere R (1986) A new approach to the adoptive immunotherapy of cancer in animals and man. *Science* **233** 1313

Rosenberg SA, Schwarz SL and Speiss PJ (1988) Combination immunotherapy for cancer: synergistic antitumor interactions of interleukin-2, alpha interferon and tumor-infiltrating lymphocytes. *Journal of the National Cancer Institute* **80** 1393–1397

Rosenberg SA, Lotze MT, Yang JC *et al* (1989) Combination therapy with interleukin-2 and alpha-interferon for the treatment of patients with advanced cancer. *Journal of Clinical Oncology* **12** 1863–1864

Rosenberg SA, Aebersold P and Cornetta K *et al* (1990) Gene transfer into humans—immunotherapy of melanoma using tumor-infiltrating lymphocytes modified by retroviral gene transduction. *New England Journal of Medicine* **323** 570–578

Rowlinson-Busza G, Bamias A, Kraus T, Evans DJ and Epenetos AA (1991) Cytoxicity following specific activation of amygdalin, In: Epenetos AA (ed). *Monoclonal Antibodies: Applications in Clinical Oncology*, pp 179–183, Chapman and Hall, London

Snell GD and Higgins GF (1951) Allelles at the histocompatability-2 locus in the mouse as determined by tumour transplantation. *Genetics* **36** 306

Spanos NP, Williams V and Gwynn MI (1990) Effects of hypnotic, placebo, and salicylic acid treatments on wart regression. *Psychosomatic Medicine* **52** 109–114

Spiegel D, Bloom JR, Kraemer HC and Gotthiel E (1989) Effect of psychosocial treatment on survival of patients with metastatic breast cancer. *Lancet* **ii** 888–890

Sternswald J, Jondal M, Vanky F *et al* (1978) Lymphopenia and change in distribution of human B and T lymphocyte in peripheral blood induced by irradiation for mammary carcinoma. *Lancet* **i** 1352–1356

Stevens VC and Crystal GD (1973) Effects of immunisation with hapten coupled hCG on human menstrual cycle. *Obstetrics and Gynaecology* **47** 485–495

Swan F, Ordonez N, Manning J *et al* (1988) Beta-2 microglobulin (B2M) cell surface expression as an indicator of resistance in lymphoma and its relation to the serum level. *Blood* **72** 258a

Talmadge JT, Phillips H, Schindler J *et al* (1987) Systematic preclincial study on the therapeutic properties of recombinant human interleukin-2 for the treatment of metastatic disease. *Cancer Research* **47** 5725–5732

Taniguchi T, Matsui H, Fujita T *et al* (1986) Molecular analysis of the interleukin-2 system. *Immunology Review* **92** 121

Temoshok L and Peeke HVS (1988) Individual behavior differences related to induced tumor growth in the female syrian hamster: two studies. *International Journal of Neuroscience* **38** 199–209

Temoshok L, Peeke HVS, Mehard CW, Axelsson K and Sweet DM (1985) Stress-behavior interactions in hamster tumor growth. *Annals of the New York Academy of Sciences* **496** 501–509

Tessler A and Catanese A (1987) Aids and germ cell tumors of testis. *Urology* **30** 203–204

Topalian SL, Solomon D, Avis FP *et al* (1988) Immunotherapy of patients with advanced cancer using tumour infiltrating lymphocytes and recombinant interleukin-2: a pilot study. *Journal of Clinical Oncology* **6** 839–853

Trainin N, Canrall C and Ilfield D (1990) Inhibition of auto sensitisation by thymic humoral factor. *nature* **245** 253–255

Tupitsyn NN, Babusikova O, Baryshnikov A *et al* (1990) Clinical significance of standard CD assessment in acute leukaemia. *Neoplasma* **37** 431

Vanky F, Wang P, Patarroyo M and Klein E (1990) Expression of the adhesion molecule ICAM-1 and major histocompatibility complex class I antigens on human tumor cells is required for their interaction with autologous lymphocytes in vitro. *Cancer Immunology Immunotherapy* **31** 19–27

Vogt P, Frei U, Repp H and Bunzendahl H (1990) Malignant tumours in renal transplant recipients receiving cyclosporin: survey of 598 first-kidney transplantations. *Nephrology, Dialysis and Transplantation* **5** 282–288

Wagner H, Hardt C, Hegg K, Rollinghoff M and Pfizenmaier K (1980) T cell derived helper factor allows in vivo induction of cytotoxic T Cell in nu/nu mice. *Nature* **284** 278

Whittle HC, Inskip H, Hall AJ, Mendy M, Downes R and Hoare S (1991) Vaccination against hepatitis B and protection against chronic viral carriage in The Gambia. *Lancet* **337** 8744

Windle R, Bell PRF and Shaw D (1987) Five year results of a randomized trial of adjuvant 5-fluorouracil and levamisole in colorectal cancer. *British Journal of Surgery* **73** 569–572

Winstanley JHR, Barraclough BR, Rudland PS *et al* (1961) Fibroblast growth factor expression in normal and malignant breast: proceedings of the 6th scientific meeting of the British Oncological Association. *British Journal of Cancer* **64** (**Supplement XV**)

Yamakido M, Ishioka S, Yanagida J *et al* (1990) The prevention of cancers in man with a biological response modifier: proceedings of the 15th international cancer congress. *Journal of Cancer Research and Clinical Oncology* **116** 84 [**Abstract B1.022.01**]

Yang LL, Maher VM and McCormick J (1982) Relationship between excision repair and the cytotoxic and mutagenic effect of the "anti" 7,8-diol-9,10-epoxide of benzo (a) pyrene in human cells. *Mutation Research* **94** 435–447

Yoshimoto M, Sakamoto G and Ohashi Y (1989) Tumour infiltrating lymphocytes in breast cancer. *Igaku No Aymi (Tokyo)* **151** 457–458

Yun T and Choi SY (1990) A case-control study of ginseng intake and cancer. *International Journal of Epidemiology* **19** 871

Zaitseva MB and Brondz BD (1990) Mechanism of MHC class II restriction in the interaction between specific suppressor and responder T cells in a proliferative response Ia interaction with a putative anti-self receptor, expressed on pre-activated responder cells. *Immunology* **70** 372–378

The authors are responsible for the accuracy of the references.

Biographical Notes

Alain Amar-Costesec received his Doctorate in Pharmacy from the University of Paris in 1960. In 1965 he joined the cell biology group at the University of Louvain. His present interest is the molecular organization of endoplasmic reticulum membrane and the intracellular localization and function of proteins corresponding to T cell recognized antigens.

Sir Walter Bodmer, Director-General of the Imperial Cancer Research Fund, read mathematics at Cambridge University and went on to do a PhD in population genetics. He spent nine years at Stanford University, California, working with Joshua Lederberg, before taking up an appointment as Professor of Genetics at Oxford University in 1970. In 1979 he became Director of Research at the Imperial Cancer Research Fund and was appointed Director-General in 1991. He is also Chairman of the Committee on the Public Understanding of Science and President of the International Human Genome Organization. His research interests centre on the expression of HLA determinants in cancer and the genetics and biology of the epithelial cells in the colon from which the majority of colorectal adenocarcinomas are derived.

Thierry Boon graduated from the University of Louvain, Belgium, and obtained a PhD at the Rockefeller University, New York, in 1970. He then worked in the laboratory of F Jacob at the Pasteur Institute in Paris and in 1975 joined the Institute of Cellular and Molecular Pathology in Brussels, Belgium. Since 1978 he has been Director of the Brussels branch of the Ludwig Institute for Cancer Research. He is also a professor in the faculty of medicine of the University of Louvain. His main research interest is the immune response against animal and human tumour cells, with particular emphasis on the analysis of genes coding for tumour rejection antigens.

Jill Brooks is a graduate in microbiology from the University of London (King's College) and is currently a PhD student in the Department of Cancer Studies, University of Birmingham.

Karl-Hermann Meyer zum Büschenfelde graduated DVM from the School of Veterinary Medicine in Hannover, West Germany, in 1955 and MD from the Medical School in Hamburg in 1960. After clinical training in internal medicine, immunology and gastroenterology in Kassel and Mainz, West Germany, he was appointed a visiting professor at the Center of Immune-Hematology, University of Geneva, Switzerland. From 1977 to 1981 he was professor and chairman of the department of medicine, Freie Universität Berlin, West Germany. Since 1981 he has been professor and chairman of the I Department of Medicine at the Johannes-Gutenberg University, Mainz, Germany. His clinical and research interests are in hepatology and gastroenterology, immunology and tumour immunology and infectious diseases.

Etienne De Plaen obtained a PhD from the University of Louvain, Belgium, in 1979. He is currently working at the Ludwig Institute for Cancer Research of Brussels, where he carries out research on genes coding for mouse tumour rejection antigens and on the mechanism of expression of DNA sequences coding for antigenic peptides.

Heather Griffin is a graduate in microbiology from the University of Sheffield and is currently a PhD student in the Department of Cancer Studies, University of Birmingham.

Günter J Hämmerling studied chemistry and biochemistry and worked in the early 1970s with HO McDevitt (Stanford, USA) on the genetic control of the immune response, which led to the discovery of IA antigens. The work on MHC antigens was continued in Cologne, Germany (with K Rajewski), and later at the Institute for Immunology and Genetics at the German Cancer Research Centre in Heidelberg, where he is a professor of theoretical medicine. His research is focused on the structure and biological function of MHC antigens, in particular on the role of MHC molecules in tumour immunology, antigen processing and peripheral tolerance.

Ann Hill, FRACP, PhD, trained as a physician in Sydney from 1979 to 1984, specializing in clinical immunology. She received her PhD from the Australian National University for a study on cellular immunity to flaviviruses and since 1990 has continued research in the Cancer Immunology and Molecular Immunology Groups at the Institute of Molecular Medicine, Oxford.

Loukas Kaklamanis, MD, graduated from the University of Patras, Greece, in 1983 and trained in pathology at the University Hospital, Patras, from 1983 to 1988. In 1989 he worked for a year at the Retroviruses National Center at the University of Athens. In 1990 he joined the Nuffield Department of Pathology at Oxford University as a research fellow.

W Martin Kast worked with Cornelis Melief on MHC regulation of T cell responses against viruses and minor histocompatibility antigens, obtaining his PhD in 1987. As a postdoctoral worker he developed the adenovirus immunotherapy model and continued his studies of immunity against Sendai virus. More recently he started studies on the T cell response against human papillomavirus type 16. Since 1991 he has been a staff member of the department of immunohaematology and blood bank at Leiden University. Dr Kast is a fellow of the Royal Dutch Academy of Sciences.

Alexander Knuth, MD, graduated from the Freie Universität Berlin, West Germany, in 1973. He received his training in internal medicine, haematology and oncology at the city hospital Moabit in West Berlin from 1974 to 1978, as a research fellow in cancer immunology with Lloyd Old and Herbert Oettgen and as a clinical fellow in haematology, oncology and immunology at the Memorial Sloan Kettering Cancer Center, New York (1978–1981). He is now an internist and medical oncologist-haematologist in the I Department of Medicine at the Johannes-Gutenberg University in Mainz, Germany. His research interest is focused on clinical and experimental cancer immunology, with particular emphasis on T lymphocytes as probes for the detection of tumour antigens.

Christophe Lurquin, PhD, trained in molecular biology at the Ludwig Institute for Cancer Research, Brussels. He received his PhD at the University of Louvain in 1990. He has been involved in the cloning of genes coding for tumour rejection antigens.

Andrew McMichael graduated in medicine from the University of Cambridge in 1968. He trained in immunology at the National Institute of Medical Research with Dr AR Williamson and Dr BA Askonas, obtaining his PhD in 1974. After two years with Dr Hugh McDevitt at Stanford University, he took up an appointment in Oxford in 1977. Since then, he has developed an interest in the role of cytotoxic T lymphocytes in human immune responses, with particular reference to the function of HLA class I antigens. He was appointed to a Medical Research Council Clinical Research Professorship in 1982.

Maria Masucci is a medical graduate of the University of Ferrara, Italy. She has worked for many years in the Department of Tumour Biology, Karolinska Institute, Stockholm, Sweden, with Professor George Klein. She is currently spending a sabbatical year at the University of Birmingham, funded by a Wellcome-Swedish MRC fellowship.

Cornelis JM Melief received his PhD in 1967 and graduated in medicine in 1970 at the University of Amsterdam. He trained in immunology at the Central Laboratory of the Dutch Red Cross Blood Transfusion Service in Amsterdam. Subsequently he spent 2 years in Boston at the haematology service of the New England Medical Center/Tufts University, where he deepened his interest in the immunogenetics of the HLA/H-2 systems and started studies of immunity against murine leukaemia viruses. From 1975 to 1985 he was head of the department of experimental cellular immunology at the Central Laboratory in Amsterdam, studying T cell response regulation in H-2 mutants, antigen presentation by dendritic cells and human T cell leukaemias. From 1985 to 1991 he was head of the department of immunology of the Netherlands Cancer Institute, where an experimental CTL therapy model with human adenovirus induced tumours in mice was developed. Since May, 1991, he has been head of the department of immunohaematology and blood bank and professor of immunohaematology at the University of Leiden.

Peter Möller is professor of general pathology and morbid anatomy in the Institute of Pathology at the University of Heidelberg, Germany. His scientific interests are human leucocyte differentiation antigens, MHC antigen expression in human tumours, B cell physiology and B cell lymphomas and leukaemias.

Denis Moss is a graduate of the University of Queensland, Australia, and has worked for many years at the Queensland Institute of Medical Research, Brisbane, where he is now senior principal research fellow.

Ruth Murray is a graduate in microbiology from the University of Leeds. She studied for her PhD in the Department of Medical Microbiology, University of Birmingham, and is currently a postdoctoral research fellow in the Department of Cancer Studies at Birmingham.

RTD Oliver graduated from the University of Cambridge and The London Hospital in 1966. He undertook postgraduate research on HLA and transplantation immunology with Hilliard Festenstein and received an MD in 1974. He trained in oncology with Gordon Hamilton-Fairley at St Bartholomew's Hospital and in urology with John Blandy at St Peter's Hospital and the Institute of Urology. He is currently on the staff of The Royal London Hospital and is reader in medical oncology at The Royal London Hospital Medical College. He runs a clinical research unit doing research in urological tumours with a special interest in germ cell tumours and the immunology of cancer.

Alan Rickinson, a graduate of the University of Cambridge, did postdoctoral work in Sydney, Australia, and then worked for several years with Professor Tony Epstein at the University of Bristol. He is now head of cancer studies, University of Birmingham.

Volker Schirrmacher, PhD, has been Professor of Immunology at the University of Heidelberg since 1976 and holds a chair in cellular immunology in the Faculty of Pharmacy. He is Head of the Division of Cellular Immunology at the German Cancer Research Centre. After graduating in biochemistry in Tübingen, he received his PhD in 1970 in Cologne in cellular immunology under Klaus Rajewsky. He spent 5 years with Hans Wigzell at the Karolinska Institute, Stockholm, and with Hilliard Festenstein at The London Hospital Medical School, London. His work at the Cancer Research Centre focuses on tumour immunology and experimental metastasis research. This includes investigations into the mechanism of cancer invasion and metastasis formation and research on the therapy of metastases by immunological means. In 1987 he was elected chairman of the German Cancer Research Association (SEK) and in 1990 became President of the International Metastasis Research Society.

Catia Traversari received a PhD in biological sciences from the University of Milan. She joined the Ludwig Institute for Cancer Research of Brussels in 1989 on a fellowship of the European Community. The aim of her research project is to isolate and characterize the gene coding for a tumour antigen of a human melanoma.

Benoît Van den Eynde graduated in medicine at the University of Louvain in 1986. His present interest is the analysis of antigens recognized on human melanoma cells by autologous CTL.

Pierre van der Bruggen obtained a PhD in agronomic sciences at the University of Louvain in 1987. He is presently involved in the genetic analysis of a human gene coding for a melanoma antigen.

Aline Van Pel received a PhD in Biology at the University of Louvain in 1974. She joined the Brussels branch of the Ludwig Institute for Cancer Research in 1978 and is now a senior member of the branch. Her main research interest is the mechanism of immune rejection of tumour cells.

Thomas Wölfel, MD, graduated from the Johannes-Gutenberg University in Mainz, West Germany, in 1982. He was a research fellow from 1984 to 1987 at the Ludwig Institute for Cancer Research in Brussels, Belgium, headed by Professor Thierry Boon. In 1987 he began clinical training in internal medicine in the I Department of Medicine at the Johannes-Gutenberg University. His research interest is the identification of target cell molecules involved in the recognition of human tumour cells by autologous cytolytic T lymphocytes.

Index

LIST OF PREVIOUS ISSUES

VOLUME 1 1982

No. 1: Inheritance of Susceptibility to Cancer in Man
Guest Editor: W F Bodmer

No. 2: Maturation and Differentiation in Leukaemias
Guest Editor: M F Greaves

No. 3: Experimental Approaches to Drug Targeting
Guest Editors: A J S Davies and M J Crumpton

No. 4: Cancers Induced by Therapy
Guest Editor: I Penn

VOLUME 2 1983

No. 1: Embryonic & Germ Cell Tumours in Man and Animals
Guest Editor: R L Gardner

No. 2: Retinoids and Cancer
Guest Editor: M B Sporn

No. 3: Precancer
Guest Editor: J J DeCosse

No. 4: Tumour Promotion and Human Cancer
Guest Editors: T J Slaga and R Montesano

VOLUME 3 1984

No. 1: Viruses in Human and Animal Cancers
Guest Editors: J Wyke and R Weiss

No. 2: Gene Regulation in the Expression of Malignancy
Guest Editor: L Sachs

No. 3: Consistent Chromosomal Aberrations and Oncogenes in Human Tumours
Guest Editor: J D Rowley

No. 4: Clinical Management of Solid Tumours in Childhood
Guest Editor: T J McElwain

VOLUME 4 1985

No. 1: Tumour Antigens in Experimental and Human Systems
Guest Editor: L W Law

No. 2: Recent Advances in the Treatment and Research in Lymphoma and Hodgkin's Disease
Guest Editor: R Hoppe

No. 3: Carcinogenesis and DNA Repair
Guest Editor: T Lindahl

No. 4: Growth Factors and Malignancy
Guest Editors: A B Roberts and M B Sporn

VOLUME 5 1986

No. 1: Drug Resistance
Guest Editors: G Stark and H Calvert

No. 2: Biochemical Mechanisms of Oncogene Activity: Proteins Encoded by Oncogenes
Guest Editors: H E Varmus and J M Bishop

No. 3: Hormones and Cancer: 90 Years after Beatson
Guest Editor: R D Bulbrook

No. 4: Experimental, Epidemiological and Clinical Aspects of Liver Carcinogenesis
Guest Editor: E Farber

VOLUME 6 1987

No. 1: Naturally Occurring Tumours in Animals as a Model for Human Disease
Guest Editors: D Onions and W Jarrett

No. 2: New Approaches to Tumour Localization
Guest Editor: K Britton

No. 3: Psychological Aspects of Cancer
Guest Editor: S Greer

No. 4: Diet and Cancer
Guest Editors: C Campbell and L Kinlen

VOLUME 7 1988

No. 1: Pain and Cancer
Guest Editor: G W Hanks

VOLUME 12 1992

Tumour Suppressor Genes, the Cell Cycle and Cancer
Guest Editor: A J Levine